The
ABSITE REVIEW:
Practice Questions

Steven M. Fiser MD

The ABSITE Review: Practice Questions

Steven M. Fiser MD
Hancock Surgical Consultants, LLC
Richmond, Virginia

This book is not intended for clinical use. Extreme care has been taken to ensure the accuracy of the information contained in this book and to devise the safest and most conservative way of practicing general surgery. However, the authors and publishers are not responsible for errors or omissions in the book itself or from any consequences from application of the information in the book and make no warranty, expressed or implied, with respect to the currency, completeness, or accuracy of the contents of the publication. Application of this information remains the professional responsibility of the practitioner. The specific circumstances surrounding any individual patient requires individual diagnosis and treatment.

Extreme care has been taken to ensure that the drug dosages herein are accurate, however illness such as renal failure and other disease states can affect dose. The reader should check the package insert for any drug being prescribed to see the current recommended indications, warnings, and precautions.

Some drugs and devices in this text have FDA clearance only for certain indications. It is the responsibility of the health care provider to ascertain the FDA status of any drug or device before use.

The American Board of Surgery Inc. does not sponsor nor endorses this book.

The author has never had access to the ABSITE exams used by the American Board of Surgery Inc. other than to take the exam. This book is meant to educate general surgery residents, not reconstruct the ABSITE.

Contents:

Cell biology	4
Hematology	6
Blood products	12
Immune System and Wound Healing	15
Transplantation	26
Infection	35
Antibiotics	44
Pharmacology	47
Anesthesia	50
Fluids and Electrolytes	61
Nutrition	68
Oncology	76
Trauma	82
Critical Care	106
Burns	124
Head and Neck	132
Adrenal Gland	141
Thyroid	146
Parathyroid	154
Pituitary Gland	160
Breast	162
Thoracic	175
Cardiac	183
Vascular	187
Gastrointestinal Hormones	202
Esophagus	205
Stomach	214
Liver	221
Biliary System	229
Pancreas	238
Spleen	248
Small Bowel	255
Colon and Rectum	263
Rectum and Anus	278
Hernias and Abdominal Wall	283
Urology	287
Gynecology	294
Neurosurgery	300
Orthopaedics	302
Pediatric Surgery	309
Skin and Soft Tissue	324
Statistics	334

Cell Biology

1. **What receptor does erythromycin bind to increase gastro-intestinal motility?
    a. Somatostatin receptor
    b. Acetylcholine and dopaminergic receptors
    c. GABA receptor
    d. Motilin receptor

    Answer d. **Erythromycin** *binds the motilin receptor.*

2. *What portion of the lipopolysaccharide complex accounts for its toxicity?
    a. Lipid A
    b. Lipid B
    c. Lipid C
    d. Lipid D

    Answer a. *Lipid A* is the toxic portion of the **lipopolysaccharide complex** found with gram negative sepsis. *Lipid A is the most potent stimulant for **TNF-alpha release**.

3. Steroid hormones:
    a. Bind a receptor on the plasma membrane and activate a plasma membrane enzyme
    b. Bind a cytoplasmic receptor, enter the nucleus, and affect transcription of mRNA
    c. Bind a receptor in the nucleus and affect transcription of RNA
    d. Do not enter the cell

    Answer b. **Steroid hormones** bind a receptor in the cell cytoplasm, enter the nucleus as a steroid-receptor complex, and then affect transcription of mRNA for protein synthesis. **Thyroid hormone** affects transcription after binding a receptor that resides in the nucleus.(steroid and thyroid hormones take 1-2 hours to have affects).

    Ribosomes synthesize proteins from mRNA (termed translation).

    DNA polymerase chain reaction – uses oligonucleotides to amplify specific DNA sequences (a tool used in research)

4. *Cells divide during what phase of the cell cycle?
    a. G1
    b. S
    c. G2
    d. M

    Answer d. Cells divide during the M phase.

Cell cycle - 4 phases
> **G1** - Most variable part, determines **cell cycle length**
> > **Growth factors** affect cell during G1
>
> **S** (synthesis) - cell is preparing for division
> > Protein synthesis, DNA replication (DNA polymerase)
>
> **G2** (G2 checkpoint) – stops cell from proceeding into mitosis if there is **DNA damage** to allow **repair;** maintains DNA stability
>
> **M** (mitosis) - cell divides

5.   *Of the following, which is the most critical component in the neovascularization of tumor metastases?
     a.   HER receptor
     b.   VEGF receptor
     c.   Neu receptor
     d.   FGF receptor

     Answer b. *One of the most critical elements in the **neovascularization** of metastases is the **VEGF** (vascular endothelial growth factor) receptor. Many new chemotherapeutic strategies target the VEGF receptor.*

6.   *All of the following are true except:
     a.   Desmosomes anchor cells to each other
     b.   Hemidesmosomes anchor cells to platelets
     c.   Gap junctions allow communication between cells
     d.   Tight junctions are water impermeable

     Answer b. Hemidesmosomes anchor cells to extra-cellular matrix

     Desmosomes and **hemidesmosomes** – anchor cells
          (cell–cell and cell–extracellular matrix molecules, respectively)
     Tight junctions – occluding junctions that occur between cells; form a
          water impermeable barrier (eg skin epithelium, bladder epithelium)
     Gap junctions – formed between cells to allow communication

7.   *All of the following are true except:
     a.   Keratin is found in hair and nails
     b.   Desmin is found in muscle
     c.   Vimentin is found in skin
     d.   The above are intermediate filaments

     Answer c. Vimentin is found in fibroblasts

     Intermediate filaments:
          Keratin (hair and nails)
          ***Desmin** (muscle tissue)*
          Vimentin (fibroblasts)

8.   *All of the following are true except:
     a.   Cholesterol increases plasma membrane fluidity
     b.   Intra-cellular calcium level is very low compared to extra-cellular level
     c.   G proteins are GTPases
     d.   The Golgi apparatus is the major site of ATP production

     Answer d. Mitochondria are the major site of ATP production

     *Cholesterol increases plasma membrane **fluidity***
     Intra-cellular calcium level is <u>very low</u> compared to extra-cellular level
     *G proteins are **GTPases***

Hemetology

9.   **All of the following are true except:
  a.   The best test for platelet function is bleeding time
  b.   FFP is the most effective way to acutely correct INR
  c.   Factor VIII is synthesized in the liver
  d.   Calcium is required for normal coagulation (pro-thrombin complex)

  Answer c. **Factor VIII is synthesized in endothelium.
  The best test for platelet function is bleeding time.

10.   *All the following are true of antiphospholipid antibody syndrome except:
  a.   Classically has an elevated PTT w/ lupus anticoagulant antibodies
       that is not corrected w/ FFP (hypercoaguable w/ elevated PTT)
  b.   Can have elevated anti-cardiolipin antibodies
  c.   Patients are prone to spontaneous abortions
  d.   Cardiolipin is a cell membrane phospholipid

  Answer d. Cardiolipin is a mitochondrial membrane phospholipid.

11.   *All of the following are true of hypercoaguable states except:
  a.   The MC congenital hypercoaguable disorder is resistance to
       activated protein C (Factor V Leiden)
  b.   The mutation for Factor V Leiden is on protein C
  c.   The MC acquired hypercoaguability disorder is smoking
  d.   Hyperhomocyteinemia Tx is w/ folate, pyridoxine cyanocobalamine

  Answer b. *For resistance to activated protein C (Factor V Leiden), the mutation is on Factor V.*

12.   **You start Coumadin on a patient with a pulmonary embolus. Three days later, he starts sloughing off skin across his arms and legs. All of the following are true of this patients most likely condition except:
  a.   This is prevented by starting heparin before Coumadin
  b.   Patients with protein C deficiency are more susceptible
  c.   The skin sloughing is caused by skin necrosis
  d.   This patient most likely has hemophilia A

  Answer d. Warfarin induced skin necrosis occurs when Coumadin is started without being on heparin 1st. It results from a relatively hyper-coaguable state because of the shorter half-life of protein C and S compared to factors II, VII, IX and X (Vit K dependent). Protein C and S decrease after Coumadin before other factors decrease, resulting in a hypercoaguable state. **Pts w/ protein C deficiency are at increased risk. It is prevented by starting heparin before giving Coumadin.*

13.   **All of the following apply to Tx of von Willebrands disease except
  a.   Type III disease does not respond to DDAVP (desmopressin)
  b.   These pts have a prolonged bleeding time
  c.   Type I and III disease have reduced quantity of circulating vWF
  d.   Type III is most common

  Answer d. Type I vWF is the most common type.

14.   **All of the following are true for hemophilia A except:
  a.   DDAVP if good for all forms of Hemophilia A
  b.   Cryoprecipitate has the highest concentration of Factor VIII compared
       to all other blood products
  c.   Factor VIII levels should be raised to 100% pre-op
  d.   These patients have a prolonged PTT

Answer a. DDAVP only works for mild forms of hemophilia A (5-25% normal activity). **Recombinant factor VIII** is the best Tx.

15. **All of the following are true of uremia induced coagulopathy except:
    a.   Occurs when BUN > 60-80
    b.   Uremia results in platelet dysfunction
    c.   Uremia stimulates von Willebrand's factor release
    d.   Treatment of choice is dialysis

    Answer c. Down-regulation of vWF is the key dysfunctional element in **uremic coagulopathy**. **Dialysis** is the Tx of choice.

16. **All of the following are true of deep venous thrombosis (DVT) except:
    a.   The MC source of pulmonary embolism (PE) is ilio-femoral DVT
    b.   The left leg develops DVT 2x more commonly than the right
    c.   IVC filters should be placed above the renal veins
    d.   Infected hemodialysis catheters w/ tip thrombosis requires removal

    Answer c. **IVC filters should be placed **below the renal veins**. If placed above renal veins, an embolus that clogs the filter will result in renal failure. HD catheters w/ infected thrombosis can't be salvaged (require removal).

17. **The best treatment for thrombolytic overdose (eg urokinase, tPA) is:
    a.   Aminocaproic acid
    b.   fresh frozen plasma
    c.   packed red blood cells
    d.   cryoprecipitate

    Answer a. Thrombolytics work by converting plasminogen into plasmin. Plasmin then degrades fibrin. ***Aminocaproic acid** works by binding plasminogen and preventing the conversion of plasminogen to plasmin. **Fibrinogen levels < 100** are associated w/ increased risk and severity of bleeding and Tx is usually indicated*

18. **All of the following are true except:
    a.   Low molecular weight heparin (LMWH) binds Anti-thrombin III (AT-III) and neutralizes Factors IIa and X
    b.   LMWH is not reversed w/ protamine
    c.   Argatroban works independently of AT-III
    d.   Drug eluting coronary stents require clopidogrel for 1 year and are at risk for thrombosis if clopidogrel is stopped early

    Answer a. LMWH (eg Lovenox) binds AT-III and inhibits **Factor Xa _only_** for its anti-coagulant effects. **Unfractionated heparin** binds AT-III and inhibits Factors **IIa and Xa**. **Argatroban** is a **direct thrombin inhibitor** and is not dependent on AT-III.

    ***Drug eluting coronary stents** require clopidogrel (Plavix) for 1 year and are at risk for thrombosis if clopidogrel is stopped early*

19. **All of the following are true except:
    a.   Prostacyclin is synthesized in endothelium
    b.   Thromboxane is released from platelets
    c.   ASA inhibits cyclo-oxygenase
    d.   Thromboxane is regenerated in platelets within 24 hours after ASA Tx

    Answer d. *Thromboxane is not regenerated in platelets as cyclo-oxygenase is irreversibly inhibited and platelets do not have nuclear material to re-synthesize cyclo-oxygenase.*

20. *Thromboxane:
    a. decreases platelet aggregation by increasing release of calcium in platelets
    b. decreases platelet aggregation by decreasing release of calcium in platelets
    c. increases platelet aggregation by increasing release of calcium in platelets
    d. increases platelet aggregation by decreasing release of calcium in platelets

    Answer c. *Thromboxane* causes platelet aggregation by **increasing Ca^{++}** in platelets. This causes exposure of the Gp IIb/IIIa receptor and platelet binding.

21. *Prostacyclin:
    a. decreases platelet aggregation and causes vasodilatation
    b. decreases platelet aggregation and causes vasoconstriction
    c. increases platelet aggregation and causes vasodilatation
    d. increases platelet aggregation and causes vasoconstriction

    Answer a. *Prostacyclin* decreases platelet aggregation and causes vasodilatation.(mediated through **increased cAMP** in platelet)

22. **All of the following are true except:
    a. HITT is caused by Ab's to platelet factor 4-heparin complex
    b. The serotonin release assay is the most sensitive test for HITT
    c. Low molecular weight heparin is the Tx of choice for HITT
    d. Argatroban is a direct thrombin inhibitor

    Answer c. **Direct thrombin inhibitors** (eg Argatroban) are Tx of choice for HITT

Coagulation Factors
  All are synthesized in **liver** _except_ **Factor VIII** (synthesized in endothelium)
    vWF (cofactor for VIII) – also synthesized in endothelium
Prothrombin complex (Xase complex)
  *X, V, **calcium**, platelet factor 3, and **prothrombin**
  Forms on platelets; **catalyzes formation of** thrombin
    Tissue factor + Factor VII initiate in the extrinsic pathway
*Thrombin (Key to **coagulation cascade**)
    1) Converts **fibrinogen** to **fibrin** (and fibrinogen degradation products)
    2) Activates **factors V and VIII**
    3) Activates **platelets**
    Generated on platelet surface (prothrombin complex above)
    Fibrin + platelets = platelet plug (hemostasis)
*Anti-thrombin III (AT-III, Key to **anticoagulation**)
    Binds and inhibits **Factors IIa** (thrombin) **IX, X,** and **XI**
    Heparin binds AT-III (increases activity 1000 x)
*Protein C - degrades **Factors V and VIII**, also degrades **fibrinogen**
*Protein S - protein C cofactor
Bleeding time – measures platelet function (_best test_ of platelet function)
*Correction of coagulopathy (↑PT or ↑INR; eg liver disease or on Coumadin)
    *FFP- effect is immediate , lasts 6 hrs, best for emergent / urgent reversal
    *Vitamin K (intravenous) - requires 6 hours to take effect

MC **congenital hypercoaguable disorder - resistance to activated protein C
MC **acquired hypercoaguable disorder – smoking
Key RFs for venous thrombosis (Virchow's triad) - stasis. endothelial injury, and hypercoaguability
Key RF for arterial thrombosis – endothelial injury

Congenital Hypercoaguable States

1) ****Resistance to activated protein C** (*MC; 5% of population*)
    *Factor V Leiden mutation (mutation is on Factor V)
2) **Hyperhomocyteinemia** (MTHFR mutation *or* folate, B6 or B12 deficiency)
3) **Prothrombin gene mutation** (G20210A)
4) **Protein C and S deficiencies**
5) **Anti-thrombin III deficiency** - **Heparin does not work in these pts*
    Have to give **AT-III** 1st (recombinant AT-III or FFP), then heparin
    FFP has highest concentration of AT-III of all blood products
    Can develop after previous heparin exposure
Tx: For all above *except* AT III deficiency and hyperhomocysteinemia→
            Tx: post-op **heparin**, then Coumadin
     For AT III deficiency → Tx: give recombinant AT III or FFP,
            heparinize, then Coumadin
     For hyperhomocysteinemia → Tx: folate, pyridoxine,
            cyanocobalamine

Anti-Phospholipid Antibody Syndrome (APAS)

Sx's: **thrombosis** (venous or arterial) *and/or* **loss of pregnancy**
Dx: high **anti-cardiolipin** *or* **lupus anticoagulant Ab's** (test x2)
Cardiolipin is a mitochondrial phospholipid
Lupus anticoagulant Ab's - prolongs coagulation reactions****Have**
    hypercoaguability w/ elevated PTT (*that does not correct w/ FFP*)
Causes – primary or from autoimmune disease (eg SLE)
Tx: **heparin**, then Coumadin after surgery (lifelong)

**Warfarin induced skin necrosis

Skin sloughs off extremities
Occurs when placed on Coumadin without being heparinized first
Due to **short half-life of proteins C and S** are decreased before
    procoagulation factors; get hypercoaguable state → **thrombosis**)
**Pts w/ protein C deficiency especially susceptible
Tx: heparin if it occurs; prevent by starting Heparin *before* Warfarin

*von Willebrand's disease (vWD)

**MC congenital bleeding disorder (AD)
MC sx – epistaxis
vWF (von Willebrand's Factor) production occurs in **endothelium**
vWF links **Gplb receptor** on **platelets** to **collagen** (main effect)
Dx: PT normal, PTT normal or slightly prolonged
    **Prolonged bleeding time (ristocetin test) – platelets can't bind
Tx: ****DDAVP** in general is 1st line tx *except* Type III
    Type III – recombinant Factor VIII-vWF complex, cryoprecipitate
Cryoprecipitate has highest **vWF + Factor VIII** of all blood products
Type I (MC type, 70%) - reduced quantity of vWF (mild sx's)
Type II - have enough vWF but doesn't work well
Type III - almost no vWF, get **severe bleeding** (**DDAVP does not work)

Platelet defect bleeding disorders - *Bernard-Soulier* (Gplb receptor
    defect), *Glanzmann's* (GpIIb/IIIa receptor defect); Dx: prolonged
    bleeding time, plts can't bind; Tx -**platelets**
H and P – best way to predict bleeding risk; **abnormal bleeding w/ tooth
    extraction or tonsillectomy** picks up 99% pts with bleeding disorder

*Hemophilia A

Factor VIII deficiency, sex linked recessive
MC Sx - hemarthrosis; others – muscle, GI tract, or brain hemorrhage
Factor VIII **crosses placenta** → newborns may not bleed at circumcision
Dx: ***prolonged PTT** and a normal PT
Tx: **Recombinant Factor VIII** (best Tx)
     Cryoprecipitate (highest concentration of Factor VIII)
     *Surgery - want levels **100% pre-op** and **50% post-op** (for 3-5 days)

Monitor PTT every 8-12 hours
Hemophiliac joint - *do NOT aspirate
Tx: **Recombinant Factor VIII**, ice, and range of motion exercises
Epistaxis, intracerebral hemorrhage or **hematuria** -
Tx: **Recombinant Factor VIII**
Spontaneous bleed – occurs at levels < 1%

Hemophilia B – Factor IX deficiency; Dx: **prolonged PTT** and normal PT
Tx **recombinant factor IX, FFP**

**Uremic coagulopathy* - occurs w/ BUN > 60-80
Uremia inhibits release of vWF is the key problem
Tx: a) **Hemodialysis* (*best Tx; reverses uremia and coagulopathy*);
hemodialysis day before procedure commonly used
b) Emergency procedure and do not have time for dialysis – give
DDAVP for acute reversal of coagulopathy; stimulates endothelial
release of *factor VIII and vWF* (30 minute time of onset, lasts 4 hrs)

Deep Venous Thrombosis (DVT)
MC DVT location – calf
MC location to result in PE – Ilio-femoral
Left leg 2x MC than right (left iliac vein compressed by right iliac artery)
Virchow's triad - venous stasis, hypercoaguability, endothelial wall injury
Dx: Duplex U/S
Tx: **Heparin**, then Coumadin (INR 2-3)
Heparin stabilizes clot and prevents extension
Phlegmasia alba dolens (swollen **white** leg) - less severe then
below; Tx: elevate leg, heparin, consider catheter thrombolysis
Phlegmasia cerulea dolens (swollen **blue** leg) Tx: leg elevation,
heparin, consider catheter-directed thrombolytics
Emergent **Fogarty balloon thrombectomy** if extremity **threatened**
(eg loss of sensation and motor function)
Coumadin contraindicated in pregnancy → Tx: enoxaparin
Post-op DVT Prevention - **Majority of adult surgery inpatient's should
receive LMWH prophylaxis* unless contraindicated* (in addition to
early ambulation and SCDs)
Sequential compression devices (SCDs) – improve venous return but
also induce **fibrinolysis** with compression (**release of tPA**)
IVC filter
**Want filter below renal veins*
**PE w/ filter in place* – comes from ovarian veins, IVC superior to
filter, or SVC route (upper extremities)

Tissue plasminogen activator (tPA)
Released from **endothelium**
Induces **fibrinolysis** by converting **plasminogen** to **plasmin**
Plasmin - degrades **Factors V** and **VIII** along w/ **fibrinogen** and **fibrin**
Lose platelet plug, get fibrin degradation products (FDPs, eg **D-dimer**)
Alpha-2 antiplasmin - natural inhibitor of plasmin, released from endothelium
Prostate surgery* can release **urokinase; induces **fibrinolysis** (*converts
plasminogen to plasmin); Sx's: bleeding;
Tx:** **aminocaproic acid** (*inhibits plasmin*)

Thrombolytics (tissue plasminogen activator (tPA), **urokinase*)
Indications – usually limb ischemia (mostly for thrombosis)
Given w/ **heparin**, usually for 8-24 hrs
Follow **fibrinogen** levels → < 100 has high bleeding risk
**Thrombolytic (eg urokinase) overdose Tx* – aminocaproic acid
Contraindications* (these are also contraindications to heparin*)
Absolute - active **internal bleeding,** recent **CVA** (< 2 months), **cranial
pathology** (eg brain tumor, subdural hematoma)

Relative - recent procedure (<10 d, surgery, biopsy, obstetric delivery) or
major trauma, heart thrombus, recent GI bleed (< 90 d), severe HTN

Unfractionated Heparin - binds AT-III and inhibits Factors **IIa** and **Xa**
Want PTT 60-90, 1/2 life 60–90 minutes
Cleared by **reticuloendothelial system** (macrophages, spleen)
S/Es: early – HITT, **long term use** - osteoporosis, alopecia
Does not cross placental barrier (Warfarin does)
Pre-op - hold heparin 6 hrs before surgery; re-start in 48 hrs if not bleeding
**See contra-indications to heparin above
Protamine – binds and reverses heparin (MC S/E – protamine reaction,
1%, anaphylactic w/ hypotension, bradycardia, Tx: Volume, epi)
Low molecular weight heparin (eg enoxaparin, fondiparinux)
Fondaparinux (Lovenox) is a selective **AT-III - Xa inhibitor**
Much smaller risk of HITT; do not need to monitor PTT
Not reversed w/ Protamine
**HITT (Heparin-induced thrombocytopenia thrombocytosis)
Anti-platelet Ab's causes **platelet destruction** and at times **thrombosis**
Forms a ****white clot**; can occur w/ just one low dose of heparin
*Caused by IgG to platelet factor4 - heparin complex
Clinical suspicion:
1) **platelet drop** < 100 or 50% baseline *or;*
2) arterial or venous **thrombosis / embolism** (eg cold leg, DVT, PE)
Dx: **ELISA for PF4-heparin Ab's**
1)   If **strongly positive**, the pt has HITT
2)   If **mildly positive**, perform [14]**C-serotonin release assay**
i.   if **positive** → pt has HITT
ii.   If **negative** → pt does not have HITT
Tx: **stop heparin, start ****direct thrombin inhibitor** *(eg Argatroban or
Bivalirudin, PTT 60-90), then Coumadin*
****Platelet transfusion is contraindicated w/ HITT** – induces thrombosis

*Prostacyclin (PGI$_2$) - released from ***endothelium**
Inhibits platelet aggregation and causes **vasodilation**
***Increases cAMP in platelets*
ASA irreversibly binds **cyclooxygenase**, but cyclooxygenase is **re-
synthesized** in endothelium (have nuclear material unlike platelets)-
result is normal PGI$_2$ production + **platelet inhibition**
*Thromboxane (TXA$_2$) - released from ***platelets**
Causes **platelet aggregation** and **vasoconstriction**
***Increases calcium in platelets* → *exposes **GpIIb/IIIa** and **GpIb** receptors
(induces **platelet binding**)*
ASA irreversibly binds **cyclooxygenase**, decreasing TXA production for
the life of the platelet (7 days, platelets do not have nuclear material –
can't re-synthesize cyclooxygenase)
ASA - stop 7 days before surgery; prolongs bleeding time
WBCs – contain nuclear material; **RBCs** – no nuclear material

Clopidogrel *(Plavix)* and **coronary stents
***There is a high risk of **stent thrombosis** (and myocardial infarction) if
Plavix is stopped early after drug-eluting stent placement*
Elective Surgery Recommendations:
****Bare metal** stents – Plavix for **6 weeks** *before elective surgery*
****Drug eluting** stents – Plavix for **1 year** *before elective surgery*
Emergency Surgery – operate on Plavix and have platelets available
Semi-Urgent Surgery – stop Plavix 5-7 days pre-op; bridge w/ short-acting
IIb/IIIa inhibitors
Clopidogrel (Plavix) is an **ADP receptor inhibitor** (↓ GpIIb/IIIa activation)

Blood Products

23. All of the following are true of acute hemolytic transfusion reactions except:
    a. Bilirubin is likely low
    b. Haptoglobin is likely low
    c. Free hemoglobin is likely high
    d. Volume resuscitation is the 1st step in this patient's management

    Answer a. Bilirubin would be elevated due to hemolysis

24. **All the following are true of transfusion related acute lung injury (TRALI) except
    a. Is caused by donor antibodies which bind WBCs and lodge in lung
    b. Tx is similar to ARDS
    c. Result in decreased capillary permeability
    d. Results in pulmonary edema

    Answer c. **TRALI *results in increased capillary permeability and is caused by **donor antibodies which bind **WBCs and lodge in lung***

25. **The most common blood transfusion reaction is:
    a. Clerical error leading to ABO incompatibility
    b. Transfusion related acute lung injury
    c. Delayed hemolysis from reaction to minor antigens
    d. Febrile non-hemolytic transfusion reaction

    Answer d. Febrile non-hemolytic transfusion reaction is the MC reaction

26. **Prevention of febrile non-hemolytic transfusion reaction involves:
    a. Heating blood to destroy the white blood cells
    b. Prophylactic antibiotics
    c. NSAID's
    d. Leukocyte filter

    Answer d. Febrile non-hemolytic transfusion reaction occurs from white blood cells in the donor blood and can be prevented by using a leukocyte filter during transfusion (the filter size is large enough to allow red blood cells through but small enough to trap white blood cells).

27. **All of the following are true of blood products except:
    a. Stored pRBCs last 3 months
    b. The MC blood product containing bacterial contamination is platelets
    c. The MC bacterial contaminant Gram negative rods
    d. Blood transfusion increases the risk of infection in pts

    Answer a. Stored pRBCs last 3 weeks. The MC blood product to contain a bacterial contaminant is platelets because they are stored at room temperature (good medium for bacterial growth: MC - GNRs, #1 E. coli)

Blood transfusion
Type O Blood (Universal donor) – contains no A or B antigens
    Males can receive Rh positive blood
    Females who are pre-pubescent or of child-bearing age should receive Rh negative blood
Type AB Blood (Universal recipient) – pt does not have A or B Ab's
Type and screen looks for **preformed Ab's** to **minor antigens**
Massive blood transfusion can result in:
    Dilution of coagulation factors - causes coagulopathy
    Hypocalcemia - manifested as hypotension, coagulopathy
    Hypothermia - causes coagulopathy by ***slowing down enzyme reactions*** (use blood warmer to help prevent);
        Best Tx for hypothermia - **warm air conduction (Bair Hugger)*

<u>Packed red blood cells</u> (PRBCs)
    1 unit pRBCs raises Hgb by 1 gm/dl
    PRBCs stored in **citrate** (CDPA) for preservation – citrate **binds Ca^{++}**
        ***Cause of *hypocalcemia* w/ *massive transfusions* ($\geq$ 10 units
            PRBCs)*
    Stored PRBCs last **3 weeks**
        <u>storage effects</u>- $\downarrow$ 2.3 DPG, $\downarrow$ pH, $\uparrow$ K^+ and $\uparrow$ lactic acid

Platelets
    Platelet transfusion indications**:**
        1) **< 10,000** - high risk **spontaneous bleeding**
        2) **< 20,000 w/ infection or bleeding risk** (eg post-op pts)
        3) **< 50,000 w/ active bleeding or pre-procedure**
        <u>Contraindications</u> – TTP, HUS, HELLP, HITT (may need to give
            platelets to control severe bleeding w/ these syndromes)
    6 units (6 pack) **–** increases platelets by **50,000**

<u>Fresh frozen plasma</u> (FFP) - contains **all coagulation factors** (includes protein
    C, protein S, and AT-III); good for deficiency of all coagulation factors (eg
    dilutional coagulopathy w/ massive transfusion, DIC, liver DZ, Warfarin, PT
    > 17 pre-procedure)

<u>Cryoprecipitate</u> - has highest levels of **Factor VIII-vWF** and **fibrinogen;** good
    for low fibrinogen (< 100); can be used for vWD and Hemophilia A

<u>CMV negative</u> (from CMV negative donors) - used for CMV sero-negative
    pregnancy, organ and bone marrow TXP candidates/recipients, AIDS, low
    birth weight infants

<u>Infectious Complications of Transfusion</u>
    Hep B - 1: 200,000, **Hep C** - 1: 2,000,000, **HIV** - 1: 2,000,000
    Blood is also tested for syphilis, HTLV, and West Nile virus
    **MC blood product w/ bacterial contaminant - **<u>platelets</u> (1:50,000)
        Platelets are stored at **room temp** - good medium for bacteria growth
        Platelets last for **5 days** at room temp
        Not refridgerated because **half-life** would be decreased
    MC bacterial contaminant – GNRs (MC ****E. coli)

<u>Other transfusion problems</u>
    Immune system – blood product transfusion *alters the immune system,*
        placing pts at increased risk of **infection**
    **Cold body temp causes *poor clotting* due to *slowing of enzymatic*
        reactions
    All blood products carry risk of **HIV** and **hepatitis** <u>except</u> $\rightarrow$ *******albumin* and
        immunoglobulins (these are heat treated)

<u>Trying to raise Hgb without giving blood</u> (eg Jehovah's Witness w/ low Hct
    before surgery); Tx: **Epoetin** and **Fe supplementation**
    Should raise hemoglobin 1-2 gm/dl / week (Hct 3-5 pts/week)

<u>Iron deficient anemia</u> (microcytic anemia) in **male** or **post-menopausal female**
    – screen for colon CA or another GI source

Transfusion reactions

**Febrile non-hemolytic transfusion reaction (1:100)
    **MC transfusion reaction
    Sx's – <u>fever and rigors</u> 0-6 hrs after transfusion
    **Preformed recipient Ab's against donor WBCs
    Causes **cytokine release**
    Tx: stop transfusion, acetaminophen (R/O infection and hemolysis)
    **WBC filters for subsequent transfusions to prevent reaction

Allergic reaction (1:150)
    MC Sx - <u>urticaria</u> (rash); rare anaphylaxis (bronchospasm hypotension)
    Reaction of **recipient Ab's to **plasma proteins** in blood product*
    **MCC - IgA deficient pt (w/ preformed Ab's to IgA) receiving IgA blood
    Tx: **Urticaria** – diphenhydramine (Benadryl), H2 blockers
          Anaphylaxis – epinephrine, fluids, possible steroids

Delayed hemolytic transfusion reaction (1:2500)
    Sx's - usually **minimal** (often goes unnoticed); mild jaundice
        Usually get sx's **5-10 days** after transfusion
    Preformed **recipient Ab's against donor RBC **minor HLA antigens***
    Tx: nonspecific; Dx impt for future transfusion (HLA match next time)

**Transfusion related acute lung injury *(TRALI, 1:15,000)*
    Sx's – hypoxia, diffuse alveolar infiltrates, fever
    Non-cardiogenic pulmonary edema **< 6 hours** after transfusion
    **<u>Donor</u> Ab's bind <u>recipient</u> WBCs and lodge in lung
        Release mediators causing ↑ **capillary permeability**
    Tx: may require intubation; Tx same as ARDS

Acute hemolytic transfusion reaction (1:250,000)
    Sx's - fever, hypotension, tachycardia, flank pain, hematuria
        Can lead to renal failure, shock and DIC
        **Anesthetized pts can present as diffuse bleeding
    Cause - **ABO incompatibility**
        Preformed recipient Ab's against donor RBCs
        Results in acute hemolysis
    Dx:
        Haptoglobin < 50 (binds Hgb, then gets degraded)
        Free hemoglobin > 5
        ↑ed **unconjugated bilirubin**
    Tx:
        Stop transfusion
        Fluid resuscitation for BP and to maintain **good UOP**
        Diuretics (lasix and mannitol)
        HCO3- (prevent Hgb precipitation in kidney and ATN)
        Pressors for refractory hypotension
    Fatal hemolytic transfusion reaction - 1: 500,000

**MCC death from transfusion reaction – *Clerical error resulting in ABO incompatibility*
**Non-immune hemolysis – from squeezing the blood bag

Immune System and Wound Healing

28. **The key growth factor in wound healing is:
     a.   PDGF
     b.   PAF
     c.   EGF
     d.   FGF

     Answer a. PDGF is the key growth factor in wound healing.

29. *All of the following participate in angiogenesis _except_
     a.   PDGF
     b.   PAF
     c.   Hypoxia
     d.   FGF

     Answer b. PAF does not have angiogenesis properties. ***Hypoxia** is the
     most potent stimulus for angiogenesis.

30. *All of the following are chemotactic for inflammatory cells _except_
     a.   IL-8
     b.   LTB-4
     c.   C5a and C3a
     d.   TGF-Beta

     Answer d. TGF-beta is not chemotactic for inflammatory cells. It is
     generally considered immunosuppressive.

31. *All of the following are the primary functions of the listed cytokine _except_:
     a.   IL-6 increase hepatic acute phase proteins
     b.   IL-8 induces PMN chemotaxis and angiogenesis
     c.   IL-10 upregulates the inflammatory response
     d.   IL-I induces fever

     Answer c. IL-10 down-regulates the inflammatory response.

32. *All of the following hepatic proteins are increased during the acute phase
     response _except_:
     a.   albumin
     b.   C reactive protein
     c.   C3
     d.   Fibrinogen

     Answer a. There is decreased synthesis of albumin, pre-albumin, and
     transferrin during the acute phase response

33. **Infections associated w/ defects in cell mediated immunity include all of the
     following except
     a.   Staph
     b.   E. Coli
     c.   Tuberculosis
     d.   Proteus

     Answer c. **Infections associated w/ **defects in cell mediated immunity**
     include **intra-cellular pathogens** (eg TB, other mycobacterium, viruses)

34. *All of the following are true of cell adhesion molecules _except_
     a.   Selectins are involved in rolling adhesion
     b.   L-selectin binds E-selectin and P-selectin
     c.   ICAM binds beta-2 integrin (CD 11/18) molecules
     d.   P-selectin is located on leukocytes

Answer d. P-selectin is located on platelets

35. *All of the following are true of complement *except*
    a. C5b, C6b, C7b, C8b and C9b form the membrane attack complex
    b. C1, C2, and C4 are found *only* in the classic pathway
    c. C1 and C2 are anaphylatoxins
    d. Factors B, D, and P (properdin) are found *only* in alternate pathway

    Answer c. *C3a, C4a and C5a are **anaphylatoxins***
    C5b, C6b, C7b, C8b and C9b** form **cell membrane attack complex

36. **All of the following are true of oxygen radicals except
    a. The primary injuring mechanism of oxygen radicals is DNA damage
    b. Cellular defense against superoxide anion primarily involves superoxide dismutase
    c. Cellular defense against hydrogen peroxide primarily involves taurine
    d. Chronic granulomatous disease results in decreased superoxide radical (O_2^-) formation due to a defect in the NADPH-oxidase enzyme system

    Answer c. **Cellular defense against hydrogen peroxide primarily involves peroxidase and catalase.*

    Chronic granulomatous disease** results in decreased **superoxide radical** (O_2^-) formation due to a defect in the **NADPH-oxidase enzyme system

37. **All of the following are true *except*
    a. LTC_4, LTD_4 and LTE_4 (slow-reacting substances of anaphylaxis) cause bronchoconstriction and vasoconstriction followed by increased permeability (wheal and flare)
    b. Thyroid hormone has a major role in inflammation and injury
    c. Dense granules have adenosine (as ATP, ADP), serotonin, calcium
    d. LTB_4 is chemotactic for PMNs and eosinophils

    Answer b. *Thyroid hormone does not have a major role in inflammation.*
    Dense granules** have **adenosine** (as ATP, ADP), **serotonin**, **calcium
    ***LTB_4** is **chemotactic** for PMNs and eosinophils*
    ***LTC_4, LTD_4 and LTE_4** (slow-reacting substances of anaphylaxis) cause bronchoconstriction and vasoconstriction followed by increased permeability (wheal and flare)*

38. *All of the following are true except
    a. The most predominate cell in the 1st 24 hrs of a wound is PMNs
    b. The most predominant cell at days 3-4 after a wound is macrophages
    c. The order of cell arrival in wound is macrophages, platelets, PMNs, fibroblasts, lymphocytes
    d. The most predominate cell type in a 7 day old wound is fibroblasts

    Answer c. The order of cell arrival in wound is platelets, PMNs, macrophages, fibroblasts, lymphocytes

39. *All of the following are true except
    a. The most predominant type of collagen in the body is Type I
    b. The most predominant type of collagen being synthesized in a healing wound in the 1st 24 hours is Type III
    c. The maximum collagen amount in a wound occurs at 3 weeks
    d. Maximum tensile strength of a wound occurs at 3 weeks

Answer d. Maximum tensile strength occurs at 8 weeks. Although the maximum collagen amount occurs at 3 weeks, remodeling and cross-linking occur to increase tensile strength, which is maximum at 8 weeks.

40. *All of the following are true except
    a. The most important cell involved in wound healing is macrophages
    b. The most predominant collagen type in cartilage is Type II
    c. Vit A prevents the negative effects of steroids on wound healing
    d. Keloids are confined to the original scar area

    Answer d. Keloids are <u>not</u> confined to original scar (hypertrophic scar tissue is). ****Best method for inhibiting keloid formation** – steroid injection following keloid excision.

41. **Peripheral nerves regenerate at:
    a. 0.01 mm/day
    b. 0.1 mm/day
    c. 1 mm/day
    d. 5 mm/day

    Answer c. ***Nerves regenerate at **1 mm/day**.*

42. **The most important factor in the healing of wounds by secondary intention is:
    a. Tensile strength of the wound
    b. Epithelial integrity
    c. Platelet activating factor
    d. Prostacyclin

    Answer b. ***The most important factor in wound healing by **secondary intention** is **epithelial integrity**.*

43. **The most important factor in the healing of wounds by primary intention is:
    a. Tensile strength of the wound
    b. Epithelial integrity
    c. Platelet activating factor
    d. Prostacyclin

    Answer a. ***Wound healing by **primary intention** is dependent on the **tensile strength** of the wound. This is created by collagen cross-linking. The sutures you place hold the wound together until appropriate collagen deposition and cross-linking can occur.*

44. **A patient with a large open gluteal laceration comes to clinic and to your surprise the wound is much smaller. This is primarily a result of:
    a. Lymphocytes
    b. Macrophages
    c. PMNs
    d. Myofibroblasts

    Answer d. *****Myofibroblasts** participate in wound contraction.*

45. **All of the following are true <u>except:</u>
    a. Natural killer are involved in T cell receptor and antigen-MHC class recognition
    b. Newborn's innate immunity has poor phagocyte chemotaxis (PMNs + macrophages), making them susceptible to cutaneous infections
    c. IL-2 is released from helper T cells and activates cytotoxic T and natural killer cells
    d. Cytotoxic T cells (CD8) attack non-self antigens attached to MHC class I receptors

Answer a. **Natural killer cells** are not involved in antigen-MHC class recognition. They attack cells w/ low expression of MHC (missing self) and cells w/ bound antibody.

***Newborn's innate immunity has **poor phagocyte chemotaxis** (PMNs + macrophages), making them susceptible to **cutaneous infections** (make sure you wash your hands)*

46. *Cachexia in patients with cancer is primarily the result of:
    a. IL-2
    b. IL-6
    c. IL-10
    d. TNF-alpha

    Answer d. **TNF-alpha promotes **cachexia** in patients with cancer.*

47. **Vitamins essential for normal bone growth include all of the following except
    a. Vit C
    b. Vit K
    c. Vit A
    d. Vit D

    Answer b. Vit K is not essential for normal bone growth.
    *****Vit C, Vit A and Vit D** are essential for normal bone growth.*

Innate Immune System (Inflammation and Complement)
Inflammation
  *****Macrophages** -**have **dominant role** in inflammation + wound healing*
      Release important **growth factors (**PDGF) + cytokines (**TNF-alpha and IL-1) to attract other inflammatory cells + fibroblasts
      Phagocytosis + remove debris (monocytes become macrophages)
  *****Order of cell arrival in wound** - Platelets, PMNs, Macrophages, Fibroblasts, Lymphocytes*
  *****Predominant cell type by day**

Days 0–2	*PMNs*
Days 3–4	*Macrophages*
Days 5 and on	*Fibroblasts*

  Inflammation is 1st step in normal wound healing
  Wound Healing: Inflammation (PDGF, PAF), **Proliferation** (PDGF, FGF, EGF), **Remodeling**
**Cell mediated immunity
  Intradermal skin test (eg PPD for TB) – tests cell-mediated immunity
  *****Infections associated w/ defects in cell mediated immunity** – intracellular pathogens (eg TB, other mycobacterium, viruses)*
Other cell types
  Mast cells – ***main cell type* involved in Type I hypersensitivity reactions
  Basophils – Type I Hypersensitivity reactions
  Eosinophils – parasitic infections, Type I hypersensitivity reactions (late)

**Cytokines
  Main cytokines released w/ inflammation - TNF-alpha (#1) and IL-1
      Vast majority of cytokines are produced by **macrophages**
  *****TNF-alpha** (tumor necrosis factor-alpha)*
      Main source - macrophages
      ↑ **cell adhesion molecules** (eg ICAM, selectins); **procoagulant**
      Activates **PMNs** and other **macrophages** → leads to **growth factor** production → **cell recruitment**
      ↑ HR, ↑ cardiac output, ↓ SVRI → high concentration can cause myocardial depression, **circulatory collapse** and **MSOF**
      ***Causes **cachexia** in pts w/ CA*

18

**IL-1
> **Main source** - macrophages
> Effects similar to TNF and synergizes TNF
> ****Induces fever** (**PGE$_2$ mediated** in hypothalamus)
>> Raises thermal set point, causing fever
>> **NSAIDs** – ↓ fever by reducing PGE$_2$ synthesis.
> **Alveolar macrophages**- cause fever w/ atelectasis by releasing **IL-1**
> **IL-6** - 1° function is ↑**hepatic acute phase proteins** (see below)
> **IL-8** - 1° function is **PMN chemotaxis** (+ other cells) and **angiogenesis**
> **IL-10** - 1° function is **down regulation inflammatory response**
>> (↓ TNF-alpha, IL-2, IL3, and interferons; down-regulates APCs)
> **Interferons** - released by **lymphocytes** in response to **viral infection**;
>> activate inflammatory cells, inhibit viral replication, upregulate MHC

****Growth factors**
> ****PDGF** (platelet-derived growth factor) - **_key factor_** in wound healing
>> Chemotactic for and activates **inflammatory cells**
>> Chemotactic for and activates **fibroblasts**
>> **Angiogenesis** and **Epithelialization**
>> Chemotactic for **smooth muscle cells**
>> Accelerates **wound healing**
> **PAF** (platelet-activating factor)
>> Activates **platelets**; PAF is a **phospholipid**
>> Chemotactic and activates **inflammatory cells**
>> ↑s **adhesion molecule** expression
>> _Not stored_, generated by **phospholipase** in endothelium, other cells
> **FGF** (epidermal growth factor) - chemotactic + activates **fibroblasts,**
>> **angiogenesis, epithelialization**
> **EGF** (epidermal growth factor) - chemotactic + activates **fibroblasts,**
>> **angiogenesis, epithelialization**
> **TGF-beta** (transforming growth factor-beta) - primarily
>> **immunosuppressive** - inhibits lymphocytes and leukocytes
> **Chemotactic factors**
>> For inflammatory cells – PDGF, PAF, IL-8, LTB-4, C5a and C3a
>> For fibroblasts – PDGF, FGF, EGF
> ****Angiogenesis factors** – PDGF, FGF, EGF, IL-8, hypoxia
>> Produced by **macrophages** and **platelets** in response to **hypoxia**
> ****Epithelialization factors** – PDGF, FGF, EGF
> **Macrophages** – main producers of **growth factors**
> **PMNs** – last 2 days in tissue (last 7 days in blood)
> **Platelets** – last 7 days

***Hepatic acute phase proteins**
> **IL-6** – most potent stimulus
> **Increased synthesis** – C-reactive protein (an opsonin, activates
>> complement), amyloid A and P, fibrinogen, haptoglobin,
>> ceruloplasmin, alpha-1 antitrypsin, and C3 (complement)
> ****Decreased synthesis** – albumin, prealbumin, and transferrin

***Cell adhesion molecules**
> **Selectins** – involved in **rolling adhesion** (1st step in transmigration
>> process); **L-selectins** (on leukocytes) bind to **E-selectin** (endothelial)
>> and **P- selectin** (platelets)
> **Beta-2 integrins** (CD 11/18 molecules)
>> Found on **leukocytes** and **platelets**
>> Involved in **anchoring adhesion** and transendothelial **migration**
>> Bind ICAM, VCAM, etc
> **ICAM, VCAM, PECAM,** and **ELAM**
>> Found on **endothelial cells**
>> Involved in **anchoring adhesion** and transendothelial **migration**
>> Bind **beta-2 integrin molecules** (above)

Complement (part of innate immune system

1) **Classic** pathway
- Activation Mechanisms
    - **a)** **Antigen–antibody complex** (IgG or IgM *only*) *or;*
    - **b)** Direct binding of **pathogen** to C1
- *Initial step* is formation of **C1 complex** (2 C1 molecules)
- *****Factors C1, C2, and C4** – found *only* in the classic pathway

2) **Alternative** pathway
- Activation mechanisms – **endotoxin, bacteria**, other stimuli activate
- *Initial step* is **C3 activation**
- *****Factors B, D, and P *(properdin)*** – found *only* in alternate pathway
- **C3 activation** – common to and convergence point for both pathways
- **Mg^{++}** required for both pathways
- **Products**:
    1) *****Anaphylatoxins** – C3a, C4a and C5a; ↑ vascular permeability bronchoconstriction, activate mast cells and basophils
    2) *****Cell membrane attack complex**: C5b-C9b(C5bC6bC7bC8bC9b) Inserted into **pathogen cell membrane**, makes hole→ cell lysis Can also **attack normal cells infected w/ bacteria**
    3) *****Opsonization**-C3b and C4b; enhances **phagocytosis of antigen**
    4) *Inflammatory cell **chemotaxis** (PMNs, macrophage) - C3a + C5a

*****Oxidants generated in inflammation** (oxidants and producers)

Superoxide anion radical (O_2^-)	NADPH oxidase
Hydrogen peroxide (H_2O_2)	Xanthine oxidase, NADPH oxidase

*******Cellular defenses against Oxidative Species** (oxidants and defense)

Superoxide anion radical	*Superoxide dismutase* (need Cu + Zn) Converts to hydrogen peroxide
Hydrogen peroxide	*Glutathione peroxidase, catalase*

*******Primary injuring mechanism of oxygen radicals** – DNA damage

Respiratory burst (macrophages, PMNs) - releases superoxide anion and hydrogen peroxide

*******Chronic granulomatous disease**
- *Defect in *******NADPH-oxidase enzyme system** in PMNs and macrophages
- *Results in *****decreased superoxide radical (O_2^-) formation*

*******Platelet granules**

Alpha granules
- Aggregation Factors– platelet factor 4, vWF, fibrinogen, fibronectin
- Beta-thromboglobulin – binds thrombin
- PDGF and TGF-beta
- Factors V and XIII
- *****Dense granules** (ASC) - Adenosine (as ATP or ADP), Serotonin, Calcium

Lipid mediators

Mainly involved in **inflammation regulation**

Initial substrate is **phospholipid essential fatty acids** (in cell membrane)
- **Phospholipids** → *(phospholipase)* → **Arachadonic acid**
- *****Glucocorticoids** inhibit *phospholipase* and production of everything below

1) **Cyclooxygenase** (COX) **pathway** (produces prostaglandins)
    - a) *PGI$_2$ (prostacyclin) and PGE$_2$*
        - Systemic and pulmonary **vasodilation** (↓ SVR, ↓ PVR)
        - ↓ **platelet aggregation**
        - **Bronchodilation**
    - b) *TXA$_2$ (thromboxane), PGG$_2$, PGH$_2$,*
        - Systemic and pulmonary **vasoconstriction** (↑ SVR, ↑ PVR)
        - ↑ **platelet aggregation**

2) **Lipoxygenase pathway** (produces leukotrienes and lipoxins)
    Are **leukocyte derived** molecules
    a) **Leukotrienes**
        **LTC$_4$, LTD$_4$, LTE$_4$ – Slow-reacting substances of anaphylaxis
           Bronchoconstriction
           Vasoconstriction followed by ↑permeability (***wheal and flare**)
        **LTB$_4$ – chemotaxis for PMNs and eosinophils
    b) **Lipoxins** - anti-inflammatory (↓ chemotaxis, ↓ transmigration)
Other Inflammation
    **Catecholamines (neural response to injury) - peak 24-48 hrs after injury
    Neuroendocrine response to injury
        Afferent nerves from site of injury stimulate ACTH, ADH, growth
           hormone, epinephrine, and norepinephrine release
    **Thyroid hormone – does <u>not</u> play a major role in injury

Wound Healing
    Wound healing phases
        1) **Inflammation** (1-10 d, see above)
        2) **Proliferation** (5 days to 3 weeks)
           a) **Granulation tissue** [= vascularized **extracellular matrix** (ECM)]
               Provisional ECM - ***hyaluronic acid** (primary component,
                  glycosaminoglycan); produced by ***fibroblasts**;
                  undergoes neovascularization (**endothelial cells**)
           b) **Epithelialization** (1-2 mm/day, requires **granulation tissue**)
               Keratinocytes (epithelial cells) from ****hair follicles (#1
                  source)** + wound edges + sweat glands **migrate** across
                  granulation tissue
           c) **Wound contraction** by ****myofibroblasts** (peaks at **10-15 days**)
           d) **Collagen Deposition** by ***fibroblasts**; provides **wound strength**
               Type I collagen predominant collagen <u>in wound</u> (although
                  **Type III is predominant type synthesized in 1st 48 hours)
        3) **Maturation and Remodeling** (3 weeks to 1 year)
           Max collagen synthesis occurs at ***3 weeks** → net amount then
               does not change although production + degradation occurs
           Type III collagen replaced w/ **Type I**
           *Cross-linking occurs along **tension lines**
           Peak strength at **8 weeks** (80% normal, most it ever gets)

        **Macrophages- essential cell in wound healing (growth factors, cytokines)
        **Accelerated wound healing – reopening a wound results in quicker
           healing the 2nd time (healing cells there already)
        **Myofibroblasts
           Fibroblast w/ smooth muscle cell components (actin / myosin)
           Communicate by **gap junctions**
           Involved in **wound contraction** and **healing by secondary
              intention**
           Perineum (more redundant tissue)- better wound contraction than leg
        Peripheral nerves – regeneration at **1 mm/day
        **Zinc – impt in many enzyme systems of wound healing
        Phosphate – important for leukocyte **chemotaxis and **phagocytosis**
           (↓ed phosphate results in ↓ed ATP)

    *Delayed primary closure - wound left open for a couple of days to make sure it
        is not infected, then close it primarily. There is a risk of abscess and
        wound infection with this method

**_Epithelial integrity_
> **_Most impt factor in healing_ **open wounds** _(secondary intention)_
> Epithelial cell **migration** occurs from ****hair follicles** (#1 source), wound
> > edges and sweat glands - dependent on **granulation tissue**
>
> Unepithelialized wounds leak serum and protein → promotes **bacteria**

**_Tensile strength_
> **_Most impt factor in healing_ **closed incisions** _(primary intention)_
> Depends on **collagen deposition** and **cross-linking**
> ****_Submucosa_** – strength layer of bowel
> ****Weakest time point for small bowel anastomosis** – 3-5 days
> At 6 weeks – wound 60% original strength
> At 8-12 weeks – wound **max tensile strength** (80% original strength)
> **Suture removal**
> > Face or cosmetic area – 1 week; Other areas – 2 weeks

Collagen
> I   ****MC type in body**
> > Skin, bone, tendons, **cornea** (not lens)
> > Primary collagen in **healing wound**
>
> II   ****_Cartilage_** → MC collagen in **cartilage**
> III   ****_Granulation tissue_**; blood vessels, fetal skin
> IV   **Basement membrane, eye lens**, glomeruli
> Many other types
> Collagen has **proline** every 3rd amino acid
> **Proline residues** undergo hydroxylation _(prolyl hydroxylase)_ and **cross-
> > linking** (requires *_Alpha-ketoglutarate, Vit C, Oxygen, and Iron_)
>
> **d-Penicillamine** – inhibits collagen cross-linking

**_Essentials for clinical wound healing_
> 1) **Moist environment** (promotes cell migration; avoid desiccation)
> 2) **Oxygen delivery** - optimal fluids, no smoking, pain control, arterial
> > revascularization if needed, supplemental oxygen
> > Want transcutaneous oxygen measurement (TCOM) **> 25 mmHg**
>
> 3) **Avoid edema** – leg elevation, light compression
> 4) **Remove necrotic tissue**, wet to dry dressings

**_Impediments to wound healing_
> 1) **Bacteria >10^5 / cm^2** (wound infection)
> 2) **Devitalized tissue and foreign bodies**
> 3) **Cytotoxic drugs** (eg cyclosporine, FK-506, 5-FU, methotrexate)
> > **Chemotherapy** – has no effect on wound healing after 14 days
>
> 4) **Diabetes**
> 5) **Albumin < 3.0** = poor nutrition = poor wound healing
> 6) ****Steroids** - Inhibit macrophages, PMNs, and fibroblasts
> > Also ↓ **wound tensile strength** from ↓ed **collagen deposition**
> > ****_Vitamin A_** _(25,000 IU qd)_ – _counteracts steroids_ for wound healing
>
> 7) **Wound Ischemia** - fibrosis (chronic scarring), pressure (sacral or
> > calcaneus decubitus ulcers), poor arterial inflow or venous outflow,
> > smoking, previous XRT, edema

Vit C, Vit A and Zinc are very important in **wound healing
**_Vitamins required for normal bone growth_ – Vit C, Vit A and Vit D

Other wound healing
> ****_Malnutrition_** – most common immune deficiency
> **Scars** – proteoglycans, hyaluronic acid, and water
> > **Scar revision** – wait for 1 year for maturation; may improve w/ age
>
> **Infants** can heal with little or no scarring
> *_Cartilage_ – no blood vessels (get nutrients and oxygen by **diffusion**)
> **Denervation** – no effect on wound healing
> **Diabetic foot ulcers** – **Charcot's joint** (2nd MTP joint) and **heel** MC sites
> > Neuropathy leads to pressure ischemia + necrosis (see Vascular chp)

Leg ulcers – 90% due to **venous insufficiency** (see Vascular chp)
Pressure sores – see Skin and Soft Tissue chp

Wound dehiscence RFs - ****deep wound infection** (*largest RF*), poor nutrition, COPD, DM, cougher; <u>Tx</u>: place **retention sutures**

Adaptive Immune System
Newborns – *innate immunity has* **poor phagocyte chemotaxis *(PMNs + macrophages); susceptible to* ***cutaneous infections → wash hands*
Newborns – have **IgG (from mother through placenta; *the only Ig that crosses placenta*) and **IgA** (from breast milk); provide humeral immunity while newborn immune system develops

<u>T cells</u> [maturation in Thymus, all have **T cell receptors** (CD3)]
    1) **Helper T cells** *(*CD4)* – interact w/ ***MHC class II** receptors (APC cells w/ attached antigen); functions -
        a) **IL-2** release - activates **cytotoxic T** and **natural killer cells**
        b) **INF-gamma** release – activates **macrophages**
        c) **IL-4** release - increases **B cell** Ab production
    Differentiate into **Effector** and **Memory Helper T cells**
    2) **Suppressor T cells** (ie regulatory T cells) - **suppress immune response** and helps prevent autoimmunity; Regulate CD4, CD8 cells
    3) **Cytotoxic T cells** (**CD8+*, activated by IL-2, cell-mediated immunity)
    Attacks antigens attached to ***MHC class I** receptors (eg viral gene protein); release <u>perforin</u> + <u>granulysin</u> (creates pores)
    Cytotoxic T cells cause <u>*nearly all*</u> of liver injury from HepB infection
    4) **Natural killer T cells** (activated by **IL-2**, cell-mediated immunity)
    Attack **host cells** that have been infected by microbes
    Do <u>not</u> use MHC-antigen complexes; Do <u>not</u> directly attack microbe;
    a) **Attack cells w/ low expression of MHC** (missing self)
        Occurs w/ cell infection (esp. viral infection)
    b) **Attack cells w/ bound Ab** (have Fc receptor)

<u>B cells</u> (maturation in Bone)
    Antibody-mediated (humoral) **immunity**
    B cell encounters antigen (+ activated by **T helper cell IL-4**), divides into many **plasma cells** (live 2-3 d), which secrete **Ab's** to antigen
    10% of plasma cells become **memory B cells**
        Can be re-activated if pathogen re-infects host
        IgG secreted (as opposed to IgM) with **re-infection** (class switching)

<u>MHC classes</u> (major histocompatibility complex or HLA classes)
    MHC class I (A, B, and C) - single chain with 5 domains
        Interacts w/ **CD8 cells** (mostly cytotoxic T cells)
        Class I MHC found on all nucleated cells (not RBCs)
        Presents **endogenous antigen** from cytosolic protein breakdown or endogenous antigen pathway (ie viral proteins produced in cell)
        Cytotoxic T cells* → recognize and attack non–self-antigens attached to **MHC class I receptors
    MHC class II (DR, DP, and DQ) - 2 chains with 4 domains each
        Interacts w/ **CD4 cells** (*exclusively* T helper cells)
        Class II MHC found on antigen presenting cells (APCs)
        APCs include dendritic cells, macrophages, and B cells
        Dendritic cells are most impt **APC** (present antigen to T cells)
        Present **exogenous antigen** (exogenous antigen pathway, eg phagocytosis of extra-cellular bacterial proteins)
        *T helper cells (T$_H$ cells) **activated** by MHC class II-antigen complex
        Then activate **macrophages** and **B cells**

Viral infection

Endogenous viral proteins produced inside cell
Are bound to **MHC class I**
MHC class I – antigen complex goes to cell surface, is recognized by
CD8 cytotoxic T cells
Cytotoxic T cell then **attacks the cell expressing the complex**

Bacterial infection (extracellular)

Dendritic cells (APCs) engulf exogenous pathogens (eg bacteria, toxins)
Migrate to T cell enriched lymph nodes
Display non-self antigen coupled to **MHC class II** molecule
This is recognized by **T Helper cells** passing through lymph node
T helper cells then activate **macrophages** and **B cells**

Adaptive Immunity for Cancer Therapy (→ **IL-2** mediated)

1) Convert harvested **lymphocytes** into **lymphokine-activated killer**
    (**LAK**) cells after exposure *in vitro* to tumor antigens
2) Converts harvested **lymphocytes** into **tumor-infiltrating lymphocytes**
    (**TILs**) after exposure *in vitro* to tumor antigens
3) Enhances endogenous T cell immune response to tumor
4) **Tumor vaccines** (ie CA antigens) are injected into the pt in an effort to
    stimulate **adaptive immunity against the tumor** (antigen engulfed
    by APCs, presented, etc)
Some success w/ melanoma for above

Antibodies (immunoglobulins)

IgM

**MC Ab in spleen*
Responsible for **primary** immune response (initial exposure to
    antigen)
Largest antibody - 5 domains and 10 binding sites (pentamer)
Activates **complement**
Opsonization for phagocytosis
Does not cross placenta
Primary Ab against **A** and **B antigens on RBCs** (ABO blood type)
    Causes **clumping** of RBCs and **thrombosis**
****Lack of IgM after splenectomy* results in *overwhelming post-
    splenectomy infection* (OPSI)

IgG

**MC Ab overall* (75% of all immunoglobulins)
Responsible for **secondary** immune response
Activates **complement** (takes 2 IgGs)
Opsonization for phagocytosis
Crosses placenta and provides protection in newborn period
    The only immunoglobulin able to do this

IgA MC immunoglobulin in **mucosal linings** (impt in mucosal immunity)
Found in **secretions**, Peyer's patches in gut, lung, saliva, breast milk
IgA **binds pathogens** to prevent adherence and invasion
    Coats bacteria so that it cannot bind to mucosal epithelium

IgD - membrane-bound receptor found on B cells

IgE - Type I Immediate Hypersensitivity Reactions, **parasite** infections

IgM and **IgG** are **opsonins**
IgM and **IgG** activate (fix) **complement** (requires 2 IgGs or 1 IgM)
Variable region – antigen recognition
Constant region (Fc portion) – recognized by macrophages, PMNs, NK
    cells, eosinophils; Fc fragment does not have variable region
All immunoglobulins have **2 binding sites** except IgM (has 10 sites)
***Polyclonal antibodies* - have multiple binding sites to the antigen at
    multiple epitopes*
**Monoclonal antibodies* - have only one binding site to only one epitope

Hypersensitivity reactions

Type I – immediate hypersensitivity reaction (**IgE** bound to mast cells)
Ex: **asthma, allergic reactions** (eg bee stings, peanuts, lymphazurin blue dye for SLNBx) and **anaphylaxis**
Provoked by **re-exposure**
Mediator - antigen interacts w/ **IgE** bound to **mast cells,** basophils
Response – degranulation of **mast cells** and basophils
Main response: *histamine* (vasodilation, bronchoconstriction)
Effects: bronchoconstriction, rhinorrhea, flushing, hypotension, dyspnea, angioedema (swelling of face, neck and throat)
Tx: **Acute airway Tx** if necessary (eg angioedema)
Anti-histamines (diphenhydramine), **steroids, epinephrine**

Type II – antibody dependent cytotoxicity (**IgG** or **IgM**)
Ex: **acute hemolytic transfusion reaction, hyperacute rejection**
Mediator – IgG or IgM; bind to **cell bound antigen** (or foreign cells w/ TXP hyperacute rejection or ABO transfusion reaction)
Response:
1) **Cell mediated immune response** to bound **IgG or IgM** via Fc receptor on macrophage, PMNs, NK cells, eosinophils
2) Bound IgM or IgG **activates complement**

Type III – immune complex deposition
Ex: serum sickness (eg anti-venom), SLE
Antigen-Ab complexes (IgG) deposited in vessel walls and induces inflammation (rash, arthralgia, fever, lymphadenopathy)
Tx: **corticosteroids, antihistamines**, possible **plasmapheresis**

Type IV – delayed type hypersensitivity reaction
Ex: PPD (TB test), contact dermatitis (eg poison ivy), chronic rejection
Mediator - **T cell** mediated immune response *(*antibody independent*)*
Takes **2-3 days** to develop (or years w/ TXP)
Response - APCs present MHC class II-antigen complex to **T helper cells** → create effector T helper cells → activate **macrophages** which destroy antigen

Other Immunology

Primary lymphoid organs – liver, bone, thymus
Secondary lymphoid organs – spleen and lymph nodes
Immunologic chimera – 2 different cell lines in one individual (eg allogenic bone marrow TXP)
Mast cells - main source of histamine in **tissues** other than stomach
Basophils - main source of histamine in **blood**
Basophils are generally not found in tissue
Angiotensin-converting enzyme (ACE) – inactivates bradykinin

Transplantation

48. *Monoclonal antibodies:
    a. Bind one epitope at one site
    b. Bind one epitope at multiple sites
    c. Bind multiple epitopes on a single antigen
    d. Bind multiple epitopes on multiple antigens

    Answer a. *Monoclonal antibodies (such as OKT3) are all identical, so they bind **one epitope** at the exact same binding site.* **Polyclonal antibodies** have multiple binding sites to the antigen at multiple epitopes.

49. **Four days after orthotopic liver TXP, your pt is noted to have a steep rise in SGOT and SGPT levels (400's) and a rise in serum bilirubin (5.2). What is the next appropriate step in this pts work-up:
    a. Liver MRI
    b. CT scan
    c. Ultrasound and biopsy
    d. Re-transplant

    Answer c. The acute rise in LFT's could be due to acute rejection, hepatic artery thrombosis or other vascular compromise, or infection (CMV, sepsis). **To start, an ultrasound to look at the vascular connections and a liver biopsy to assess for rejection and CMV infection are needed.** Blood cultures for infection are also indicated.

50. *All the following are contra-indications to living donor kidney transplant except:
    a. Duplicated Urinary Collecting System
    b. DM
    c. HIV
    d. Hep B

    Answer a. Duplicated urinary systems or collecting systems are not a contra-indication to living related donor kidney TXP

51. *All of the following mechanisms are true except:
    a. Cyclosporin binds cyclophilin protein, which inhibits calcineurin and inhibits genes for cytokine synthesis (primarily **IL-2**)
    b. Azathioprine inhibits purine synthesis by way of 6-mercaptopurine which in effect inhibits T cells.
    c. Sirolimus binds the FK binding protein and inhibits cyclophilin protein
    d. Tacrolimus binds FK binding protein and inhibits cyclophilin protein

    Answer c. Sirolimus binds the **FK-binding protein** and that complex binds the **mammalian target of rapamycin** (mTOR). That complex inhibits response to **interleukin-2** (IL-2) and blocks activation of T- and B-cells. The tacrolimus-FK binding protein complex binds calcineurin protein.

52. **Three weeks after kidney TXP, your pt presents w/ poor urine output and a creatnine of 2.0. You give a fluid challenge without an increase in urine output. U/S which shows a 4 x 4 x 4 cm hypoechoic mass and moderate hydronephrosis. The graft appears to have good perfusion. All of the following apply to the management of this patient's condition except
    a. Percutaneous drainage is the 1st option in this pts management
    b. Peritoneal window should be performed if it recurs
    c. This complication usually occurs weeks after transplant (3-4)
    d. This complication is related to bleeding

    Answer d. This pt has a lymphocoele that is obstructing his ureter. This Cx usually occurs 3-4 weeks after TXP. **Initial Tx is percutaneous drainage. If the fluid recurs, a **peritoneal window** should be performed* *to allow drainage into the peritoneum.* A **urine leak** usually would occur early post-op (hrs to days, not at 3 weeks)

53. *Two months after kidney TXP, a pt develops respiratory sx's requiring admission to the ICU. CXR shows diffuse infiltrates and bronchial washings show cells w/ inclusion bodies. Creatnine has risen from 1.4 to 2.0 The most appropriate Tx is:
    a. Gangciclovir
    b. Acyclovir
    c. Bactrim
    d. Penicillin

    Answer a. CMV infection is common among transplant pts and forms characteristic *inclusion bodies* in cells *Ganciclovir* is used to treat *CMV infection.*

54. *All of the following are true of hyperacute rejection except:
    a. It is MC due to ABO incompatibility
    b. Is a Type II hypersensitivity reaction
    c. Successful Tx usually requires organ removal and re-transplantation
    d. Steroids are usually sufficient Tx

    Answer d. Hyperacute rejection is most often due to ABO incompatibility and involves pre-formed recipient Ab's to donor antigens. Hyperacute rejection signs intra-op include the organ turning blue and mottled with interstitial hemorrhage, cyanosis, gross edema and graft rupture. Tx is immediate removal of organ + re-transplantation (or just removal if kidney)

55. *The most common malignancy following transplantation is:
    a. Lung cancer
    b. Prostate cancer
    c. Breast cancer
    d. Skin cancer

    Answer d. *The MC malignancy following transplantation is **squamous cell skin cancer**.*

56. *A cross-match is performed by:
    a. Mixing donor lymphocytes with recipient serum
    b. Mixing recipient lymphocytes with donor serum
    c. Mixing donor plasma with recipient serum
    d. Mixing recipient plasma with donor serum

    Answer a. *A **crossmatch** is performed by mixing donor lymphocytes (which contains the antigen) with recipient serum (which contains the antibody). A **positive cross-match** means that the recipient has preformed antibodies to donor antigens. Hyperacute rejection would likely occur if the transplant were to ensue.*

57. *The principal cells involved in acute rejection is:
    a. B cells
    b. T cells
    c. Macrophages
    d. Platelets

    Answer b. *The principle cells involved in **acute rejection** is **T cells**.*

58. *Post-transplant lymphoproliferative disorder has been most commonly linked to:
    a. HSV
    b. RSV
    c. EBV
    d. Influenza viruses

Answer c. **Ebstein barr virus** has been implicated in development of post-transplant lymphoproliferative disorder.

59. **A 35 yo man POD #10 from a cadaveric renal transplantation develops a rise in creatnine. A fluid and lasix challenge has no effect The appropriate next step is:
   a. Emergent re-operation
   b. Angiography
   c. OKT3
   d. Ultrasound

   Answer d. **Elevated creatnine or decreased urine output (or any other signs of rejection) is an indication for U/S following kidney TXP. The U/S assesses vascular supply to the graft, looks for ureter compression, and can identify fluid collections consistent w/ either urine leaks, lymphocoeles, hematomas, or seromas. Kidney Bx can be performed at the same time.

60. *In the previous pt, U/S shows flow acceleration and narrowing at the level of the arterial anastomosis. The next appropriate step is:
   a. Emergent re-operation
   b. Angiography
   c. OKT3
   d. Biopsy

   Answer b. Angiogram with angioplasty and stent placement is the Tx of choice for a tight arterial anastomosis following kidney TXP.

61. *Instead of the above, the U/S is normal. The most appropriate next step is:
   a. Emergent re-operation
   b. Angiography
   c. OKT3
   d. Biopsy

   Answer d. If there is no mechanical problem w/ the graft, Bx should be performed.

62. *Biopsy in the above pt shows tubulitis. This is consistent with:
   a. Acute rejection
   b. Urinary tract infection
   c. Chronic rejection
   d. Renal vein thrombosis

   Answer a. Lymphocytic **tubulitis** is consistent w/ **acute rejection**. A more severe acute rejection would involve vasculitis. Pulse steroids are indicated. You should follow creatnine and likely re-biopsy after 5-7 days.

63. *Five days after kidney TXP, your pt has poor UOP despite fluid challenge and lasix. U/S shows a large fluid collection anterior to kidney. You aspirate the fluid and the creatnine is 20 (serum creatnine 0.8). The next step in management is:
   a. Explant the kidney
   b. Try to repair the cysto-ureteral anastomosis
   c. Place a stent and percutaneous drainage
   d. Nothing

   Answer c. *The most appropriate Tx for a **urine leak** (in most instances) is percutaneous drainage and placement of a ureteral stent across the anastomosis. Trying to redo the anastomosis is usually unsuccessful.

64. *New proteinuria in a patient following kidney transplant is most consistent with:

a. Acute rejection
b. Urinary tract infection
c. Chronic rejection
d. Renal vein thrombosis

Answer d. *New proteinuria is consistent w/ **renal vein thrombosis**.*

65. **All of the following are true except
    a. Cystic fibrosis requires <u>double</u> lung transplant
    b. Chronic allograft vasculopathy is the MCC of death after heart TXP
    c. Diabetic ESRD is MC indication for combined kidney-pancreas TXP
    d. Bronchiolitis obliterans is the MCC of acute death after lung TXP

Answer d. Reperfusion injury is the MCC early death after lung TXP.
***Bronchiolitis obliterans** is the MCC late death and MCC of overall death after lung TXP.*
***Chronic allograft vasculopathy** is the MCC of late death and MCC of overall death after heart TXP*

66. *The MCC of acute death in a living related kidney donor is:
    a. Pulmonary embolism (PE)
    b. Hemorrhage
    c. Myocardial infarction
    d. Infection

Answer a. *The MCC of acute death in a living related kidney <u>donor</u> is **PE**.*
*The MCC of death in a kidney TXP <u>recipient</u> is **myocardial infarction***

67. **All of the following are true of liver TXP except;
    a. Acute hepatic artery thrombosis after liver TXP usually resolves without Tx.
    b. Post-op lamivudine and HBIG reduce HepB re-infection to 20%
    c. HepC is the MC indication for liver TXP and is the disease most likely to recur (re-infects almost all liver allografts)
    d. Primary sclerosing cholangitis recurrence is 20% after liver TXP

Answer a. ***Acute hepatic artery thrombosis** usually requires re-TXP.*
***Post-op lamivudine and HBIG** reduce **HepB re-infection** to 20%*

68. **A 50 yo man on cyclosporine and s/p kidney TXP 3 months ago undergoes a difficult cholecystectomy requiring a biliary T-tube. Five days post-op he has an acute rise in creatnine and poor UOP. Given the most likely Dx, the most appropriate next step is
    a. Removal of T-tube
    b. Antibiotics
    c. Steroids
    d. Ganciclovir

Answer c. ***Cyclosporin** undergoes significant **entero-hepatic recirculation**. A biliary T-Tube would remove 90% of cyclosporine and the pt would be subject to acute rejection, which would be treated w/ steroids.*

69. *All the following are true of renal TXP donor and recipient compatibility except:
    a. HLA-DR is the most important antigen in donor/recipient matching
    b. A blood type O recipient is compatible w/ a blood type AB donor
    c. Time on list + HLA matching are used to decide kidney allocation in the US
    d. Better matching results in better long term function

Answer b. A blood type AB recipient is compatible w/ a blood type O donor.***HLA-DR** is the most important antigen in donor/recipient matching*

Transplant immunology

Major transplant antigens – <u>ABO</u> blood type and <u>MHC</u>

MHC (Major Histocompatibility Complex)

Major factor leading to acute and chronic rejection

HLA (Human Leukocyte Antigen) is the MHC form in humans

HLA class I antigens: HLA -A, –B, and -C

HLA class II antigens: HLA -DP, -DQ, and -DR

HLA -A, -B, and -DR used for kidney allocation

***HLA-DR** – *most impt antigen* in donor/recipient matching*
Better matching of HLA = better long term function
Identical twin (paternal) organ TXPs do not undergo rejection

Time on list + HLA matching - *criteria used for cadaveric kidney allocation in US*

ABO blood compatibility

Generally need **ABO compatibility** for TXP

Would cause **hyperacute rejection**

Recipient **AB blood type** (has no A or B Ab's) – can receive Type A, Type B, Type AB, or Type O organs

Recipient **O blood type** (has Ab's to A + B antigens) - need Type O organ

Crossmatch (lymphocyte crossmatch)

Detects **recipient preformed Ab's** by mixing recipient serum w/ donor lymphocytes → would result in **hyperacute rejection** (termed *positive crossmatch*)

Rejection

1) **Hyperacute rejection** (minutes to hours after TXP)

Preformed recipient Ab's to donor antigens

This should have been identified w/ the **crossmatch**

MC problem – ABO blood type incompatibility

Results in:

1) **Type II Hypersensitivity Reaction**

2) **Complement** activation (Ab binding) + **vessel thrombosis**

Sx's – organ turns blue and mottled, hemorrhages, edema, rupture

Tx: **remove organ** and **emergency re-transplantation** (if kidney, just remove organ)

2) **Acute rejection** (1 week to 6 months)

Recipient T cells (cytotoxic + T helper) against donor HLA antigens

Can occur w/ living related donors

T cells need **1 week** for APC recognition, to differentiate and to mount a response (reason for 1 week delay after TXP)

Tx: ↑ **immunosuppression** (eg pulse steroids, thymoglobulin, organ preserved in 95%)

3) **Chronic rejection** (months to years)

Specifically a chronic immune response to transplanted tissue

***Acute rejection is a RF for chronic rejection*

Major etiology - MHC

Effectors: **T cells** (Type IV hypersensitivity), **B cells** (Ab production)

***Different from chronic allograft vasculopathy*

Tx: ↑ **immunosuppression** (eg pulse steroids, thymoglobulin, ↑ maintenance drugs) → <u>not</u> effective long term

Re-transplantation is the only definitive tx

4) **Chronic Allograft Vasculopathy**

Fibrosis or accelerated atherosclerosis of **internal blood vessels** of transplanted tissue

Chronic rejection of **blood vessels**

***Main mechanism of chronic rejection after Heart TXP*

Tx: ↑ **immunosuppression** (eg pulse steroids, thymoglobulin, ↑ maintenance drugs) → <u>not</u> effective long term

Re-transplantation is the only definitive tx

Immunosuppressive Drug Classes

1) **Calcineurin Inhibitors**
   - *****Cyclosporin** (Neoral, CSA)
     - Binds *****cyclophilin protein**, inhibits genes for cytokine synthesis (<u>**IL-2**</u>, IL-4, INF-gamma) and blocks activation of **T-cells** and **B-cells**
     - S/Es: nephrotoxicity, hepatotoxicity, HUS, tremors, <u>seizures</u>
     - Undergoes **hepatic metabolism** and **biliary excretion**
       - ******Undergoes **enterohepatic re-circulation** *(reabsorbed in gut)*
         - *Biliary drain decreases levels and causes acute rejection*
     - Trough level 200–300
   - *****Tacrolimus** (Prograf, FK-506)
     - Binds *****FK binding protein**; similar action as CSA (ie inhibits genes for <u>**IL-2**</u>, IL-4, INF-gamma), 50 x more potent
     - S/Es: similar to CSA, less lipid, HTN and cosmetic problems
     - Hepatic metabolism (highly metabolized) - enterohepatic recycling much less of an issue
     - Trough level 10–15
     - *******Generally, less acute rejection episodes than cyclosporin*
2) **mTOR inhibitors**
   - *****Sirolimus** (Rapamycin)
     - Binds *****FK-binding protein** similar to tacrolimus
       - ******However inhibits **mammalian target of rapamycin** *(mTOR)*
     - Inhibits **response to IL-2**, blocks activation of T- and B-cells
       - ******Is <u>**not**</u> **nephrotoxic** (chief advantage over CSA, tacrolimus)
3) **Anti-proliferative agents**
   - *****Mycophenolate** (MMF, Cellcept) –
     - *Inhibits de novo **purine synthesis**, which **inhibits T cells**
     - S/Es: myelosuppression, GI intolerance
     - **Keep WBCs > 3**
4) **Steroids**
   - Inhibit **macrophages** and genes for *******cytokine synthesis* *(IL-1, IL-6)*
   - **S/Es – **Cushing's syndrome
5) **Antibodies**
   - *****Daclizumab** (Zenapax)
     - *****Monoclonal anti -IL-2 receptor Ab** *(are <u>not</u> cytolytic)*
     - Used w/ **induction** *(decreases acute rejection)*
       - ****** <u>Low risk</u> of **infection** and **PTLD** compared to other agents
     - S/Es - should <u>not</u> be combined w/ other cytolytic Ab's (eg ATG below) → ↑ infection and ↑ mortality
   - *****Anti-thymocyte globulin** (thymoglobulin, ATG, Rabbit Ab's)
     - *****Polyclonal Ab's** directed against antigens on T cells (CD2, CD3, CD4, and CD8)
     - **Complement dependent** opsonization of T cells (*is **cytolytic**)
     - Used for **induction** or refractory **acute rejection**
     - Keep **WBCs > 3**
     - S/Es: **PTLD, Myelosuppression, Cytokine release syndrome** (SIRS reaction, pre-tx pt w/ steroids and antihistamines)

Malignancy related to TXP Immunosuppression

- *******MC malignancy following TXP* - skin cancer (MC squamous cell CA)
- *******Post-transplant lymphoproliferative disease* (PTLD)
  - Sx's – fever, adenopathy, mass lesions; usually in 1st year or TXP
  - 2nd MC malignancy following TXP
  - **Highest risk** – small bowel TXP (10%; lot of lymphoid tissue)
  - *******Epstein-Barr virus* (EBV) mediated **B cell** proliferation
  - RFs – cytolytic Ab's (eg thymoglobulin)
  - **Mechanism** - calcineurin inhibitors, anti-T cell Ab's, and anti-proliferative agents decrease **suppressor T cell population** so **B cell** proliferation after **EBV** infection goes unchecked → can progress to Non-Hodgkins Lymphoma (**B cell**)

Dx: FNA or tissue Bx
Tx: Significant **lowering or withdrawal of immunosuppression**
Rituximab (anti-CD 20, depresses B cells), **CHOP-R** (± XRT)
for NHL

**Cytomegalovirus infection (CMV)
Transmitted via **leukocytes** (use leukoreduced or CMV negative blood)
*CMV is the MC infection in TXP recipients
Causes PNA, gastritis, colitis, ophthalmitis, and mononucleosis
*MC manifestation - febrile mononucleosis (sore throat, adenopathy)
*Most deadly form - CMV pneumonitis
Dx: **Bx** - characteristic **cellular inclusion bodies*; CMV **serology**
Tx: ****Gangciclovir** (inhibits DNA polymerase)
S/Es – CNS toxicity, bone marrow suppression
Reduce immunosuppression if possible
CMV-IVIG (CMV immunoglobulin) - given for severe infections and
after TXP for CMV negative recipient and CMV positive donor;
S/Es – N/V, flushing
Varicella (Zoster) – dissemination can be life-threatening
Tx: acyclovir, IVIG, ↓ immunosuppression
HSV – Tx: acyclovir

Kidney transplantation
MC indication - ESRD from diabetes
**Not a contraindication - HIV infection
Donor Kidney (cadaveric or living donor)
Can store **48 hours**
UTI in donor – can still use kidney
Acute ↑ in creatinine (1.0–3.0) – can still use kidney
Attach to **iliac vessels** w/ **ureteral-bladder anastomosis**

Cx's	
MCC Postop Oliguria	ATN (**path** - dilation and loss of tubules)
MCC Postop Diuresis	High urea and glucose pre-TXP
*MCC new Proteinuria	Renal vein thrombosis (Dx – U/S)
MCC Postop Diabetes	S/E of CSA or FK, steroids

*Urine leaks (MC complication)
Sx's: ↓ed UOP early (1st week), ↑Cr
Dx:**Duplex U/S** - hypoechoic mass early, aspirate fluid (high Cr)
Tx: ****percutaneous drainage + stent** (best Tx)
*Renal artery stenosis (or thrombosis) – MC vascular Cx
Sx's: ↓ed UOP, ↑Cr
Dx: **Duplex U/S** – shows flow acceleration, narrowing at
anastomosis
Tx: ****PTA + stent** (also Tx for **renal vein stenosis**)
**Lymphocele - MCC of external compression (MC 3 wks after
TXP); Sx's: ↓ed UOP late (compression of ureters); ± pain
Dx: **Duplex U/S** - hypoechoic mass, hydronephrosis from ureter
compression, good graft perfusion, fluid has normal Cr
Tx: **1st** – percutaneous drainage
2nd- If that fails need ***intra-peritoneal marsupialization*
(peritoneal window - 95% successful) → drains
through window in peritoneum and re-absorbed
*Acute rejection
MC from 1 week to 6 months
Dx: **Duplex U/S** and **renal Bx**
Path – **tubulitis** (**vasculitis** w/ severe form)
Tx:pulse steroids, other immunosuppressive drugs, Daclizumab
Repeat Bx after tx to make sure rejection is cleared
Chronic rejection – usually don't see until after 1 year; no good Tx
*MCC mortality after kidney TXP – myocardial infarction
5-year graft survival – 75% (cadaveric 70%, living donors 80%)
Median survival – 15-20 years (Kidney TXP extends survival **15 yrs**)

**S/P kidney TXP, now w/ ↑Cr or poor UOP post-op →
  DDx – acute rejection, vascular problem, urine leak w/ compression,
    lymphocele (late)
  Initial Tx - fluid challenge and/or lasix trial, check bladder catheter
  Dx and Tx: ****Duplex U/S w/ biopsy (best test)** - checks for vascular
    problem, urine leak, acute rejection
    Empiric ↓ in CSA or FK (these can be nephrotoxic)
    Pulse steroids (often empiric); further Tx based on cause
Living kidney donors
  MC Cx – wound infection (1%); ***MCC of death** (0.05%) – fatal PE
  The remaining kidney hypertrophies
  **Donor w/ dual collecting systems is <u>not</u> a contraindication to TXP

Liver transplantation
  MC indication for liver TXP – chronic hepatitis from <u>Hep C</u>
    Children – biliary atresia
  Some Hepatocellular CA can undergo TXP
    Cannot have mets or vascular invasion; _No_ cholangiocarcinoma
    Not contraindications – HIV, portal vein thrombosis, recipient age
  Donor Liver (cadaveric or living related)
    Can store **24 hours**
    Macrosteatosis (cadaveric)
      Extracellular fat globules in liver allograft
      Best overall predictor of **primary non-function**
      If 50% of cross section is macrosteatatic in potential donor,
        there is a 50% chance of primary non-function
    Living related
      *MC for adult donation - right portion of liver
      *MC for pediatric donation – left lateral (segments 2 and 3)
      Donor liver regenerates to 100% in **6-8 weeks**
  Cx's
    **Liver failure or problems post-op, **Dx: Duplex U/S (finds
      vascular problems, fluid collections) _and Bx_
    Biliary Leak (MC complication): Tx: **percutaneous drainage** and
      ERCP w/ sphincterotomy and **stent** (across leak if possible)
    Biliary stenosis (dilated ducts on U/S)- Tx ERCP dilatation and stent
    Primary non-function total bilirubin >10, bile output < 20 cc/12 hr
      PT and PTT 1.5x normal; After 96 hrs: lethargy, ↑ed LFTs,
        renal failure, respiratory failure
      Tx: **re-transplantation**
    **Vascular Cx's
      Early Hepatic artery thrombosis
        **MC early vascular Cx
        Sx's: ↑ LFTs, ↓ed bile output, **fulminant hepatic failure**
        Tx: Can try angio w/ PTA ± stent or reop
              MC will need **emergent re-transplantation** for
                ensuing fulminant hepatic failure
      Late Hepatic artery thrombosis results in biliary strictures and
        abscesses (<u>not</u> fulminant hepatic failure)
      MCC hepatic abscess after liver TXP - hepatic artery
        thrombosis
    Cholangitis – see **PMNs** around portal triad, ***_not_** mixed infiltrate
      (DDx vs. acute rejection)
    **Acute rejection
      T cell mediated against **blood vessels**, MC in 1st 2 months
      Sx's: fever, jaundice, ↓ bile output
      Dx: ↑ WBCs, ↑ LFTs, and ↑ PT; get duplex U/S + Liver Bx
      Path (portal triad shows): **Portal venous lymphocytosis**
        **Endothelitis (<u>mixed</u> infiltrate, not just PMNs)
        Bile duct injury
      Tx: **pulse steroids**; other immunosuppressive agents

Chronic rejection
Very low chronic rejection w/ liver TXP – only *5%*
    Path - disappearing bile ducts
RFs high number of acute rejection episodes (biggest RF)
S/P liver TXP, now w/ ↑ed LFTs or ↓ed bile output early post-op → *Dx:* ****Duplex U/S w/ Liver Bx *(best test; will Dx vascular problem, acute rejection, primary non-function, bile leak)]*

5-year survival – 70%
    Median Survival – 15-20 years
    ETOH – 20% will start drinking again (recidivism)
Living Liver Donor – 10% complication rate (MC bile leak), Mortality < 1%
Hepatitis B Recipient - *Tx:* ****HBIG *(hepatitis B immunoglobulin) and* ****lamivudine** *(protease inhibitor) post-op to prevent re-infection →* *reduces re-infection rate to 20%*
**Hepatitis C Recipient
    ***Disease most likely to recur in the new liver allograft*
    Re-infects *essentially all* grafts; re-infection is usually indolent

Heart transplantation
Indications - life expectancy <1 year; can store heart for **6 hours**
Persistent pulmonary hypertension after heart TXP (↑s mortality)
    Tx: inhaled nitric oxide, ECMO if severe
MCC early mortality (< 1 year) – infection
**MCC late mortality (> 5 years) – chronic allograft vasculopathy
    (accelerated atherosclerosis of small coronaries– can't use CABG)
**MCC mortality overall – *chronic allograft vasculopathy*
Acute rejection – **peri-vascular infiltrate** w/ increasing grades of **myocyte inflammation** and **necrosis**
High risk of **silent MI** due to **vagal denervation** after heart TXP
Median Survival – 10 years

Lung transplantation
Indications - life expectancy <1 year; can store lung for **6 hours**
**Absolute indication for double-lung TXP – cystic fibrosis
Exclusion criteria for using donor lungs – aspiration, moderate to large contusion, infiltrate, purulent sputum, PO_2 < 350 on 100% FiO_2
MCC early mortality (< 1 year) – reperfusion injury (primary graft failure)
**MCC late mortality *(> 1 year) – bronchiolitis obliterans*
**MCC mortality overall – *bronchiolitis obliterans*
Acute rejection – peri-vascular lymphocytosis
Chronic rejection – bronchiolitis obliterans
Median survival – 5 years

Pancreas transplantation
MC indication – type I diabetes and ESRD (usually combined w/ kidney)
Need **donor celiac artery, SMA** (arterial blood for both) and **portal vein** (for venous drainage); attached to **iliac vessels**
Most use **enteric drainage** for pancreatic duct - 2nd portion of duodenum
**Successful pancreas/kidney TXP *results in:*
    Stabilization of retinopathy
    ↓ **neuropathy** w/ ↑ nerve conduction velocity
    ↓ **autonomic dysfunction** (gastroparesis)
    ↓ **orthostatic hypotension**
    ***No reversal of vascular disease*

Infections

70. *Six hours after emergency partial colectomy following a penetrating farming accident, your pt is confused, has a fever of 41ºC and develops gray, foul smelling drainage from his wound. You feel crepitus around his wound. All of the following are true except:
    a. GPRs on gram stain would be consistent w/ the most likely diagnosis
    b. Alpha toxin is the greatest source of morbidity and mortality
    c. This pt requires emergent re-exploration and debridement
    d. The pt requires broad-spectrum abx's *only*

    Answer d. This presentation is classic for **clostridium perfringens** infection. The pt needs emergent **wound debridement**. This pt is at high risk for **myonecrosis** and **fasciitis**.

    Beta-hemolytic group A strep (necrotizing fasciitis) can also cause early invasive wound infection. **Fournier's Gangrene** refers to a perineal necrotizing fasciitis (esp in diabetics) that is polymicrobial. ****Emergency wound debridement** is the first step in Tx for all these infections (preserve the testicles if possible for Fournier's)

71. **All of the following are true except:
    a. Enterococcus is sensitive to most cephalosporins
    b. Proteus produces urease
    c. Staph Aureus in the MC organism in VAP
    d. The MC fecal bacteria is bacteriodies fragilis

    Answer a. Enterococcus is resistant to all cephalosporins.
    The MC fecal bacteria is **bacteriodies fragilis

72. All of the following are true of post-op fever except:
    a. Fever within 48 hours is MC due to atelectasis
    b. Fever after 48 hours is MC due to urinary tract infection
    c. Fever after day 5 is MC due to wound infection
    d. Abscess is MC within 3 days

    Answer d. **Abscess is MC between days 7-10*

73. **All of the following are true in prevention of surgical site infection (SSI) except:
    a. Antibiotics given at least 30 min to 2 hours prior to incision are used to prevent wound infection
    b. Blood glucose should be maintained between 80-120 in diabetics
    c. PaO2 should remain high during the operation (use of 100% FiO2)
    d. Warm IV fluids is the best method for preventing hypothermia

    Answer d. ***Warm air conduction (eg Bair Hugger) is the best method for preventing hypothermia.*

    Pre-op Antibiotics are used to prevent **wound infection

74. **All of the following are true of ventilator associated pneumonia (VAP) except:
    a. Initial Tx should include vancomycin for empiric Tx of MRSA
    b. BAL aspirates > 10,000 CFU suggests VAP
    c. Routine ventilator circuit changes are indicated
    d. VAP is the MCC of infectious death in surgical pts

    Answer c. ***Routine circuit changes are not indicated (only w/ contamination).*

75. **All of the following are true of infections except:

a. The internal jugular vein line site has the lowest infection rate
b. Central lines are the MCC of blood stream infections
c. UTI is the MC acquired hospital infection
d. Bacteremia generally occurs 1 hour before fever

Answer a. **Subclavian lines** *have the lowest infection rates.*

76. **A 55 yo man develops severe abdominal pain, fever and profuse foul diarrhea after being hospitalized for pneumonia. His BP is low (80/30, HR 120) and he is diffusely tender but does not have peritoneal signs. His WBCs are 52. You start aggressive fluid resuscitation. All of the following are true of this pts likely condition except:
    a. IV vancomycin is the treatment of choice
    b. ELISA for toxin A + B is the most rapid test for C. difficile colitis
    c. Toxic colitis requiring resection can occur
    d. Vancomycin PO is treatment of choice in pregnant women

    Answer a. Given recent antibiotics for pneumonia, severe diarrhea, and extremely elevated WBCs, the most likely diagnosis in this patient in **pseudomembranous colitis**. **Flagyl** is the treatment of choice. IV vancomycin is not effective for Clostridium difficile colitis.
    Pregnant women *should receive* PO **vancomycin** *as there is no systemic absorption.*
    ELISA for toxin A + B *is the most rapid test for C. difficile colitis*

77. *All of the following are true except:
    a. Spontaneous bacterial peritonitis (SBP) is MC poly-organismal
    b. IV albumin increases survival in pts w/ SBP
    c. Fungal infection of peritoneal dialysis catheters requires removal
    d. Peritoneal fluid w/ WBCs > 500 or PMNs > 250 suggest SBP

    Answer a. *SBP is MC* mono-organismal *(MC - E. coli)*
    Poly-organismal *infections suggest secondary bacterial peritonitis (eg perforated viscous)*
    Peritoneal fluid w/ **WBCs > 500** *or* **PMNs > 250** *suggest SBP*

78. *All of the following are true except:
    a. Elevated anti-HBs Ab's only suggests previous HepB infection
    b. High anti-HBc, anti-HBe and anti-HBs Ab's and no HBs antigens suggests pt had infection, recovery and subsequent immunity
    c. HepC is the most common viral infection leading to liver TXP
    d. Combined HepB + HepD infection has the highest mortality for viral hepatitis

    Answer a. *Elevated* **anti-HBs Ab's** *only suggests HepB immunization.*
    High anti-HBc, anti-HBe and anti-HBs Ab's and no *HBs antigens suggests pt had infection, recovery and subsequent immunity*
    HepC is the most common viral infection leading to liver TXP

79. **All of the following are true of HIV except:
    a. CMV colitis complications (bleeding, perforated ulcer) are the MC indication for laparotomy in HIV pts
    b. The MC CA in HIV pts requiring surgery is lymphoma
    c. Kaposi's sarcoma is MC treated non-operatively
    d. The MC solid organ lymphoma in HIV pts is colon

    Answer d. **The MC solid organ lymphoma** *in HIV pts is* **stomach** *(usually NHL, presents as bleeding or perforation).*
    CMV colitis cx's *(bleeding, perforation) are the MC indication for* **laparotomy** *in HIV pts*
    The MC HIV **CA** *requiring laparotomy is* **lymphoma**-*bleeding, perforation*

*Clostridial Myonecrosis
    MC organism – clostridium perfringens (anaerobic) – farm wounds
    Can cause ****rapid, early wound infection** *(*can occur after surgery)*
    Sx's: acute onset of pain, fever, mental status changes (lethargy)
        Bullae, crepitus (deep), skin discoloration (bronze)
        Gray dish-water fluid from wound
        **Pain may be *out of proportion* to cellulitis *(deep infection)*
    Path: ****Large GPRs** (long bacilli) and **very few PMNs**
        Alpha toxin – inserts into cell membrane, creating gap and cell lysis
            Is the major of source of **morbidity and **mortality***
    Dx: <u>Clinical Dx</u> enough to initiate **surgical exploration**
        X-ray – gas dissecting into muscle
    Tx: ****Take to OR for debridement immediately** *(muscle and fascia)*
        High dose **PCN G** + **Clindamycin**

*Necrotizing fasciitis
    Rapidly spreading infection involving **superficial** and/or **deep fascia**
        leading to **soft tissue** and **muscle necrosis**
    RFs – DM, peripheral arterial disease, cirrhosis, ETOH, poor hygiene
    Can present within **6-8 hrs** of **trauma or surgery** (*rapid* wound infection)
    Sx's: N/V, fever, mental status changes (lethargy)
        Edema, bullae, crepitus, drainage, erythema (can be purple)
        If **deep** → overlying skin can initially look **normal** w/ *pain out of*
            proportion to apparent cellulitis
    Path   **Type I** - <u>Poly-microbial</u> (GPCs GNRs, anaerobes); surgery related
            Type II - <u>Mono-microbial</u> (2 types)
                1) **Streptococcus pyogenes** (Group A beta hemolytic)
                    'Flesh eating strep'; MC monomicrobial cause
                    Release **exotoxins** (A + C → SIRS syndrome)
                        Major of source of **morbidity** and **mortality**
                        Infection → **Fever** → **SIRS** → **MSOF** → **death**
                2) **MRSA** – also have **exotoxins**
            *Wound Bx for Type II – **GPCs** w/ <u>paucity</u> of PMNs
    Dx: ***Clinical Dx enough to initiate surgical exploration**
    Tx: ****Take to OR for fascial and muscle debridement** <u>*immediately*</u>
        Broad spectrum abx's until organisms isolated
        Strep pyogenes – high dose PCN G + clindamycin
        MRSA – vancomycin

*Fournier's Gangrene
    A type of **necrotizing fasciitis** that affects perineal region (50% mortality)
    RFs – **DM** *(classic)*, immunocompromised, poor hygiene, malnutrition
    Path – **polymicrobial** (GPCs, GNRs, anaerobes)
    Sx's: Pain and redness in scrotum, penis, labia, perineum, crepitance
        Foul smelling gray discharge
    Tx: **Immediate radical fascial + soft tissue debridement*
        (preserve <u>testicles</u>); **broad spectrum Abx's** (aerobes + anaerobes)

*Staph Aureus (coagulase <u>positive</u>)
    Have **exoslime biofilm - adhere to prosthetic material*
    *Resistance to PCN – *beta-lactamase*
    MRSA (methicillin resistant staph aureus) – ***have altered **penicillin***
        binding protein; Tx: vancomycin
Staph Epidermidis (coagulase <u>negative</u>)
    Have **exoslime biofilm - adhere to prosthetic material*
Enterococcus faecalis - common in gut (95% of population)
    *Resistant to <u>all</u> cephalosporins
    Vancomycin resistant enterococcus (VRE)
        **Mutation in cell wall binding protein Tx: Synercid or Linezolid
Pseudomonas aeruginosa - **alginate mucoid layer** (biofilm), colonize tubes

MC organism in SSI (surgical site infection) – staph aureus
MC organism in VAP (ventilator associated pneumonia)
and nosocomial PNA – staph aureus
MC organism in line infections and CRBSI (catheter-related blood
stream infection) – staph epidermidis
MC organism overall in gut *- Bacteroides fragilis*
MC organism in anaerobic peritoneal infections (eg abscess) –
bacteroides fragilis
MC GNR in gut (colon); MC aerobic organism in gut – E coli
MC organism in UTI (80%), biliary tract infections (cholangitis) and
pyogenic liver abscess – E. Coli
MC organism in struvite kidney stones – proteus mirabilis (*have urease
production*)
MC lung infection w/ cystic fibrosis - Pseudomonas aeruginosa
MC organism in severe burn wound infections - Pseudomonas aeruginosa
MC colonizer of indwelling catheters - Pseudomonas aeruginosa

Anaerobes outnumber aerobic bacteria in colon (1000:1); need low oxygen
content (lack superoxide dismutase and catalase, vulnerable to oxygen
radicals)

*Gut Flora
Stomach - almost sterile, few GPCs, some yeast
Proximal small bowel - 10^5 bacteria, mostly GPCs
Distal small bowel - 10^7 bacteria; GPCs, GPRs, GNRs
Colon - 10^{11} bacteria; 99% anaerobes; few GNRs and GPCs
**MC fecal bacteria - bacteriodies fragilis
**MC organism overall in gut - bacteroides fragilis

*Fever Source	MC Time Frame (post-op day)
Atelectasis	1-2
UTI	3-5
Wound infection, medications, DVT	5-7
Abscess	7-10

*MC fever source within 48 hours	Atelectasis
*MC fever source 48 hours – 5 days	Urinary tract infection
*MC fever source after 5 days	Wound infection

Nosocomial Infections
Infections acquired in hospital (> 48 hours after admission or up to 30 d
after discharge); 35% of all nosocomial infections can be prevented
**Hand washing before each pt contact most effective way of preventing
transmission
Judicious use of abx's also impt
Nosocomial Infections: SSI, VAP, CRBSI, UTI (MC)
**Highest risk pt group for nosocomial infections overall – burn
patients; also highest specifically for UTI, VAP and CRBSI

Surgical Site Infections (SSI, wound infections)
Comorbidity RFs - advanced age, COPD, renal failure, liver failure, DM,
malnutrition, immunosuppression, obesity
Methods to decrease SSI
1) Pre-op – avoid operating if active infection; stop tobacco use
(poor healing); clippers to remove hair (not shaving); shower
night before w/ abx soap; appropriate skin prep
2)**Abx's 30 min to 2 hrs prior to incision and for 24 hrs afterward
(maintain levels during procedure); 1st or 2nd generation
cephalosporins usual; decreases wound infection risk 5 x
**Preop abx's are given to prevent wound infection(SSI)
3) **Maintain blood glucose 80-120 in diabetic pts

4) Keep **PaO₂ high** during operation (use 100% FiO2)
5) Keep ***pt warm* (*best method* - warm air conduction)
2) **OR staff** - exclude infected staff, sterile technique, mask, cap
3) **OR** - doors closed; impervious drapes, sterile instruments, avoid
flash sterilization; <u>avoid hypothermia</u> (70ºF ideal)
4) **Procedure** - avoid unnecessary trauma, ensure hemostasis,
obliterate dead space, sterile dressing for 24-48 hrs

SSI Incidence

Clean (eg umbilical hernia)	2%
Clean contaminated (elective bowel rsxn w/ prepped bowel):	4%
Contaminated (stab wound to colon w/ repair)	8%
Gross contamination (perforated appendix):	30%

MC organism in SSI – staph aureus; others – staph epidermidis, E. coli
MC GNR in SSI – E. coli
MC anaerobe in SSI – bacteriodies fragilis
Dx of SSI – need ≥ 10^5 bacteria (less if foreign body present)

MC infection in surgical pt – UTI (MC - E. coli)
    Early removal of bladder catheters ↓s UTI
    Best tx of UTI - removal of bladder catheter (usually also give abx's)

Prevention of Hypothermia - *Warm air conduction* (*best*; Bair Hugger)
    Effects of hypothermia - ↑ infection, poor coagulation, ↓ C.O.

Ventilator Associated Pneumonia (VAP)
    MCC infectious death in surgical pts (25% mortality)
    RFs – *prolonged intubation* (#1), advanced age, pre-existing lung
        disease, immunosuppression, malnutrition, ARDS
    From *aspiration* of exogenous or endogenous microbes in **oropharynx**
    Sx's: **fever** or low temp, purulent sputum, and hypoxia
    Dx: ↑ **WBCs**, CXR – ***new unilateral infiltrate***
        Tracheal aspiration or **broncho-alveolar lavage** (BAL) – send for
            cultures; BAL or aspirate > **10,000** (10^4) CFUs/ml = **pneumonia**
    Do <u>NOT</u> reduce VAP
        1) Gut decontamination
        2) **Routine ventilator circuit changes (only change if contaminated)
    VAP pathogens
        Staph Aureus - MC organism overall in VAP
        GNRs - MC class of organism in VAP
    Tx: **Vancomycin** (cover MRSA) + (3rd generation cephalosporin,
        fluoroquinolone, or anti-pseudomonal PCN); usually 2 weeks of abx's
    Hospital acquired PNA (or **aspiration** PNA while in hospital)
        Pathogens – same as VAP pathogens; Tx – same as VAP

Line infections
    Sx's of line infection: ↑WBCs, fever, chills, site erythema
        Can lead to CRBSI (see below)
    MC organism – staph epidermidis
        others – staph aureus (#2), enterococcus (#3) yeast (#4), GNRs
    Central line w/ lowest risk of infection – subclavian
        Internal jugular lines higher risk than subclavian
        Femoral lines higher risk compared to subclavian and jugular
        Contraindications to subclavian line – coagulopathy or low
            platelets (incompressible area), pts in whom a PTX would be
            life-threatening
    ↑ed length of time catheter is present → ↑ed line infection risk
    Prevention: Wash hands, **chlorhexidine** for skin preparation, full barrier
        precautions when inserting (mask, shield, gown), subclavian
        preferred site, remove when unnecessary
    Tx (suspected line infection):

*Send **peripheral blood cultures***
Assess patient
>   **Pt very ill** → change sites
>   **Site looks bad** (eg erythema) → change sites
>   **If not ill and site OK** → change over wire, send tip (5 cm)
>   >   → **tip cultures > 15 colonies** → change sites
>   >   → **positive blood cultures** → change sites
>   A **positive blood culture** (ie CRBSI)) requires 14 d of abx's
>   **Does pt need the line?** → maybe get rid of it altogether

Blood stream infection (BSI, bacteremia)
>   ***MCC BSI** – central line*
>   These pts _do not_ necessarily have sepsis
>   >   Represents spectrum of DZ (**Line infection** → **CRBSI** → **Sepsis**)
>   >   ****Sepsis** = SIRS + infection
>   ***MCC CRBSI** – staph epidermidis (coagulase negative staph)*
>   Tx: **D/C central line** if present; **empiric abx's** (2 weeks; include vancomycin for MRSA until cultures back)

Gram-negative sepsis
>   **MC organism** – E. coli
>   ***Endotoxin** (LPS – lipopolysaccharide, **lipid A** portion) is released*
>   >   ****Lipid A** is the most potent trigger of **TNF-alpha** release
>   >   **TNF-alpha** (from macrophages) → activates inflammatory, complement, and coagulation cascades (microthrombi), leads to **SIRS**
>   ***Hyperglycemia** occurs w/ sepsis*
>   >   **Early:** ↓ insulin, ↑ glucose (impaired utilization)
>   >   **Late:** ↑ insulin, ↑ glucose (due to insulin resistance)

Community aspiration pneumonia
>   MC site - ****superior segment of RLL**
>   **MC organism** – strep pneumonia; Others – staph aureus, anaerobes
>   Tx: (3rd gen cephalosporin *or* fluoroquinolones) ± (clindamycin *or* flagyl)
>   **Lung abscess** can form (MC location – superior segment of RLL)

Abscess
>   90% of **abdominal** abscesses contain **anaerobes**
>   >   **MC anaerobe infection** – bacteriodies fragilis
>   80% of **abdominal** abscesses contain both **anaerobes** and **aerobes**
>   **MC time frame:** 7–10 d after operation
>   Tx: ****Drainage** _(most impt;_ usually percutaneously for intra-abdominal)
>   >   **Abx's indicated for:** diabetics, cellulitis, sepsis (fever, high WBCs), hardware (eg mechanical valves, hip replacements)
>   >   **Broad spectrum coverage** (include ***Flagyl** for anaerobes)
>   ****Special abscesses**
>   >   ****Lung abscess** – ***95% are treated w/ **abx's alone*** (rarely need drainage); MC related to aspiration
>   >   ****Pancreatic abscess** – need open drainage *(safest answer)*
>   >   >   Percutaneous drainage generally does not work for these
>   >   ****Splenic abscess** – Tx: splenectomy *(safest answer)*
>   >   >   Mortality rate 30%, MC source **– endocarditis or IVDA**
>   >   **Peri-rectal or peri-anal abscess** – open drainage
>   >   **Epidural abscess** – open drainage
>   >   **Retropharyngeal abscess** – _airway emergency_, open drainage
>   >   >   Can lead to **mediastinitis**
>   >   **Parapharyngeal abscess** – watch airway, open drainage
>   >   >   Can lead to **mediastinitis**
>   >   **Liver abscess –** variety of causes and Tx (see Liver chp)
>   >   ****Suppurative Flexor Tenosynovitis** (flexor tendon sheath in finger)
>   >   >   *Tx: need **axial longitudinal drainage***

**Pseudomembranous Colitis (Clostridium difficile Colitis)
Normal colonic flora altered by **abx's**, allowing overgrowth of C. difficile
Can occur after a **single dose of abx's*
*RFs: co-morbidities, long hospital stay, nursing home, age
Sx's: **Pain, cramping** and **foul diarrhea** - watery, green, mucoid (±.blood)
   Fulminant colitis (ie sepsis and/or perforation) or **toxic megacolon**
    (colon > 6 cm on KUB + sepsis) occur in 1%
Toxins A + B cause **diarrhea** (both kill mucosal cells, A more damaging)
Dx: 1) ****Stool ELISA for toxin A** *(enterotoxin, best)* or **toxin B** *(cytotoxin)*
    Takes 2-6 hrs; **repeat** if initially negative (false negative rate
     15%) and suspicion high
   2) Stool **cytotoxin assay** (<u>gold standard</u>; but takes 24-48 hours)
    *Often have **very high WBCs** (30-40)*
   Fecal leukocytes - not specific; Stool cultures - takes long time
  Colonoscopy - mucosal **inflammation**, yellow **pseudomembranes**
Tx: **Fluid resuscitation** (lose fluid from diarrhea); <u>Avoid</u> anti-motilities
  Abx's (if clinical suspicion high, tx empirically while waiting for Dx)
   IV – Flagyl
   Oral – Flagyl or vancomycin (very expensive).
   Pregnancy – **PO vancomycin (<u>no</u> systemic absorption and
    very effective)
  Lactobacillus, stop or change other abx's
  *Fulminant colitis (sepsis and/or perforation) requires **total
   abdominal colectomy* w/ ileostomy *(life-saving)*

*Fungal infection
  *MC organism in fungemia (fungus BSI) – Candida albicans
   RFs – prolonged abx's
   Empiric Tx: Anidulafungin (Eraxis, *best Tx*) or liposomal amphotercin
  *Candiduria – typically from colonization of catheter
   **Tx: remove catheter, likely <u>do not</u> need to Tx w/ anti-fungals
  *Actinomyces (<u>not</u> a true fungus) - pulmonary sx's MC
   Can cause **tortuous abscesses** in neck, chest, and abdomen
   Often **confused w/ CA** (eg tortuous abscess in cecum)
   Path –**yellow sulfur granules*
   Tx: **drainage + **PCN-G***
  *Nocardia (<u>not</u> a true fungus) - pulmonary and CNS sx's
   Tx: **drainage + *bactrim** (sulfonamides)

*Spontaneous bacterial peritonitis (SBP, primary bacterial peritonitis)
  Occurs in pts w/ **cirrhosis** and **ascites**
  Mortality rate – 30%
  RFs – ascites fluid total protein < 1, previous SBP, current GI bleed
  Sx's: **Fever and abd pain** (peritonitis) ± N/V; **encephalopathy** may be the
    only sx → Pts w/ encephalopathy need **paracentesis to R/O SBP**
  Dx (fluid): WBCs > 500 <u>or:</u>; **PMNs > 250 <u>or:</u>; **positive cultures**
  Path: From **impaired host defenses** (intrahepatic shunting + impaired
    bactericidal activity in ascites); <u>not</u> transmucosal migration
   MC organism – ****E. coli** (50%), others - pneumococci, klebsiella
   Should be **mono-microbial* → if not, worry about bowel perforation
    or abscess (would need exploratory laparotomy)
  Tx: **3rd generation cephalosporin** - usually respond in 48 hrs
    If not getting better - confirm your dx by repeating paracentesis
     or laparotomy if suspected bowel perforation or abscess
   *IV albumin – ↑s survival w/ SBP (1.5 gm/kg at Dx, 1 gm/kg HD #3)
   Liver TXP <u>not</u> an option w/ active SBP
   Need **weekly prophylactic abx's** after episode of SBP (norfloxacin)
   Pts w/ **bleeding esophageal varices should also receive
    prophylactic abx's for SBP (high risk)*
   *Polymicrobial infection (likely viscous perforation) → laparotomy

Secondary bacterial peritonitis
  Intra-abdominal source (eg perforated viscus)
  Polymicrobial – *Bacteroides fragilis, E. coli, Enterococcus*
  Tx: **laparotomy** to find source
Peritoneal dialysis catheter infections
  Sx's: cloudy fluid, abd pain, fever
  MC organism – staph aureus (70% GPC's)
  Tx: *Intravenous* – **vancomycin + gentamicin**
       Peritoneal – **vancomycin + gentamicin**
       70% catheter preservation rate
       Fecal peritonitis requires **laparotomy** to find perforation
       Need to **remove catheter w/ certain organisms (eg **fungus,
           pseudomonas, TB**)*

TIG **(tetanus immune globulin)** – give only to pts w/ contaminated wounds who
  lack appropriate immunizations (inject near wound)

**Viral hepatitis
  **HepB (DNA)
      The only **DNA** hepatitis virus (**s** = surface, **e** = envelope, **c** = core)
      Infection - Anti-HBc **IgM** highest in first 6 mos, then **IgG** takes over
      **HepB Vaccination - have increased anti-HBs Ab's only
      Ex.:A pt w/ ↑ed **anti-HBc, anti-HBe** and **anti-HBs** Ab's and no HBs
          antigens→ pt had infection, recovery and subsequent immunity
  HepD (RNA) - **cofactor** for HepB
      ***In combination w/ HepB, has the **highest overall mortality rate** of
          all the hepatitis infections (20%; from ↑ed cirrhosis + CA)*
  No surgery in setting of **acute hepatitis** (viral or ETOH, high mortality)

**Human Immunodeficiency Virus (HIV)
      Loss of **cell mediated immunity** due to low **T helper cell** (CD4+) counts
          Then susceptible to **opportunistic infections**
      RNA virus that has a **reverse transcriptase** to make DNA that gets
          incorporated into host genome
      Testing- ELISA (looks for Ab), then Western Blot (detects HIV protein)
      Tx: **HAART** (Highly Active Anti-Retroviral Tx) $\geq$ 3 drugs in $\geq$ 2 classes
      Post-exposure prophylaxis (eg needle stick from HIV pt)
          1)   **Begin HAART Tx immediately** (within 1 hour)
          2)   Usually **4 weeks** of tx; ELISA at time of exposure and 4 weeks
      **Opportunistic infections
          MC reason for laparotomy in HIV pts
          **MC infection leading to laparotomy in HIV pts – CMV colitis
              CMV colitis – MC intestinal manifestation of AIDS
                  Sx's: bleeding or perforation from **ulcers**
                  Tx: ganciclovir; surgery w/ perforation or refractory bleed
      **Neoplastic disease
          2nd MC reason for laparotomy in HIV pts
          ***MC malignancy requiring laparotomy – lymphoma (due to
              bleeding or perforation)*
          **Lymphoma w/ HIV (usually NHL, 70% B cell) – usually solid organ
              **MC solid organ lymphoma w/ HIV – stomach (rectum is #2)
              Tx: CHOP-R (± XRT) – see Spleen chp
          *Kaposi's sarcoma– see purple nodule w/ ulceration
              **MC CA in pts w/ AIDS
              Rarely need surgery (want to palliate these)
              Rarely cause of death w/ AIDS *unless* intestinal hemorrhage
              Tx: **HAART Tx** usually shrinks AIDS Kaposi's Sarcoma
                  Local Tx – XRT, intra-lesional vinblastine, cryosurgery
          Anal CA (squamous cell CA) - ↑ed in HIV due to HPV

Condyloma accuminata – can grow very rapidly w/ HIV (felt to be low grade verrucous CA w/ HIV) – Tx: laser fulgration usual

GI bleeds w/ HIV:
- **Lower GI bleeds** more common than upper GI bleeds
- **Upper GI bleeds** – <u>Kaposi's sarcoma</u> (MC)
- **Lower GI bleeds** – <u>CMV</u> (MC)

Bactrim or Pentamidine used for prophylaxis against PCP

Infections

Brown recluse spider bites (necrosis from vasculitis)
- Tx: oral ****Dapsone** *(**avoid surgery early),* WTD dressings TID
- **Late** – possible resection and STSG for large ulcers

Acute infectious arthritis w/ sepsis
- **Etiology** – gonorrhea, staph, strep (check cultures)
- Tx*: *open drainage* and **3rd gen. cephalosporin + vancomycin**

Diabetic foot infections – GPCs, GNRs, anaerobes
- Tx: broad-spectrum abx's (eg Unasyn, Zosyn)

**Impetigo, erysipelas, cellulitis, folliculitis, furuncle, carbuncle
- **MC organism* – <u>staph</u>; others - strep
- **Folliculitis** – infection of hair follicle
- **Furuncle** – boil (abscess of hair follicle); Tx: drainage ± antibiotics
- **Carbuncle** – a multi-loculated furuncle (often w/ sinuses); ↑ed in **DM**

Increased infection risk in **diabetics** due to →
1) **PMN dysfunction** (glycosylation ↓s chemotaxis)
2) **↓ed blood flow** – arteriopathy (narrowing of small blood vessels)
3) **Glycosylation of RBCs** impairs oxygen delivery
4) **Neuropathy** – pts don't realize the wound (delayed Dx)

Dx osteomyelitis
- ***Needle **Bone Bx** (best Dx test)* – not swabs of fistula or openings
- ****Tagged WBC scan** - ****Highest sensitivity** for osteomyelitis but not specific (false positive w/ soft tissue inflammation)

Antibiotics

80. *All of the following are true except:
    a. Erythromycin is considered bacteriostatic
    b. Mechanism of action for fluoroquinolones is inhibition of DNA gyrase
    c. Mechanism of action of rifampin is inhibition of the 50s ribosome
    d. Mechanism of action for metronidazole is oxygen radical production

    Answer c. Rifampin inhibits RNA polymerase

81. **All of the following are true except
    a. MRSA MC develops from plasmids to beta-lactamase
    b. Aminoglycoside resistance is from decreased active transport due to modifying enzymes
    c. PCN resistance is from plasmids for beta-lactamase
    d. Ceftriaxone can cause gallbladder sludging and cholestatic jaundice

    Answer a. Resistance is from **mutation in cell wall binding proteins**

82. *All of the following are true except:
    a. The most likely antibiotic to cause erythema multiforme is bactrim
    b. Carbapenems can induce seizures
    c. Cilastatin increases the half-life of carbapenems
    d. Extended spectrum PCNs are implicated in tendon ruptures

    Answer d. Fluoroquinolones are implicated in **tendon ruptures**

83. *Appropriate vancomycin peak and trough values are:
    a. Peak 20-40, trough 5-10
    b. Peak 5-10, trough < 1
    c. Peak 40-80, trough 20-40
    d. Peak < 1, trough 5-10

    Answer a. The appropriate peak (20-40) and trough (5-10) values for **vancomycin** are important in patients with renal failure.

    The appropriate peak (5-10) and trough (< 1) values for **gentamicin** are important in patients with renal failure.

84. *A patient on gentamicin has a peak level of 80 and a trough of <1. The most appropriate management is:
    a. Continue current dosing
    b. Decrease dose but maintain frequency
    c. Decrease dose and decrease frequency
    d. Maintain dose and decrease frequency

    Answer b. To decrease the **peak** level of a drug, one needs to decrease the dose of the drug (the peak level is taken 1 hour after dosing). To decrease the **trough** of a drug, you need to increase the interval at which the drug is given (decrease frequency or longer time between doses).

Mechanism of action
   Inhibitor of DNA gyrase (topoisomerase) - Quinolones (levofloxacin)
   Inhibitor of RNA polymerase - Rifampin
   Produces oxygen radicals that breakup DNA - Metronidazole (Flagyl)
   Sulfonamides – has a PABA analogue which inhibits purine synthesis
   Trimethoprim – inhibits dihydrofolate reductase (inhibits purine synthesis)
   Bacteriostatic antibiotics:
       Chloramphenicol, tetracycline, clindamycin, macrolides
       (erythromycin) - all above have reversible ribosomal binding
       Bactrim

Other antibiotics considered *bacteriocidal*
Aminoglycosides – have irreversible binding to ribosome and are considered **bactericidal**

Plasmids
>*Transfer of plasmids* – MC method of antibiotic resistance
>**MC type** - Beta lactamase plasmids

Mechanisms for antibiotic resistance
>*PCNs, cephalosporins, monobactams and carbapenems resistance* – beta lactamase type plasmids; *Exception*– MRSA (see below)
>**Gentamicin** resistance - modifying enzymes leading to **decreased active transport** into cell
>*Methicillin-resistant Staph aureus (MRSA)*
>>Resistance develops from **mutation in cell wall binding proteins**
>*Vancomycin-resistant Enterococcus (VRE)*
>>Resistance develops from **mutation in cell wall binding proteins**

Extended Spectrum Penicillins (eg ticarcillin, piperacillin)
>S/Es: *platelet inhibition*; high salt load (same for extended- below)

Carbapenems (eg meropenem, imipenem, ertapenem)
>**Cilastatin** – prevents renal hydrolysis of drug and increases half-life
>S/Es: **seizures**

Cephalosporins
>Cephalosporins are <u>not</u> effective for Enterococcus
>10% w/ PCN allergy have cephalosporin allergy
>*Third-generation* (eg ceftriaxone, ceftazidime, cefepime)
>>**S/Es: cholestatic jaundice**, sludging in gallbladder (ceftriaxone)

Vancomycin (glycopeptides)
>*Resistance develops from change in **cell wall binding sites***
>S/Es: HTN, *Redman syndrome* (histamine release), nephrotoxicity, ototoxicity

Bactrim
>S/Es (numerous): teratogenic, allergic reactions, renal damage, Stevens-Johnson syndrome (**erythema multiforme**), hemolysis in G6PD-deficiency

Quinolones (eg ciprofloxacin, levofloxacin, trovafloxicin)
>Same efficacy PO and IV
>S/Es: *tendon ruptures* (esp w/ concomitant steroid use)

Aminoglycosides (eg gentamicin, tobramycin, amikacin)
><u>Not</u> effective for anaerobes (needs O_2 to work)
>*Resistance due to modifying enzymes leading to **decreased active transport***
>S/Es: reversible **nephrotoxicity**, irreversible **ototoxicity**

Macrolides (eg erythromycin)
>**Erythromycin** also binds motilin receptor and is pro-kinetic for bowel
>S/Es: **Nausea** (PO, MC S/E) and Cholestasis (IV)

Metronidazole (flagyl) - Anaerobes
>Active agent – ferredoxin (**creates oxygen radicals that disrupt DNA**)
>S/Es: disulfiram-like reaction, **peripheral neuropathy** (chronic use)

Appropriate drug levels
>**Vancomycin** – peak 20–40 ug/ml; trough 5–10 ug/ml
>**Gentamicin** – peak 6–10 ug/ml; trough <1 ug/ml
>**Peak too high** → decrease amount of each dose
>**Trough too high** → decrease frequency of doses (increase time interval between doses)

MRSA Tx: vancomycin
VRE Tx: Synercid or Linezolid

**Peri-operative antibiotics - *prevent surgical site infections*
Need to be given between 30 minutes and 2 hours before incision

*Antiseptic – antimicrobial that kills and inhibits organisms on body (skin)
(eg chlorhexidine, betadine)
Disinfectant – antimicrobial that kills and inhibits organisms on inanimate
objects
Sterilization – all organisms killed (eg autoclave)

*Common antiseptics in surgery
Iodophors (eg Betadine) – GPCs, GNRs, <u>poor</u> fungi
*Chlorhexidine gluconate (eg Hibiclens) – GPCs, GNRs, and fungi
<u>Better coverage</u> overall compared to betadine type drugs

<u>**Anti-fungals**</u>
1) **Anidulafungin** (Eraxis)
1st line *therapy for suspected* **Candidemia
Inhibits **cell wall synthesis** (*inhibits* **glucan synthase**)
S/Es → **Very few S/Es** and equally effective as amphotercin
*Spontaneous degradation, safe w/ renal or hepatic disease

2) **Amphotercin** (polyene)
*Creates channels w/ **ergosterol** *in cell wall (increases cell*
membrane permeability, causes cell lysis)
S/Es: renal toxicity, hypotension, fever, ↑ LFTs, anemia, ↓ K+
S/Es less w/ **liposomal variant** (liposomal amphotercin B)
Used less since introduction of less toxic drugs w/ equal efficacy

85. *A drug that is given demonstrates first order elimination kinetics. All of the following are true except:
   a.   A fixed ratio of the drug is eliminated over time
   b.   Increasing the dose will increase the amount eliminated
   c.   The enzyme and elimination systems involved in removing the drug are likely not saturated
   d.   Zero order elimination kinetics is exponential.

   Answer d. *Zero order elimination kinetics* eliminates a fixed amount of the drug regardless of the dose. This is considered linear and the elimination systems involved in removal of the drug are likely saturated.
   First order elimination kinetics a fixed ratio of the drug is eliminated over time. Increasing the amount of the drug in the body will increase the amount eliminated.

86. *All of the following are complications of ketorolac (Toradol) except:
   a.   Bleeding
   b.   Renal failure
   c.   Ulcers
   d.   Peripheral neuropathy

   Answer d. **Side effects of **ketorolac** (and other NSAIDS) include **bleeding, renal failure** (/ caution in pts > 65 or elevated Cr), and **ulcers**.*

   Peripheral neuropathy is a side effect of **metronidazole, not ketorolac.*

87. **All of the following are true except:
   a.   Drugs that readily distribute into fat have a high volume of distribution
   b.   Hoffman elimination relies on kidney metabolism
   c.   Tachyphylaxis is tolerance to a drug after only a few doses
   d.   Hydrophilic drugs are more likely to be excreted in unaltered form

   Answer b. ***Hoffman elimination* does not rely on organ metabolism. These drugs can be used in pts w/ liver or kidney failure without toxic buildup of metabolites (eg **cisatracurium** undergoes Hoffman elimination)*

   Drugs that readily distribute into fat have a **high volume of distribution*

88. **All of the following are true except:
   a.   Over-diuresis w/ lasix can result in metabolic alkalosis
   b.   The cytochrome p-450 system is the primary mechanism for most drug metabolism
   c.   Over-diuresis w/ acetazolamide can result in metabolic acidosis
   d.   Furosemide doses > 100 mg can result in ototoxicity

   Answer a. Over-diuresis w/ spironolactone Tx results in hyperkalemia.
   *****Furosemide** doses > 100 mg can result in **ototoxicity***

Pharmacokinetics
Absorption
Sublingual and **rectal meds** – do not pass through liver first so do not undergo first pass metabolism (****higher bioavailability**)
Skin – *high lipid solubility* increases absorption through epidermis
CSF– absorption usually restricted to non-ionized, lipid-soluble drugs
*Kinetics
0 order kinetics – constant amount of drug eliminated regardless of dose (increasing dose will not increase amount eliminated)
Enzyme and elimination systems saturated

1st order kinetics – amount of drug eliminated is proportional to dose (increasing does will increase amount eliminated)
Enzyme and elimination systems are likely not saturated
Need 5 half-lives for drug to reach steady-state

1) *Volume of distribution* = amount of drug in body divided by amount of drug in plasma (blood)
   *Drugs w/ a high volume of distribution have higher concentrations in the **extra-vascular compartment** (eg fat) compared to intravascular compartment*

2) **Bioavailability** = fraction of unchanged drug reaching systemic circulation [100% for IV drugs, less for other routes (eg PO)]

**Drug Effects

Hyperactive – effect at an unusually low dose
Tachyphylaxis – tolerance after only a few doses
Potency – dose required for effect
Efficacy – ability to achieve result without untoward effect
Tolerance – progressive decline in potency w/ continued usage
Addiction – psychological compulsion to take drug
Physical dependence – physiological effects occur when drug is stopped

Drug metabolism

Converts **lipophilic** (more lipid soluble) compounds into more readily excreted **hydrophilic** polar products (more water soluble)
99% of the time this is associated w/ **detoxification** of drug

1) **Primary system** – hepatocyte **smooth endoplasmic reticulum** _and_ **cytochrome P-450** mono-oxygenase system
   Phase I - demethylation, oxidation, reduction, hydrolysis
   Phase II (conjugation reactions)
   Glucuronic acid (MC) and **sulfates** attached to drug
   Forms **water-soluble metabolite** (usually inactive) → then undergo excretion
   Drugs excreted in bile may become **deconjugated** in intestines w/ **reabsorption**, some in active form (eg cyclosporin) → process is termed **entero-hepatic recirculation**
   Pt w/ biliary drainage tube that bypass intestines will not have this reabsorption [eg kidney TXP pt requiring bile duct T-tube has acute rejection episode (↑ Cr, ↓ UOP) due to low cyclosporin levels] Tx: **pulse steroids**

2) *Hoffman degradation* (does not rely on organ metabolism)
   These drugs can be used in pts w/ liver or kidney failure without worry about toxic buildup of metabolites (eg **cisatracurium**); Drug is metabolized in blood

Drug Elimination

Kidney – most impt organ for eliminating most drugs (glomerular filtration and tubular secretion)
Biliary system – may have entero-hepatic recirculation (see above)
Polar drugs (ionized) – more **water soluble** and more likely to be eliminated in unaltered form
Non-polar drugs (non-ionized) – more **lipid soluble** and more likely to be metabolized before excretion

Important drug interactions

Albumin – largely responsible for binding drugs (PCNs, Warfarin 90% bound)
Sulfonamides (eg bactrim) – displace unconjugated bilirubin off albumins in newborns; cause **kernicterus** (brain damage)

GI Drugs

Promethazine (Phenergan, anti-emetic) – dopamine receptor blocker
   S/Es: tardive dyskinesia, Tx: diphenhydramine (Benadryl)
Metoclopramide (Reglan, prokinetic) – dopamine receptor blocker
Erythromycin – can act on **motilin receptor** (pro-kinetic)

Loperamide – slows gut motility by binding the **opioid receptors**
Ranitidine, famotidine – histamine H_2 receptor blockers; ↓ stomach acid
Megestrol (Megace) – increases appetite in pts w/ advanced CA
Magnesium- used for torsades de pointes (ventricular tachycardia)
Diuretics
   1)**Loop diuretics** [eg furosemide (Lasix), bumetanide (Bumex)]
      Over-diuresis causes **metabolic alkalosis** and **hypokalemia**
      Lasix S/Es – **ototoxicity** (keep dose ≤ 100 mg),
   2) **Thiazide** [eg hydrochlorothiazide (HCTZ)]
      Over-diuresis results in **metabolic alkalosis**

   3) **Carbonic anhydrase inhibitor** [eg acetazolamide (Diamox)]
      Over-diuresis results in *metabolic acidosis*, hypokalemia
   4) **Potassium sparing diuretics** (eg spironolactone)
      Over-diuresis results in **metabolic acidosis** and hyperkalemia
Anti-Inflammatory Drugs (NSAIDs)
   Non-selective COX inhibitors
      Types – naproxen, ketorolac, ibuprofen, indomethacin, ASA
      Inhibit both **constitutive** (COX-1) and **inducible** (COX-2)
         cyclooxygenase and **prostaglandin** synthesis (all reversible
         except ASA)
      S/Es (dose-dependent):
         1) *GI bleeding* (gastric ulcers and gastritis)
            **Inhibition of prostaglandin synthesis leads to decreased
              mucus and HCO_3^- secretion (↓ed protection)**
            PPIs and **misoprostol** can be given for protection
         2) *Renal insufficiency*
            **Inhibition of prostaglandin synthesis leads to
              vasoconstriction of renal afferent arterioles**
            PGEs usually keep the arterioles vasodilated
            Refrain from use in pts w/ ↑ed **creatinine**
   ASA (*irreversible* non-selective COX inhibitor)
      S/Es (ie poisoning) – HA's, N/V
      1st – respiratory alkalosis, **2nd** – metabolic acidosis
   Selective COX-2 inhibitors (celecoxib)
      Inhibit inducible form of cyclooxygenase (COX-2)
      Expressed at sites of inflamed tissue
      Fewer ulcers and less renal failure than non-selective COX inhibitors
      S/Es: ↑ **risk of cardiovascular events** (2-3 x, eg MI, stroke)
   Misoprostol – PGE_1 derivative
      A **prostaglandin** used to prevent ulcers in pts on chronic NSAIDs
Infliximab (Remicade) - **Ab's** to **TNF-alpha**, given IV
   Used for **inflammatory bowel** (Crohn's Disease, Ulcerative Colitis)
   Contraindications – allergy to rodents, active infection, CHF
   S/Es: **Infection Risk** (MC serious complication)
      MC serious infection → **tuberculosis
      ↑ed re-activation and ↑ed incidence of acquiring TB
      PPD placed before starting drug
      When treating pts w/ Infliximab who have a positive PPD,
         isoniazid should be started as well
Gadolinium (Gd) – used in MRI as a contrast agent
   Do not use in pts w/ *renal insufficiency* (GFR < 60), get buildup of Gd
   S/Es: 1) **Acute renal dysfunction**
         2) **Nephrogenic systemic fibrosis** (fibrosis of skin, joints, eyes,
            organs); from Gd^{+++} deposition
Xigris (Drotrecogin alfa activated)
   Activated protein C – used to prevent microthrombi in pts w/ sepsis
   Mechanism of action - *fibrinolysis*; S/Es: bleeding
   Indications (*many* requirements): used in really sick septic pts
   Contraindications – active bleeding, recent surgery / trauma, bleeding risks

Anesthesia

89. **All of the following are true except:
    a. The MCC of post-op hypoxia is atelectasis (alveolar hypoventilation)
    b. The MCC of post-op hypercarbia is poor minute ventilation
    c. The most effective way to prevent peri-operative hypothermia is warm IV fluids
    d. Bipolar cautery is the safest method of electrical surgical dissection

    Answer c. ***The most effective way to prevent peri-operative hypothermia is warm air conduction (eg Bair Hugger).*

    *** **Bipolar cautery** is the safest method of electrical surgical dissection.*
    ***The MCC of post-op **hypoxia** is **atelectasis** (**alveolar hypoventilation and collapse)*
    ***The MCC of post-op **hypercarbia** is poor minute ventilation*

90. *Severe hallucinations are a common side effect of:
    a. Ketamine
    b. Etomidate
    c. Propofol
    d. Sodium thiopental

    Answer a. **Severe hallucinations are a side effect of **ketamine**.*

91. **All of the following are true of rapid sequence intubation in a pt w/ CHF and small bowel obstruction except:
    a. Pre-oxygenation is the first step
    b. Paralytic is given before induction
    c. Cricoid pressure can help reduce risk of aspiration in pts w/ small bowel obstruction
    d. Etomidate is fast acting, has the least amount of cardiovascular side effects, and works well as an induction agent for RSI.

    Answer b. *The induction agent is given before the paralytic.** **Cricoid pressure** can help reduce risk of aspiration in pts w/ small bowel obstruction. ** **Etomidate** is a fast acting induction agent, has the least amount of cardiovascular side effects, and works well for RSI. **<u>Nitrous oxide</u> should be avoided in pts w/ bowel obstruction as it diffuses into closed spaces and increases risk of perforation.*

92. *Prior to performing a lung resection, the anesthesiologist attempts to intubate the patient but he is not sure if the tube is in the trachea. The best determinant of esophageal versus tracheal intubation is:
    a. Breath sounds
    b. Gastric sounds
    c. Opinion of the anesthesiologist
    d. End tidal CO2

    Answer d. **The most sensitive test as to whether or not the endotracheal is placed correctly is **end tidal CO2.***

93. *Histamine release is characteristic of:
    a. Meperidine
    b. Fentanyl
    c. Sufentanil
    d. Morphine

    Answer d. **Morphine has a characteristic histamine release which can cause **hypotension**.*

94. **Seizures in pts w/ acute renal failure is characteristic of which drug:
    a. Meperidine
    b. Fentanyl
    c. Sufentanil
    d. Morphine

Answer a *******Meperidine*** *in acute renal failure can result in buildup of normeperidine analogues which can cause* ***seizures****.*

95. An overdose of fentanyl is treated with:
    a. Flumazenil
    b. Narcan
    c. Neostigmine
    d. Edrophonium

Answer b. All narcotic agent (morphine, fentanyl, Demerol, sufentanil, etc.) overdoses can be treated with **Narcan** (naloxone).

96. All of the following are contra-indications to succinylcholine except:
    a. Renal failure
    b. Burn patients
    c. Spinal cord injury
    d. Elderly

Answer d. Succinylcholine in not contra-indicated in elderly

97. **Malignant hyperthermia is MC is related to a defective receptor (ryanodine receptor) on the sarcoplasmic reticulum that controls calcium release. The 1st sign of malignant hyperthermia after succinylcholine in an intubated patient is:
    a. Fever
    b. Rigors
    c. Increase in end-tidal CO2
    d. Tachycardia

Answer c. *Increase in* ***end-tidal CO2***

98. **The most appropriate step in the treatment of malignant hyperthermia is:
    a. Dantrolene
    b. Dopamine
    c. Dobutamine
    d. Lasix and potassium

Answer a. Malignant hyperthermia can be triggered by either succinylcholine or inhalation anesthetics (sevoflurane, isoflurane, halothane, enflurane, etc.). ****Dantrolene** is the most effective Tx*

99. **Cisatracurium is metabolized by:
    a. Liver
    b. Kidney
    c. Plasma cholinesterase
    d. Hoffman degradation

Answer d. ****Cisatracurium** undergoes **Hoffman degradation** (degraded in blood) which makes it ideal for pts with either renal failure or liver failure.*

100. **Two days after a severe inhalational injury, you have trouble oxygenating your pt so you decide to paralyze her with pancuronium. The MC side effect is:
    a. Fever
    b. Hypotension
    c. Increased intracranial pressure
    d. Tachycardia

Answer d. ***The MC S/E of pancuronium is **tachycardia**.*

101. *All of the following are true except
    a. Neck muscles and face are the 1st to relax w/ paralytics
    b. Diaphragm muscles are last to relax w/ paralytics and 1st to recover
    c. Non-depolarizing paralytics can be reversed w/ Neostigmine
    d. Depolarizing paralytics can be reversed w/ atropine

    Answer d. Depolarizing paralytics cannot be reversed (are metabolized by pseudocholinesterases). Pts w/ **atypical pseudocholinesterases** have prolonged paralysis>

    ***Neck muscles** and face are the 1st to relax w/ paralytics*
    ***Diaphragm muscles** are last to relax w/ paralytics and 1st to recover*

102. *A severe overdose of Ativan (lorazepam) is treated with:
    a. Flumazenil
    b. Narcan
    c. Neostigmine
    d. Edrophonium

    Answer a. Severe overdoses of benzodiazepines (Ativan, Valium, Versed) are treated with **flumazenil**.

103. *Of the anesthetics listed below, the one most likely to cause allergic reaction is:
    a. Lidocaine
    b. Bupivicaine
    c. Mepivicaine
    d. Procaine

    Answer d. ****Amide type** *local anesthetics (all have "i" in 1st part of their name) such as lidocaine, bupivicaine, and mepivicaine rarely cause allergic reactions.* ****Ester type** *local anesthetics, such as procaine, cocaine, and tetracaine are more likely to cause allergic reactions because of their PABA analogue.*

104. **All of the following are true of local anesthetics except:
    a. These agents work by increasing the action potential threshold in peripheral nerves
    b. Work better in acidic environments
    c. Can cause seizures
    d. The first sign of lidocaine toxicity is peri-oral paresthesias

    Answer b. ***Local anesthetics work by raising the **action potential threshold** (makes it harder to have an action potential occur so the pain sensation is not transmitted).* ***Local anesthetics work* <u>poorly</u> *in **acidic environments** (which makes it hard to anesthetize infected wounds).* ***The first sign of lidocaine toxicity is peri-oral paresthesias.*

105. **All of the following are contraindications to spinal anesthesia except:
    a. cirrhosis
    b. hypertrophic cardiomyopathy
    c. elevated ICP
    d. INR 1.3

    Answer d. INR of 1.3 is not a contra-indication to spinal anesthesia

106. **A pt undergoing lung resection has an epidural placed containing morphine and bupivicaine. All of the following are true concerning the epidural except:

a. Respiratory depression is most likely due to the morphine
b. Hypotension and bradycardia are most like due to the bupivicaine
c. Epidurals are well tolerated in patients with hypertrophic cardiomyopathy
d. Spinal headaches can often be treated with a blood patch

Answer c. Hypertrophic cardiomyopathy is a contraindication to epidurals because they cause a decrease in afterload, which can be catastrophic in patients with dilated cardiomyopathy (the ventricle will collapse on itself usually at the level of the septum).

Hypotension and bradycardia which occur with epidurals are almost always related to the local anesthetic (bupivicaine) placed in the epidural.

Interestingly, although morphine can cause hypotension when given systemically, it does not occur with epidural infusion (likely because the CSF does not contain histamine releasing mast cells). Respiratory depression is related to morphine in epidurals. Many centers place Dilaudid (hydromorphone) in epidurals to avoid this side-effect.

107. *A 65 yo man on dialysis for renal failure undergoes an elective abdominal aortic aneurysm repair. This patients ASA class is:
    a. II
    b. III
    c. IV
    d. V

    Answer c. This pt is class IV.

108. **Which of the following represents the highest cardiac risk for pts undergoing non-cardiac surgery:
    a. Recent MI
    b. Previous stroke, now functional
    c. S3 gallop
    d. Peripheral arterial disease

    Answer c. **S3 gallop represents uncompensated CHF, which is the highest risk factor on the Goldman criteria (11 points). **Creatnine > 2 is also a cardiac RF for pts undergoing non-cardiac surgery.

109. All of the following are true of myasthenia gravis except
    a. The ocular muscles are the most commonly involved muscles
    b. Myasthenia Crisis can be precipitated by stress and is usually treated with steroids, Mestinon, plasmapheresis, and possible intubation
    c. The most accurate and sensitive test for myasthenia gravis is the EMG "jitter" test
    d. Surgery is indicated for myasthenia crisis

    Answer d. Surgery is not indicated for myasthenia crisis (should be treated medically).

110. **The most common reaction to iodine is
    a. nausea
    b. Hypotension
    c. Loss of consciousness
    d. Cardiac arrest

    Answer a. **MC reaction to iodine – **nausea**
    MC life-threatening reaction – **dyspnea

111. **All of the following are true except:

a. The ACS NSQIP collects outcome data to measure and improve surgical quality in U.S
b. GAP protection seeks structured handoffs and checklists for pt transfers and transfer of pt care between caregivers
c. A sentinel event is an unexpected occurrence involving death or serious injury, or the risk thereof; hospital undergoes root cause analysis to prevent
d. A time-out should just verify the pt and procedure

Answer d. ****The *time out* before the incision is made should include the following:** verifying <u>patient</u>, <u>procedure</u>, <u>position</u> <u>site + side</u>, and availability of <u>implants</u> or <u>special requirements.</u>

The **ACS NSQIP collects risk-adjusted outcome data to measure and improve surgical quality in U.S. Outcomes are reported as observed vs. expected ratios.

****GAP protection** seeks structured handoffs and checklists for pt transfers and transfer of pt care between caregivers

A **sentinel event is an unexpected occurrence involving death or serious injury, or the risk thereof; hospital undergoes root cause analysis to prevent

**Induction
Can use either **inhalational agent** (MC sevoflurane) or **IV agent** (MC Propofol)
Inhalational agents (volatile anesthetics)
   Effects of inhalational anesthetics
      Anesthesia (unconsciousness), **Amnesia**, **± Analgesia**-↓ pain
      Blunt **hypoxic respiratory drive**
      Most have ***myocardial depression*, **increased cerebral blood flow**, and **decreased renal blood flow**
      Short acting (5-10 min) – redistributes into body fat, muscle
   Types
      Sevoflurane (MC used) – high cost, fast onset, less myocardial depression, less laryngospasm
      Desflurane - pungent odor, irritates airways, <u>not</u> used to induce
      Isoflurane - pungent odor, irritates airways, <u>not</u> used to induce
      Enflurane - S/Es: *seizures* (not used in pts w/ epilepsy)
      Halothane – slow
         Highest myocardial depression + arrhythmias
         Least pungent (good for children)
         Halothane hepatitis- fever, eosinophilia, jaundice, ↑ LFTs
      ****Nitrous oxide** (NO_2) – fast, minimal myocardial depression
         Used as a carrier gas for sevoflurane or desflurane
         ***Diffuses into closed air spaces*- avoid w/ bowel obstruction or PTX

**IV agents
   **Etomidate – few hemodynamic effects; fast acting (unknown mech)
      ***Least cardiovascular effects* of all IV agents (good for pts w/ pre-existing cardiac condition such as **CHF or angina**)
      Often used for **rapid sequence intubation**
      Good anesthetic + amnesic properties, <u>not</u> **analgesic**
      S/Es: continuous infusion leads to *adrenal suppression*
   Propofol – very rapid distribution and **on/off** (unknown mechanism)
      Good anesthetic and amnesic properties, <u>not</u> **analgesic**
      Metabolized in **liver** and by **plasma cholinesterases**
      S/Es: *hypotension*, resp depression, pain at injection site
      Do not use in pts w/ **egg** or **soybean allergy**

Avoid in children - <u>prolonged use</u> associated w/ **metabolic acidosis + death** (rhabdomyolysis, ARF, cardiac failure)
Avoid in obstetrics, Parkinson's Disease
Ketamine – dissociation of thalamic and limbic systems
Places pt in cataleptic state (**amnesia, analgesia**)
No respiratory depression
Good for **children**
S/Es: **hallucinations**, catecholamine release ($\uparrow$ CO_2, tachycardia), $\uparrow$ airway secretions, $\uparrow$ cerebral blood flow
Contraindicated in pts w/ **head injury**

Rapid sequence intubation - used in pts w/ $\uparrow$ed risk of **aspiration**
RFs for aspiration - recent oral intake, GERD, delayed gastric emptying (gastroparesis), pregnancy, **bowel obstruction**
Sequence:
1) **Pre-oxygenation** (tight fitting mask)
2) **IV induction agent** (eg <u>Etomidate</u>, Propofol)
3) **IV paralytic** (eg <u>succinylcholine</u> or rocuronium)
4) **cricoid pressure** to reduce risk of aspiration w/ intubation

Best indicator of successful tracheal intubation – ET-CO2 (end tidal CO2)
ET-CO2 specifically reflects exchange of CO2 from blood to alveolus
1) **Sudden $\uparrow$ ET-CO2** → MCC - **hypoventilation**
Tx: $\uparrow$TV or $\uparrow$RR
2) **Sudden $\downarrow$ ET-CO2** → MCC - **became disconnected from the vent**
Others (associated w/ hypotension) – PE, CO2 embolus
Endotracheal tube – should be placed 2 cm above the carina
MC PACU complication – nausea and vomiting

Dexmedetomidine (Precedex)
Provides anesthesia + analgesia <u>without</u> decreasing respiratory drive
Good for **early extubation protocols** (eg cardiac surgery)
Mechanism – CNS alpha-2 receptor agonist

Narcotics (opioids)
Types - morphine, fentanyl, meperidine (Demerol), codeine, hydromorphone (Dilaudid), oxycodone (Percocet), hydrocodone (Vicodin), oxycontin, oxymorphone, dextropropoxyphene (Darvocet)
All act on **μ-opioid receptor** in **CNS**
All are reversed w/ Narcan (naloxone)
Effects: profound **analgesia** (euphoria), **respiratory depression** ($\downarrow$ CO_2 drive), **blunt sympathetic response**
Liver metabolism and **kidney excretion**
1) *Morphine*; S/Es: miosis, $\downarrow$cough, $\uparrow$constipation, **histamine release** (mild $\downarrow$BP)
2) **Meperidine** (Demerol)
S/Es: miosis, <u>tremors</u>, <u>fasciculations</u>, <u>seizures</u>; <u>No</u> histamine release
Avoid **high doses**
Avoid in pts w/ **renal failure**
→ get buildup of **normeperidine analogue** (→ **seizures**)
Avoid in pts on **MAOIs** (monoamine oxidase inhibitors)
→ leads to **serotonin syndrome** ($\uparrow\uparrow$ serotonin release in CNS - severe fever, tachycardia, seizures, shock, coma)
3) **Fentanyl** – 80x strength of morphine
Does <u>not</u> cross react w/ morphine allergy; <u>No</u> histamine release
4) **Sufentanil, remifentanil** – very fast-acting, short half-lives
Careful w/ opioid + benzodiazepine combinations (have **synergistic effect**)
Methadone – binds CNS **μ-opioid receptor**, less euphoria

**Muscle relaxants *(paralytics)*
- ***Diaphragm** – last muscle to go down and 1st muscle to recover from paralytics
- ***Neck muscles and face** – 1st to go down and last to recover from paralytics

Depolarizing agent (only agent is **succinylcholine**)

Succinylcholine – fast, short-acting; fasciculations, *__many__* S/Es

1) ****Malignant hyperthermia**

Defect in calcium metabolism

Calcium released from sarcoplasmic reticulum causes **muscle excitation–contraction syndrome**.

Sx's:
- ****1st sign** is ↑ **end-tidal CO_2**
- Then **fever**, tachycardia, **rigidity**, acidosis, hyperkalemia, hypoxia
- **Rhabdomyolysis** can lead to **myoglobin release**

Tx:
- ****Dantrolene** *(best Tx)* – inhibits Ca release and decouples excitation complex
- **Cooling blankets, HCO_3, glucose**, supportive care

Can also be caused by ***inhaled anesthetics** *(volatile)*

Mechanism - **ryanodine receptor defect** on sarcoplasmic reticulum

Local anesthetics do <u>not</u> trigger the reaction (consider for future surgeries)

2) ****Hyperkalemia**

Depolarization releases **potassium**

Don't use in pts w/ **severe burns, neurologic injury, neuromuscular disorders, spinal cord injury** (all have up-regulation **of ACh receptors** in muscle which dramatically ↑s potassium release)

Don't use in **massive trauma pts** (↑ potassium from muscle injury)

Don't use w/ **acute renal failure**

3) Open-angle **glaucoma** can become closed-angle glaucoma.

4) **Atypical pseudocholinesterases** – prolonged paralysis (Asians)

5) **Increased intracranial pressure** (ICP)- avoid w/ head injury

*Metabolism - degradation by **plasma pseudocholinesterases**

*Non-depolarizing agents

Inhibit neuromuscular junction by competing w/ ACh at ACh receptor (competitive antagonist); not as fast as depolarizing agent

Types

1) **Rocuronium** - fast acting, intermediate duration (good for RSI); **Metabolism** – <u>hepatic</u>

2) ****Pancuronium** - slower acting, long duration (good in **ICU**)
   - <u>No</u> hypotension
   - **Metabolism** – <u>renal</u>
   - ****MC S/E: **<u>tachycardia</u>**

3) ***Cisatracurium** – slower acting, intermediate duration
   - Good in pts w/ *liver or renal failure*
   - ****Metabolism** – ****<u>Hoffman degradation</u>**
   - S/Es: <u>Histamine release</u> (hypotension)

*Reversing drugs for non-depolarizing agents

*Neostigmine – blocks **acetylcholinesterase**, ↑s ACh

Edrophonium – blocks **acetylcholinesterase**, ↑s ACh

Atropine or glycopyrrolate (ACh antagonists) given w/ neostigmine or edrophonium to counteract effects of generalized acetylcholine overdose (salivation, diarrhea)

Benzodiazepines
Effects: anxiolytic, anticonvulsant, amnesic, respiratory depression
   Not analgesic
Metabolism – hepatic
Mechanism- bind GABA receptor (most prevalent inhibitory brain receptor)
1) **Versed** (midazolam) – short acting, contraindicated w/ pregnancy
2) **Ativan** (lorazepam) – long acting
3) **Valium** (diazepam) – long acting; lot of metabolites, not used as a drip
   Benzodiazepines Overdose Tx - flumazenil
      Competitive inhibitor; may cause seizures and arrhythmias;
         Contraindicated in pts w/ elevated ICP or status epilepticus

Local anesthetics
Mechanism – increase **action potential threshold**, preventing Na influx
Infected tissues – hard to anesthetize secondary to *acidosis*
Length of action: bupivacaine > lidocaine > procaine
Epinephrine allows higher doses to be used, stays local
   No epinephrine w/ arrhythmias, unstable angina, uncontrolled HTN,
      poor collaterals (penis and ear), uteroplacental insufficiency
Neuro blockade: sensory > motor
Allergic reactions
   Amides (all have an "i" in first part of name) – lidocaine,
      bupivacaine, mepivacaine; *rare* **allergic reactions**
   Esters – tetracaine, procaine, cocaine; ↑ed **allergic reactions**
      (bronchospasm, pruritis), secondary to *PABA analogue*
Max Dosage:
   Lidocaine max dosage – 5 mg/kg (w/ epi 7 mg/kg)
      Can use 0.5 cc/kg of 1% lidocaine
   Bupivicaine max dosage – 2 mg/kg (w/ epi 3 mg/kg)
   After max dose, can re-administer after 2 hours
Lidocaine toxicity progression:
   1st sx → **Peri-oral paresthesias** (tingling, numbness)
   2nd sx → Visual and auditory **hallucinations**
   Sedation, unconsciousness, SZs, resp depression, arrhythmias,
      and cardiovascular collapse
   Neuro S/Es occur at lower doses than cardiovascular S/Es

Epidural anesthesia
Epidural (outside dura)
   *Causes **sympathetic denervation** and **sensory blockade***
   Pain receptors affected much more than motor receptors
      Does not provide good paralysis
      Good for control of **post-op pain**
   Finding epidural space – loss of resistance w/ injection
   Bloody tap – insert at new level
   Block height is 3-4 levels above site of insertion
      T-5 epidural – affects cardiac accelerator nerves
   Contraindications to epidural and spinal anesthesia
      Hypertrophic cardiomyopathy (↓ afterload causes LV
         outflow tract collapse); also **AS** and **MS**
      Cyanotic heart disease (↓ afterload shunts blood away from
         lungs)
      Aortic stenosis (↓ afterload impairs coronary blood supply)
      Liver DZ (cirrhosis; bleeding risk → epidural hematoma)
      Systemic infection or at site (worry about epidural abscess)
      Coagulopathy (INR > 1.5, low plts, uremia, heparin- bleed risk)
      Anatomic abnormalities (spina bifida, meningomyelocele)
      Elevated ICP
      Severe hypovolemia (can worsen hypotension)

Epidural Cx's:
- **Morphine** component - **resp depression** (esp high spinal)
  - Tx: Turn off epidural, airway management
  - Avoid respiratory depression by using **Dilaudid**
- **Lidocaine** component - **↓ heart rate + ↓ blood pressure**
  - Tx for hypotension and bradycardia:
    1) Turn epidural down
    2) Fluids, phenylephrine, atropine
    3) Make sure hypotension not due to another source (eg bleeding)
- **Urinary retention** (all pts need bladder catheter)
- *Spinal headaches* – HA gets worse <u>sitting up</u>
  - Tx: rest, increased fluids, caffeine, analgesics
  - *Blood patch to site if persists >24 hours*
- **Epidural Hematoma**
  - **Classic Sx's:**
    1) **sudden localized back pain** at epidural site
    2) **within 1-2 hours → motor + sensation loss** ± loss of bladder and bowel function
  - Dx: **emergent MRI**; Tx: decompressive **laminectomy**
- **Decreased motor in legs**
  - Usually **unilateral**
  - MC from medication overdose (leg should feel <u>warm</u>)
  - Tx: Turn down epidural and monitor, if no recovery, emergent MRI to R/O epidural hematoma
- **Benefits of epidural** – ↓ pain, ↓ resp cx's (eg PNA), ↓ myocardial infarction, ↑ TV, ↑ return of bowel function, no survival difference

Spinal anesthesia – *sensory <u>and</u> motor blockade*
- Sensory blockade is above motor blockade
- *Can perform **any surgery below umbilicus** w/ spinal anesthesia <u>alone</u>* (eg C-sections, hernia, ortho, hysterectomy, appendectomy)

Caudal block- through sacrum, good for pediatric hernias, perianal surgery

*ASA class (American Society of Anesthesiologists)
- Class I – healthy patient
- Class II – mild disease without limitation (HTN, DM, obesity, smokers)
- Class III – severe disease (stable angina, previous MI, moderate COPD)
- Class IV – disease is a severe constant threat to life (unstable angina, renal or liver failure, severe COPD)
- Class V – moribund patient (eg ruptured AAA, saddle pulmonary embolus)
- Class VI – organ donor

<u>**Revised Cardiac Risk Index**</u> (modified; Circulation 1999; 100:1043-1049)
Each risk factor is assigned one point (6 points max):
1. **High-risk procedures** (Intra-peritoneal, Intra-thoracic, major vascular)
2. Hx of **ischemic heart disease** (MI, pos. stress test, angina, Q waves)
3. **Hx of CHF** *(pulmonary edema, **S3**)*
4. Hx of **cerebrovascular disease** (TIA or stroke)
5. Preop Tx w/ **insulin** (ie diabetic)
6. *Preop **creatinine > 2.0***

RISK OF MAJOR CARDIAC EVENT

# of points	Class	Risk of Major Cardiac Event
0	I	0.5%
1	II	1%
2	III	7%
3 or more	IV	11%

Major cardiac events - MI, pulmonary edema, cardiac arrest
Beta-blocker – *most effective agent to prevent intra-op and post-op cardiac events*
Wait **6-8 weeks after MI** for elective surgery (10% mortality if < 6-8 weeks)

Aortic and **lower extremity vascular procedures** considered **high risk**
CEA considered **moderate risk**
Largest risk factor for cardiac complications – uncompensated CHF
*(as evidence by JVD, high CVP or **S3 gallop**; 11 points on*
Goldman criteria); Recent MI (#2) – 10 points

Non-invasive cardiac testing [eg dobutamine-thallium, stress-thallium
(walking), adenosine-thallium scans]
Looking for areas of **ischemia** (ie decreased thallium uptake) w/:
1) the heart under **stress** (eg Dobutamine or walking) *or*
2) **coronary vasodilatation** (eg adenosine or dipyridamole)
*Termed **reversible ischemia***
Positive stress test = chest pain, ST changes, hypotension, or areas of
reversible ischemia → all indications for **coronary angiogram**

Coronary Angiogram Indications (invasive testing)
1) **Positive non-invasive cardiac testing**
2) ***Acute ST elevation MI*** (STEMI) – standard is 90 minutes ER door to
PTCA time (termed door to balloon time); ***STEMIs should undergo***
PTCA/stenting *if technically feasible*
3) **Non-ST elevation MI** - usually cath before discharge

Myasthenia Gravis
Sx's: ***ocular muscles MC involved***; general skeletal involvement (90%)
Dx: **EMG** *(best test,* Jolly test) – shows **jitter** (non-uniform NMJ destruction)
Path: ***Ab's to ACh receptors at NMJ*** → ACh receptors get destroyed
Myeloid cells in thymus may serve as Ag source
Tx: **Cholinesterase inhibitors** (#1; pyridostigmine, Mestinon)
S/Es – salivation, diarrhea, bradycardia
Cholinergic crisis – too much ACh (see below)
Steroids, **Plasmapheresis** (removes Ab's), **IVIG**
Thymectomy
Indications – <u>thymomas</u> or <u>severe</u> myasthenia gravis (80% get
improvement)
Thymus receives branches from **inferior thyroid artery** and **internal**
mammary artery
***Myasthenia Crisis** (too little ACh)
Respiratory Failure - caused by infection, stress, sepsis
NO surgery – no role for emergency thymectomy
Tx: ***pyridostigmine***, plasmapheresis, steroids; may need to intubate
***Cholinergic Crisis** (too much ACh)
Overdose of cholinesterase inhibitor
Causes too much ACh at NMJ – results in **depolarization blockade**
Effects – paralysis, respiratory failure, salivation, sweating
May need intubation to allow it to wear off

***Iodine Allergy**
MC reaction to iodine – ***nausea*** (others include urticaria, itching, heat)
MC life threatening reaction – ***dyspnea*** (others hypotension, arrest)

Advanced oral directives
Advanced oral directives take precedence in cases where the pt is
otherwise not able to make informed decisions about their care.
The next order of precedence is **living will**
Followed by **durable power of attorney** (eg wife or husband)

National Surgical Quality Improvement Program (NSQIP) - seeks to collect outcome data to measure and improve surgical quality in the U.S. Outcomes are reported as observed vs. expected ratios.

JCAHO prevention of wrong site / procedure / patient protocol
1) pre-op verification of **patient** and **procedure**
2) **operative site** and **side** (marking if left or right or multiple levels; must be visible after the pt is prepped)
3) **time out** before incision made (verifying <u>patient</u>, <u>procedure</u>, <u>position site + side</u>, and availability of <u>implants</u> or <u>special requirements</u>)

Promoting Culture of Safety
1) confidential system of reporting errors
2) emphasis on learning over accountability
3) flexibility in adapting to new situations or problems

RFs for retained object after surgery (MC sponge) – emergency procedure, unplanned change in procedure, obesity, towel used for closure

Sentinel Event (JCAHO) – unexpected occurrence involving death or serious injury, or the risk thereof; hospital undergoes **root cause analysis** to prevent and minimize future occurrences (Ex. **wrong site surgery**)

Safest electrosurgical setting - <u>bipolar cautery</u>, use to avoid lateral thermal injury and arcing (**short circuit** created between tips of instrument)

GAP protection technique - gaps in care (eg change in care-giver, divisions of labor, shift changes, transfers) can lead to loss of information and error: prevention – **structured handoffs** and **checklists** (face to face if possible); standardizing orders; reading back orders if verbal

MCC post-op hypoxemia – <u>alveolar hypoventilation</u> (causes **atelectasis**) get V/Q shunt

MCC post-op hypercarbia – <u>poor minute ventilation</u>

Fluids and Electrolytes

112. *A 60 yo woman undergoes parathyroidectomy for a parathyroid adenoma. Seven days post-op she develops peri-oral tingling and numbness and has noticed a twitching in her face. All of the following are true except:
    a. Bone hunger likely accounts for her problem
    b. The treatment is calcium
    c. A magnesium level is important in this patient
    d. This is caused by hypercalcemia

    Answer d. *This pt has* **hypocalcemia** *likely from* **bone hunger.**

113. **All of the following are true except
    a. The MCC of significant hypo-phosphatemia is renal failure
    b. The MCC of significant hypo-calcemia is previous thyroid surgery
    c. The MCC of significant hypo-magnesemia is massive diuresis
    d. The MCC of significant hypo-kalemia is over-diuresis

    Answer a.
    MCC of significant **hypo-phosphatemia is **re-feeding syndrome**.*
    The MCC of significant **hypo-calcemia is **previous thyroid surgery***
    The MCC of significant **hypo-magnesemia is **massive diuresis***
    The MCC of significant **hypo-kalemia is **over-diuresis***

114. **A 35 yo woman suffering from Crohn's disease is admitted to the hospital for control of a high output fistula. She was started on TPN some time ago. She now has weakness, muscle cramps, tremors, confusion, and has hyper-reflexes. She has also been having short runs of supra-ventricular tachycardia. This is associated with which of the following metabolic disorders?
    a. Hyperkalemia
    b. Hypomagnesemia
    c. hypermagnesemia
    d. Hypercalcemia

    Answer b. **Hypomagnesemia**. *The sx's are similar to hypocalcemia. 50% of pts w/ hypomagnesemia also have hypokalemia or hypocalcemia.*

115. *A 55 yo pt w/ severe pancreatitis and hyperlipidemia has a Na of 125. All of following are true except:
    a. This pts hyponatremia is most likely from over-resuscitation
    b. This pts hyponatremia is most likely from hyperlipidemia
    c. There is no specific treatment for this pts for hyponatremia
    d. Tx of the underlying pancreatitis corrects the problem

    Answer a. This pt has **pseudo-hyponatremia** as a result of **hyperlipidemia** associated w/ pancreatitis. The elevated lipids draw fluid into the intravascular compartment creating pseudohyponatremia. No specific Tx (other than treating the underlying disorder) is necessary.

116. *The composition of lactated ringers is:
    a. Na 154, Cl 109, K 4, Ca 2.7, HCO3 28
    b. Na 130, Cl 103, K 4, Ca 2.7, HCO3 28
    c. Na 154, Cl 109, K 4, Ca 4, HCO3 28
    d. Na 130, Cl 109, K 4, Ca 2.7, HCO3 28

    Answer d. Lactated ringers has Na 130, Cl 109, K 4, Ca 2.7, HCO3 28

117. *A ventilated patient has the following arterial blood gas values: pH 7.50, CO_2 55, HCO3 35. This condition is most likely caused by:
    a. Poor minute ventilation
    b. Aggressive NG tube suctioning

c.   Renal failure
d.   Severe sepsis

Answer b. The ABG presented suggests a **metabolic alkalosis**. Of the items listed, NGT suctioning is most likely to cause a metabolic alkalosis.

118. *A ventilated patient has the following arterial blood gas values: pH 7.50, CO 24, HCO3 18. This condition is most likely caused by:
    a.   Low minute ventilation
    b.   NGT suctioning
    c.   Renal failure
    d.   High minute ventilation

Answer d. The ABG presented suggests a **respiratory alkalosis**. Of the items presented, high minute ventilation is them most likely cause. You correct this by either decreasing respiratory rate or decreasing tidal volume.

119. *A ventilated patient has the following arterial blood gas values: pH 7.25, CO2 70, HCO3 35. This condition is most likely caused by:
    a.   Poor minute ventilation
    b.   NGT suctioning
    c.   Renal failure
    d.   Severe sepsis

Answer a. The ABG presented is most c/w a **respiratory acidosis**. Of the items listed, poor minute ventilation is most likely to give you a respiratory acidosis. You correct this by either increasing respiratory rate or tidal volumes.

120. *A ventilated patient has the following arterial blood gas values: pH 7.26, CO 28, HCO3 18. This condition is most likely caused by:
    a.   Poor minute ventilation
    b.   NGT suctioning
    c.   Renal failure
    d.   High minute ventilation

Answer c. The ABG presented is most consistent with **metabolic acidosis**. Of the items listed, **renal failure** is most likely to give you a metabolic acidosis.

121. **The initial Tx of choice for hyperkalemia w/ arrhythmias after succinylcholine is:
    a.   Insulin and glucose
    b.   Calcium gluconate
    c.   Kayexalate
    d.   Dialysis

Answer b. Although all of these agents are used for **hyperkalemia**, a pt that is having arrhythmias as a result of the hyperkalemia should receive ****Calcium gluconate** 1st to stabilize cardiac muscle cell membranes.

122. **Re-feeding syndrome results in all of the following except:
    a.   Hypokalemia
    b.   Hypomagnesemia
    c.   Hyponatremia
    d.   Hypophosphatemia

Answer c. *Re-feeding syndrome* can result in **low K, Mg and PO4**. It occurs in the severely malnourished when they start receiving nutrition. Re-feeding syndrome is prevented by starting nutrition at a low rate initially (10-15 kcal/kg/day). ****Phosphate is replaced w/ potassium phosphate**

123. **Which of the following abnormalities can cause prolonged ventilation:
    a.   Hypokalemia
    b.   Hypomagnesemia
    c.   Hyponatremia
    d.   Hypophosphatemia

    Answer d. Hypophosphatemia can result in prolonged ventilation due to relative **ATP insufficiency** (need PO4 to convert ADP to ATP). Phosphate deficiency also results in encephalopathy and ↓ed WBC phagocytosis.

124. **The following are the initial fluids used to Tx each dehydration category except:
    a.   Sweat loss (eg marathon runner that collapses on hot day) – normal saline bolus
    b.   Gastric loss from pyloric stenosis – normal saline bolus
    c.   Small bowel fistula – normal saline bolus
    d.   Large bowel fistula – lactated ringers

    Answer c. The initial fluid of choice for dehydration due to small bowel fistula is lactated ringers. ***Normal saline** should be used for excessive sweat loss dehydration*

125. **All of the following are true except:
    a.   Hyperosmolar hyperglycemic non-ketotic syndrome can result in cerebral edema, seizures, coma and respiratory arrest
    b.   DKA results in hypokalemia
    c.   DKA occurs almost exclusively in Type I DM
    d.   Initial Tx for DKA is fluid hydration and insulin

    Answer b. DKA results in hyperkalemia.

Total body water
Protein – main determinant of intravascular and interstitial compartment _oncotic_ pressure
Na^+ – main determinant of intracellular and extracellular _osmotic_ pressure
*Volume overload: MCC → iatrogenic; 1st sign is *weight gain*
    3rd space fluid (edema) is in the *interstitial space*
*Normal saline (NS, 0.9%) - Na 154 and Cl 154
    *3% saline - Na 513, Cl 513
    0.45% saline - Na 77, Cl 77
*Lactated Ringer's (LR; ionic composition of plasma)
    Na^+ 130, Cl^- 109, K^+ 4, Ca^{++} 2.7, lactate 28
Plasma osmolarity = (2 x Na) + (glucose/18) + (BUN/2.8)
    Normal: 290 ± 10
Normal K^+ requirement: 0.5 - 1.0 mEq/kg/day
Normal Na^+ requirement: 1 - 2 mEq/kg/day
Hemodialysis (HD) can remove **K, Ca, Mg** and **PO4**; also **urea + Cr**

Volume replacement
*Maintenance IVFs:
    4 cc/kg/hr for 1st 10 kg
    2 cc/kg/hr for 2nd 10 kg
    1 cc/kg/hr for each kg after that
**The best indicator of adequate volume replacement → *urine output*
Open abdominal operations - fluid loss is **0.5–1.0 L/hr** unless there is a measurable blood loss
Usually do not replace blood lost unless it's **> 500 cc**
Insensible fluid losses – 10 cc/kg/day (75% sweat, 25% respiratory, hypotonic)
IV replacement after major adult GI surgery
    During operation and 1st 24 hours → use lactated ringers
    After 24 hours → switch to D5 ½ NS with 20 mEq K^+.

5% dextrose stimulates **insulin release** (↑glucose and amino acid uptake, protein synthesis, prevents protein catabolism)

D5 ½ NS @ 125/hr provides 150 gm glucose per day (525 kcal/day)

**Moderate to Severe Dehydration (related fluid loss / replacement)
1) ****Sweat** (eg marathon runner)   ****NS bolus**
2) ****Gastric** (eg gastric outlet obstruction w/ profuse N/V)   ****NS bolus**
3) ****Pancreatic. biliary, or small bowel** (eg high output fistula)****LR bolus**
4) **Large intestine** (eg C. diff colitis w/ severe diarrhea)   ****LR bolus**
   **Never bolus normal saline with K added (cardiac arrest)

	Fluid Secretion (cc/d)	Electrolyte Loss	*Maintenance IVFs
Sweat	300 - 500	**Water**, some NaCl	**1/2 NS** (if excessive loss)
Saliva	Normally negligible	**K** (highest K concentration in body)	**1/2 NS w/ 20 mEq K** (if excessive loss)
Stomach	1000-2000	**H+ and Cl-**	**D5 1/2 NS w/ 20 mEq K**
Pancreas	500-1000	**HCO3-**	**LR****
Biliary System	500-1000	**HCO3-**	**LR****
Small Intestine	Fluid absorption unless fistula	**HCO3-, ± K+**	**LR**** (eg fistula)
Large Intestine	Fluid absorption unless diarrhea	**K+**	**LR***** (eg diarrhea)

*Above are **maintenance,** not resuscitation IVFs for dehydration (see above)
May need additional **HCO3- replacement
***May need additional **K** replacement
GI losses – should generally be replaced **cc for cc**
Urine output – keep at least 0.5 cc/kg/hr; not replaced, sign of normal post-op diuresis

<u>Sodium</u> (nl 135 - 145)
Hypernatremia
Synonymous w/ **dehydration** 99% of the time
MCC – poor fluid intake (95%); over-diuresis, diabetes insipidus
Sx's: irritability, restless, ataxia, weakness, seizures
Tx: **D5 water**
Correct slowly to avoid *__brain swelling__ (< 0.7 meg/L/hr)

Hyponatremia
Synonymous w/ **fluid overload** 99% of the time
MCC – iatrogenic (1st sign – **weight gain**), others - *SIADH*
Sx's: N/V, headaches, delirium, seizures, stupor, coma
Tx: ****Water restriction and Diuresis (best Tx)**
Correct Na slowly to avoid *__central pontine myelinolysis__ (≤ 0.5 mEq/L/hr)
***Pseudo-hyponatremia** – from **hyperglycemia** (eg DKA) or **hyperlipidemia** (eg acute pancreatitis); Tx: nothing, need to Tx <u>underlying illness</u>*

Potassium (nl 3.5 - 5.0)

    Kidneys regulate serum K^+

    **Hyperkalemia

        MCC – renal disease (80%),

        EKG – initial peaked T waves deteriorates to ventricular fibrillation

        Tx:

            1) ****calcium gluconate** (1 amp, heart membrane stabilizer)
                → *1st drug to give*

            2) **10 U insulin** and **1 ampule of 50% dextrose**
                K driven into cells w/ glucose

            3) 1 amp **sodium bicarbonate**
                Alkalosis causes K to enter cell in exchange for H

            4) others - Kayexalate, Lasix, Albuterol, Dialysis (if refractory)

        *Pseudohyperkalemia – hemolysis of blood sample

    **Hypokalemia

        MCC – **diuretics; poor intake (eg TPN), GI loss (NG tube, diarrhea)

        EKG – T waves disappear

        Tx: **potassium chloride* (10 mEq ↑s serum K by 0.1 mEq/L)

        ***May need to **correct magnesium** before you can correct potassium*

Calcium

    Normal total   8.5 - 10.5 mg/dl (2.0 - 2.5 mmol/L)

    Normal ionized   4.5 - 5.5 mg/dl (1.0 - 1.5 mmol/L)

    Ca absorbed in GI tract (**calcium binding protein**) + reabsorbed in kidney
    (regulated by **PTH**); Ca also *excreted* into GI tract

    Hypercalcemia

        Hyperparathyroidism and **malignancy** account for 90% of all cases
            of hypercalcemia (see Parathyroid chp)

        *MCC hypercalcemia – *hyperparathyroidism (MC- parathyroid
            adenoma)*

        *MC malignant cause of hypercalcemia – *small cell lung CA*

        *MCC hypercalcemic crisis – *previous primary hyperparathyroidism
            undergoing another procedure*

        Sx's: lethargy, weakness, N/V, hypotension, arrhythmias, short QT
            kidney stones, stomach ulcers, ↓ DTRs (deep tendon reflexes)

            Ca > 13 mg/dl (ionized > 6) → symptoms

            Ca > 15 mg/dl (ionized > 7) → risk for cardiac arrest

        Tx ****Hypercalcemic Crisis** (Ca 13-15):

            1) *1st *Rapid volume infusion-* Normal Saline at 200-300 cc/hr
                <u>Do not use lactated ringers</u> (contains Ca)

            2) *2nd *Lasix (Do <u>not</u> use thiazide diuretics - reabsorb Ca)*

            3) **Dialysis** if refractory to above

            4) **If malignancy* → **Bisphosphonates (alendronate)*,
                calcitonin, mithramycin, glucocorticoids

            5) **If hyperparathyroidism** → parathyroidectomy after recovery

        Just to re-state:

        No lactated ringers (contains Ca)

        No thiazide diuretics (these retain Ca)

    Hypocalcemia

        MCC – ***previous thyroid surgery* (iatrogenic injury to parathyroid
            glands results in hypoparathyroidism); others – massive blood
            transfusion (citrate), pancreatitis

        Ca < 8 (ionized < 4) → symptoms

        Sx's: **1st sx – Peri-oral tingling**

            Chvostek's sign (tapping facial nerve causes face twitching)

            Trousseau's sign (carpopedal spasm after occluding arm blood
                flow)

            Laryngospasm and hyper-reflexia

            Prolonged QT on EKG → can get ventricular arrhythmias

Tx: PO **calcium carbonate** if mild sx's; IV **calcium gluconate** if severe sx'; IV **calcium chloride** if coding, Vit D
May need to correct **Mg before being able to correct calcium
***Hypo-proteinemia** (↓ed albumin) causes **artificially low Ca**
For every 1 g decrease in protein, add 0.8 to Ca level
Can occur after surgery for **hyperparathyroidism**
Caused by ***bone hunger** (<u>early</u>, bone repleting lost supply) or
***failure of parathyroid remnant or graft** (<u>late</u>)
Remember to give Ca after parathyroid surgery

Magnesium (nl 2.0 - 2.5 mg/dl)
*Hypermagnesemia
MCC – renal failure combined w/ Mg intake (eg laxatives, antacids)
Sx's: lethargy, weakness, N/V, hypotension, arrhythmias, ↓ DTRs
> 10 → complete heart block; **> 13** → risk for cardiac arrest
Tx: ***calcium** (best Tx, competitive Mg antagonist), diuretics, dialysis
Hypomagnesemia
MCC

Symptomatic – diuretics (massive diuresis)
Asymptomatic - 70% of all ICU pts have low Mg^{++}
Sx's start when **Mg < 1**
Sx's: (similar to hypocalcemia) irritability, confusion, hyper-reflexia,
SZs, prolonged QT, V-Tach (torsades de pointes), V-Fib
Tx: **magnesium**

Phosphate (nl 2.5 - 4.5 mg/dl)
Hyperphosphatemia
MCC – renal failure
Sx's: Majority asymptomatic; May have sx's associated w/
hypocalcemia (see above)
Tx: **sevelamer chloride** (Renagel, phosphate binder in gut), low
phosphate diet (eg avoid dairy), **dialysis** (removes PO4)
**Hypophosphatemia
Usually due to **PO4 shift** from **extra-cellular to intracellular**
MCC – ****re-feeding syndrome** (often in setting of ETOH abuse)
Sx's: ****Failure to wean from the ventilator** (↓ ed ATP production)
Muscle weakness (lack of PO4 for ATP production)
Infection risk (impaired leukocyte chemotaxis due to ↓ ATP)
Tx: ****potassium phosphate**

**Acid-Base

	pH	pCO$_2$	HCO$_3$
Normal values			
Respiratory acidosis	↓	↑ (1° problem)	↑
pH 7.35-7.45 (**7.<u>4</u>**)			
Respiratory alkalosis	↑	↓ (1° problem)	↓
CO2 35-45 (**<u>40</u>**)			
Metabolic acidosis	↓	↓	↓ (1° problem)
HCO3⁻ 22-26 (**<u>24</u>**)			
Metabolic alkalosis	↑	↑	↑ (1° problem)

$$H^+ + HCO_3^- \ = \ H_2CO_3 \ = \ H_2O + CO_2$$
(bicarb)   (carbonic acid)

***Lung** controls pH through **pCO2** regulation (rapid process)
***Kidney** controls pH primarily through **HCO3-** regulation (carbonic anhydrase
mediated, slow → days)
Henderson-Hesselbach equation: $pH = pK + \log [HCO_3^-] / [0.03 \times CO_2]$
Ratio of base to acid (HCO$_3^-$ to CO$_2$) of 20:1 = pH of 7.4

<u>Reparatory Alkalosis</u> - from hyper-ventilation (↓s pCO2, eg PE causes hypoxia and hypocarbia); Chronic cases associated w/ hypokalemia

<u>Respiratory Acidosis</u> - from hypo-ventilation (eg COPD exacerbation; ↑ pCO2)

Metabolic alkalosis
**Mechanism of hypochloremic, hypokalemic, metabolic alkalosis w/ paradoxical aciduria *(gastric fluid loss)*
Loss of Cl⁻ and H ion from stomach (**hypochloremic alkalosis**)
Water loss causes kidney to reabsorb Na (+ water) in exchange for K⁺ (Na/K ATPase) resulting in **hypokalemia**
K⁺/H⁻ exchanger activated (reabsorbs K, excrete H)→ **paradoxic aciduria**

Metabolic acidosis
Gain of acid or **loss of HCO3-**
2 types (anion gap and non-anion gap)
Anion Gap = Na⁺ − (HCO3⁻ + Cl⁻)
{normal < 10-15}, the gap is <u>created</u> by unmeasured anions
Etiologies
1) **Anion gap** metabolic acidosis (MUDPILES); *All are gaining acid <u>and</u> unmeasured anions* (eg DKA, ethylene glycol, renal failure, lactate acid)
2) **Non-anion gap** metabolic acidosis
All gaining HCL or losing NaHCO3
GI losses of HCO3- (eg ileostomy, small bowel fistula)
Dilutional (rapid infusion of HCO3- deficient fluids)
**Lactulose
Hyperparathyroidism (gain HCL)
Tx: treat underlying pathology (keep **pH >7.25 w/ HCO3** to avoid myocardial depression)

Diabetic Ketoacidosis (DKA)
Precipitants (I's) - **i**nsulin deficiency, **i**nfection / inflammation, intoxication (ETOH, drugs), ischemia / infarction (MI, stroke), iatrogenic (steroids)
Occurs almost <u>exclusively</u> in type I DM
Glucose cannot be taken up by cells due to lack of insulin (↑ glucose, ↑ ketones from fatty acid oxidation in the liver)
Sx's: polydipsia, polyuria, dehydration, N/V, abd pain, Kussmaul's respirations, **acetone breath**, mental status changes (**somnolence**)
Dx: anion gap **metabolic acidosis**; ketones in urine, ↑ glucose (> 500)
↓ed Na⁺ (**pseudohyponatremia**)
K⁺ usually elevated initially
Tx: **Hydration, Insulin, HCO3-**

**<u>Hyperosmolar Hyperglycemic Non-ketotic Syndrome</u> - in Type II DM; severe elevated glucose levels causes cerebral edema, seizures, coma and respiratory arrest; Tx same as DKA

Nutrition

126. *A patient receives a 1000 cc bag of TPN which contains 10% dextrose and 7% protein. In addition, this patient receives 250 cc of a 20% fat emulsion solution. How many calories does this approximately represent?
   a.   1020 calories
   b.   1420 calories
   c.   1820 calories
   d.   2220 calories

   Answer a.
   A 1000 cc bag of 10% dextrose is equal to 100 gm of dextrose (0.10 x 1000 = 100 gm), which is 340 calories (100 gm x 3.4 calories/gm).

   A 1000 cc bag of 7% protein is equal to 70 gm of protein (0.07 x 1000 = 70 gm), which is 280 calories (70 gm x 4 calories/gm).

   A 250 cc bag of 20% fat emulsion is equivalent to 50 gm of fat (0.20 x 250 = 50), and 50 gm of fat is equivalent to 400 calories (50 gm x 8 calories/gm).

   Then just add them up 340 + 280 + 400 = 1020 calories.

127. *All of the following are true except:
   a.   Intestinal medium and short chain fatty acids enter the circulation through lymphatics
   b.   Chylomicrons contain primarily triacylglycerides (TAGs)
   c.   Linoleic acid is an essential fatty acid
   d.   Lipoprotein lipase is located on endothelium and clears chylomicrons from blood

   Answer a. ****Intestinal medium and short chain fatty acids enter the circulation through the portal vein.** **Conversely, chylomicrons and long chain fatty acids enter the circulation through lymphatics (terminal lacteals) and enter the thoracic duct.*

128. *All of the following are true of carbohydrate metabolism except:
   a.   The first enzyme in carbohydrate digestion is amylase
   b.   Skeletal muscle contains the majority of the body's glycogen stores
   c.   Skeletal muscle is abundant in glucose-6 phosphatase
   d.   The body's glycogen stores are depleted 18-24 hrs after fasting

   Answer c. Skeletal muscle *lacks* **glucose-6 phosphatase**, thus glucose from glycogen breakdown *stays in muscle* (glucose-6 *can't* be released)
   The body's **glycogen stores** are **depleted 18-24 hrs after fasting
   *****Skeletal muscle** contains the majority of the body's glycogen stores*
   *****Fat** is the main energy source after 24 hrs of starvation or major stress*

   The first enzyme in carbohydrate digestion is **salivary amylase

129. *All of the following are true of protein metabolism except:
   a.   The first enzyme in protein digestion is pepsin
   b.   Leucine is both a branched chain and essential amino acid (AA)
   c.   Glutamine is the most common AA in the blood stream and tissues
   d.   Pancreatic proteases are not required for protein absorption

   Answer d. Pancreatic proteases are required for protein absorption
   *****Leucine** is both a branched chain and essential amino acid (AA)*
   *****Glutamine** is the most common AA in the blood stream and tissues*

130. **All of the following are true except:

a. The primary nutrition source of colonocytes short chain fatty acids (butyrate)
b. The primary nutrition source of small bowel is glutamine
c. The primary nutrition source of most cancer cells is glutamine
d. During prolonged starvation, the brain switches from using glucose to using glutamine

Answer d. Brain switches from glucose to ketones w/ starvation.
  ***The primary nutrition source of **colonocytes** is **short chain fatty acids** (eg butyrate or butyric acid).*
  The primary nutrition source of **small bowel** is **glutamine
  The primary nutrition source of most **cancer cells** is **glutamine

131. *Which of the following lab values is most predictive of post-op mortality?
  a. Low sodium
  b. Low potassium
  c. Low transferrin
  d. Low albumin

Answer d. ****Low albumin** has been directly correlated with increased morbidity and mortality following operative procedures.

132. **Over-feeding patients in the intensive care unit is most likely to result in:
  a. Prolonged intubation
  b. Hypoglycemia
  c. Renal failure
  d. Hypokalemia

Answer a. ****Overfeeding** can lead to high carbohydrate build-up and increased CO_2 production. This makes the lungs work harder to get rid of the CO_2, which can tire pts out and result in **prolonged ventilation**.

133. **All of the following are true except:
  a. Respiratory quotient is CO_2 production over O_2 consumption
  b. A respiratory quotient < 0.7 indicates starvation
  c. The respiratory quotient of fat = 0.7
  d. Excess carbohydrates are converted to amino acids

Answer d. ** **Over-feeding** results in conversion of carbohydrates to fat. This conversion causes an increase in CO_2 production compared to O_2 consumed, thus RQ will increase. Conversely, **under-feeding** results in breakdown of fat and glycogen stores which does not increase CO_2. Oxygen consumption increases during starvation. In this situation, the RQ will decrease. **The **respiratory quotient of fat = 0.7**

134. *Ileal resection can result in all of the following except:
  a. Decreased B_{12} and folate uptake, resulting in megaloblastic anemia
  b. Decreased bile salt uptake which can cause osmotic diarrhea (bile salts) and steatorrhea (↓ fat uptake) in colon
  c. Increased bile salt uptake which can result in the formation of gallstones
  d. Ca oxalate kidney stones (hyperoxaluria)

Answer c. Ileal resection does <u>not</u> result in increased bile salt resorption. It does result in decreased bile salt uptake and the formation of **gallstones**.

135. *The strongest layer of the bowel wall is:
  a. Mucosa
  b. Submucosa
  c. Muscularis
  d. Serosa

Answer b. The strongest layer of the bowel wall is the **submucosa**. This is where you want your sutures when doing a hand sewn bowel anastomosis. The time point at which small bowel is weakest is **3-5 days**.

136. **A 35 yo woman suffering from Crohn's disease on chronic TPN is admitted for hair loss, skin lesions on her extremities and peri-orificial areas, diarrhea, and wasting of body tissues. This is associated with which of the following?
    a.   Copper deficiency
    b.   Zinc deficiency
    c.   Phosphate deficiency
    d.   Chromium deficiency

    Answer b **Zinc deficiency** *is associated w/ poor healing, hair loss, diarrhea, extremity and peri-oral skin lesions and body wasting.*

137. **All of the following are true except:
    a.   Glutamine is the MC substrate for gluconeogenesis
    b.   Fatty acids cannot be used for gluconeogenesis
    c.   Glutamine is to MC amino acid released from catabolism of skeletal muscle
    d.   Steatorrhea from obstructive jaundice can result in deficiency of fat soluble vitamins (A, D, E, K) which can result in complications such as bleeding (ie lack of Vit K)

    Answer a. **Alanine** *is the MC substrate for* **gluconeogenesis.**

    Glutamine *is to MC amino acid released from catabolism of skeletal muscle and is the primary amino acid used in the urea cycle.*
    Steatorrhea *from obstructive jaundice (eg pancreatic tumor) can result in deficiency of fat soluble vitamins (A, D, E, K) which can result in cx's such as bleeding (ie lack of Vit K).*
    Fatty acids are not used for gluconeogenesis because acetyl CoA (breakdown product of fatty acids) cannot be converted to pyruvate.

138. **All of the following are part of the metabolic syndrome except:
    a.   Obesity
    b.   Hypothyroidism
    c.   Insulin resistance
    d.   Elevated triglycerides

    Answer b. Hypothyroidism is not part of the metabolic syndrome.

Calories

Fat	9 kcal/g
Protein	4 kcal/g
Oral carbohydrates	4 kcal/g
Dextrose	3.4 kcal/g

Caloric need
  Need 25 kcal/kg/day (resting energy expenditure) *plus* stress factor
    20% protein (1-1.5 g protein/kg/d), 20% essential amino acids
    30% fat (impt for essential fatty acids)
    50% carbohydrates
  Typical 70 kg adult male needs 1500-1750 calories/d
  Majority of surgery pts can go NPO for **7 days** safely
  Stress Factor (trauma, surgery, or sepsis) - ↑ kcal requirement **20%–60%**
    Protein requirement w/ stress
  Burns (start nutrition early in burn pts)
    Calories   25 kcal/kg/day + (30 kcal/day x % burn)
    Protein   1-1.5 g/kg/day + (3 g x % burn)

Energy expenditure

Much of the energy expenditure is used for **heat production**

Harris-Benedict equation calculates BMR from **weight, height, age**, and **gender**

Fat and cholesterol digestion

Triacylglycerides (TAGs), **cholesterol** and **lipids** are digested

Broken down by pancreatic **lipase, cholesterol esterase, phospholipase**, and **bile salts** → form **micelles** and **free fatty acids** (FFAs) in the intestinal lumen

**Micelles

Aggregates of bile salts, **long-chain FFAs, monoacylglycerides, and cholesterol*

Also contain **fat-soluble vitamins** (A, D, E, K)

Enter enterocyte by **fusing w/ membrane**

Bile salts – help form **micelles** (↑s absorption area for fats)

*Medium- and *short-chain FFAs* – enter enterocyte by simple diffusion (not in micelles)

Micelles and **medium- + short- chain FFAs** enter **enterocytes**

TAGs are re-synthesized in intestinal cells- placed in **chylomicrons**

Chylomicrons then enter ****lymphatics *(terminal lacteals →* *thoracic duct)*; chylomicrons contain - **90% TAGs**, + 10% phospholipids, proteins, and cholesterol

Long-chain FFAs – enter ****lymphatics along w/ chylomicrons

Medium- and **short-chain FFAs – enter ****portal system** *(same as amino acids and carbohydrates)*.

LDL receptor on cells at **clathrin coated pits**- bind LDL, then endocytosis

The majority of **body cholesterol** is **synthesized in liver;* 95% of cholesterol released into the bile is **reabsorbed** (termed entero-hepatic recirculation)

Essential fatty acids – **linolenic (omega 3) and **linoleic** (omega 6)

Needed for **prostaglandin** synthesis (long-chain fatty acids)

Important for immune cells

Carbohydrate digestion

Carbohydrates are the body's key source of **energy**

Glucose is prime energy source for **brain**

Glucose either 1) enters **glycolysis pathway** to produce **energy** (ATP) *or* 2) is stored as **glycogen**

Digestion begins w/ **salivary amylase*, then pancreatic amylase and intestinal brush border disaccharidases (maltase, sucrase, lactase)

Disaccharides

Sucrose = fructose + glucose

Lactose = galactose + glucose

Maltose = glucose + glucose

Transport

Glucose and **galactose** – absorbed by secondary active transport (Na$^+$ gradient); released into **portal vein**

Fructose – facilitated diffusion; released into **portal vein**

Glucose ingestion causes **insulin release** from **beta cells** in **pancreas**, which results in cellular uptake of circulating glucose

Primary storage area for glucose (glycogen) – skeletal muscle (#1), liver

Glucagon - has opposite effect of insulin, causes breakdown of glycogen to glucose

Cellulose (fiber) – non-digestible carbohydrate chains

Protein digestion

Digestion begins w/ **stomach pepsin*, then pancreatic proteases (eg trypsinogen, chymotrypsinogen, and pro-carboxypeptidase)

Pepsin not required; **pancreas proteinases required for digestion*

Trypsinogen is released from pancreas and activated by *enterokinase* released from duodenum

Other pancreatic proteases then activated by trypsin

Trypsin can also **autoactivate** other trypsinogen molecules

Protein broken down to amino acids, di-peptides, and tri-peptides

Absorbed by **secondary active transport** (Na^+ gradient) into enterocytes (primarily **jejunum**) and released as free amino acids into <u>portal vein</u>

Then taken up by various cells under the influence of **insulin**

During **stress**, protein shunted to **liver** for **gluconeogenesis**

Liver is prime regulator of **amino acid** (AA) **production** and **breakdown**

Nonessential AAs – those that begin with **A, G or C,** plus **serine, proline, tyrosine,** and **histidine**

Essential AAs – leucine, isoleucine, valine, lysine, methionine, phenylalanine, threonine, tryptophan

Branched-chain AAs (all <u>essential</u> AAs)- leucine, isoleucine, valine ("LIV")
Can be metabolized in muscle (only AAs metabolized <u>outside</u> liver)
Impt source of **protein calories** (energy source) w/ **liver failure**

**Glutamine
*MC AA in bloodstream and tissue
**MC AA released from muscle during catabolism
Can be used as an **energy source** (TCA cycle, see below)
Can be used for **gluconeogenesis** (see below)
Primary AA used in the **urea cycle** (see below)

Limit protein intake in pts w/ **liver failure** to avoid **ammonia buildup** and worsening **encephalopathy**

Limit protein intake for pts w/ **end stage kidney DZ** (to limit urea buildup)

<u>Nitrogen balance</u> (N balance)

6.25 g of protein contains 1 g of nitrogen

N balance = (N in – N out) = ([protein/6.25] – [24 hr urine N + 4 g])

Positive N balance (anabolism) – more nitrogen ingested (in form of protein) than excreted (in form of urea)

Negative N balance (catabolism) – more nitrogen excreted than taken in

Total protein synthesis for a healthy, normal 70-kg male is **250 g/day**

Liver - responsible for **AA production** and **breakdown**

Majority of protein breakdown from skeletal muscle is in the form of **glutamine (#1) and alanine

**<u>Normal Major Fuel Source</u> *(non-stress, non-starvation)*

Stomach, **small bowel enterocytes, ***pancreas, spleen* - glutamine

Liver - ketones (acetoacetate + butyric acid; from FFA breakdown)

**Large bowel colonocytes - <u>short</u> chain fatty acids [eg butyrate]

Heart - <u>short</u> chain fatty acids

Skeletal muscle, brain, kidney - glucose

Peripheral nerves, adrenal medulla, RBCs, PMNs - <u>obligate</u> glucose use

**MC primary fuel for <u>neoplastic cells</u> - glutamine (glucose #2)

Glutamine, ketones, and **short chain FFAs** – can enter TCA cycle for NADP, NADPH and FADH production → eventual ATP production

**<u>Respiratory quotient</u> *(RQ)*

Ratio of CO_2 produced to O_2 consumed (RQ = CO_2 / O_2)

Measures **energy expenditure** (metabolic cart, indirect calorimetry)

*RQ > 1 = lipogenesis (<u>overfeeding</u>; sx's - ↑ RR, ↑pCO2)

↑ed metabolic rate

High carbohydrate intake leads to **CO_2 buildup** (eg ****failure to wean from ventilator**; lungs working hard to get rid of CO2)

CO2 produced when **excess carbohydrates** are converted to **fat**

Tx: ↓ carbohydrates and caloric intake

RQ < 0.7 = **fat oxidation** and **ketosis** (starvation)
↓ed **metabolic rate**
Fat breakdown does not ↑CO_2 and O_2 consumption ↑s w/ starvation
Tx: ↑ carbohydrates and caloric intake

Pure fat metabolism	RQ = 0.7
Pure protein metabolism	RQ = 0.8
Pure carbohydrate metabolism	RQ = 1.0
Balanced Feeding	RQ = 0.825

Cori cycle - glucose is utilized and converted to **lactate** in muscle
Lactate then goes to liver and is converted back to **pyruvate** and eventually **glucose** via gluconeogenesis
Glucose is then transported back to muscle

Urea cycle (90% of all nitrogen loss) - **Glutamine** is principal NH_3^+ donor to remove **excess NH_3^+** from body in form of **urea**; reactions occur and urea is formed in **liver;** urea removed by **kidney**

Preoperative nutritional assessment
Approximate half-lives

Albumin	18 days
Transferrin	8 days
Prealbumin	2 days

Normal albumin level: 3.5 - 5.5; **Normal pre-albumin** level: 15 - 35
Acute indicators of nutritional status – ****pre-albumin (#1), transferrin, retinal binding protein, total lymphocyte count
*Preoperative signs of severe malnutrition
Acute weight loss > 20% in 6 months
**Albumin < 2.5 – strong RF for cx's and mortality after surgery
Preop enteral nutrition (for at least 7 days) decreases **mortality in severely malnourished pts*

Normal Post-operative phases

Catabolic phase	post-op days 0 - 3 (negative nitrogen balance)
Anabolic phase	post-op days 3 - 6 (positive nitrogen balance)
Diuresis phase	post-op days 2 - 5

Enteral Tube Feeds (TFs)
Standard TFs (Jevity, 1-1.5 kcal/cc)
*Diarrhea Tx: slow rate, add fiber (bulk) to slow transit time, use **less concentrated** feeds (prevent osmotic diarrhea)
*High gastric residuals (stomach feeds) **Tx:** Reglan or erythromycin
*Renal formulation (Nepro) – low in K and PO_4; low protein
Try to feed gut (rather than use TPN) to avoid **bacterial translocation (bacterial overgrowth and increased permeability due to starved enterocytes)*
**Early enteral feeding improves survival in sepsis and in pancreatitis

TPN composition (total parenteral nutrition)
20% calories as **protein** (1-1.5 g protein/kg/day, 20% essential AAs)
Usually a 5-10% AA solution (↓ protein w/ liver or renal failure)
30% calories as **fat** (lipids, 500 cc of 10% lipid solution - contains 550 kcal)
10% lipid solution has 1.1 kcal/cc, 20% lipid solution has 2 kcal/cc
50% calories as **dextrose** (consists of a 15-25% dextrose solution)
Additives:
Electrolytes
Na^+ (2 mg/kg/day), K^+ (1 mg/kg/day), Ca^{++}, Mg^{++}, PO_4^-, Cl^-
*Acetate – buffer to ↑ pH of solution (prevents met. acidosis)
Vitamins
**Need to add Vit K separately – Not normally added to TPN

Trace minerals
Zinc deficiency *can lead to poor wound healing*
ETOH abuse – ↑ thiamine and folate
Total volume = 2-3 liters / day usual (apx. rate → 100-150 cc/hr)
Indications for TPN – short gut, high output fistulas, when enteral feeding can't be used
Central line TPN – glucose based; maximum glucose administration – **3 g/kg/hr**
Peripheral line parenteral nutrition (PPN) – fat based (high glucose concentration damages peripheral veins)
Stopping TPN – cut rate in 1/2 for 1-2 hours 1st (avoids hypoglycemia)
Short term TPN – complicated by issues associated w/ **indwelling catheters** (line sepsis, pneumothorax, etc.)
Long term TPN – can eventually lead to **cirrhosis**

Post-op Nutrition

Pts can tolerate about **7 days** w/o eating; if longer than that, place a **feeding tube** or start **TPN**; enteral feeding is preferred
PEG –when regular feeding not predicted to occur for **> 4 weeks**

Response to Starvation and Major Stress (eg major surgery, trauma, sepsis)
Glycogen stores
Depleted *after 18-24 hours of starvation or major stress*
2/3 stored in **skeletal muscle** (#1 *glycogen storage area*), 1/3 in **liver**
Liver is the source of systemic glucose in times of stress
Skeletal muscle lacks **glucose-6-phosphatase** (found only in **liver**); Glucose-6-phosphate stays in muscle after breakdown from glycogen and is utilized there (*cannot* be released into circulation)
Body **switches to fat** after glycogen stores run out (fat is largest potential energy source)
Adipose stores
Fat is main energy source w/ **starvation** and **major stress**
Fat is broken down to acetyl-CoA or succinyl-CoA which enter Kreb's
Krebs cycle produces NADPH, NADH, and FADH from **FFAs, lactate** (pyruvate) and **AAs** (AAs and pyruvate converted to acetyl-CoA 1st)
Electron transport chain – NADPH, NADH, and FADH are used to produce **ATP**; occurs on <u>inner</u> **mitochondrial membrane**
Gluconeogenesis
Precursors – **#1 alanine** (*primary substrate for gluconeogenesis, simplest precursor*). lactate, pyruvate, glycerol, other AAs
Gluconeogenesis primarily occurs in **liver**
Occurs to much greater degree w/ **major stress** than w/ starvation
Fatty acids are *not* **used in gluconeogenesis because Acetyl-CoA** *cannot be converted back to pyruvate*
Simple Starvation
↓ed **metabolic rate** (↓ insulin, ↑ glucagon)
Fat is major energy source, ↑↑ **ketone production**
Protein conserved - gluconeogenesis doesn't occur until late
Major stress
↑ **catecholamines, cortisol** and **cytokines** → all ↑**metabolic rate**
↓ insulin and ↑ glucagon
Fat is main energy source, however significant *protein breakdown* and **gluconeogenesis** occur (*catecholamine + cortisol effect*)
Hepatic urea formation and **negative nitrogen balance** also occur w/ protein breakdown
Brain – switches to <u>ketones</u> as energy source (from fatty acid breakdown)
Metabolic Syndrome (need 3)– obesity (waist circumference > 40 inches men, > 35 inches women), insulin resistance (fasting glucose > 100), elevated TAGs (> 100), reduced HDL (< 50), HTN (> 130/85) – all related to obesity

**Re-feeding syndrome

Occurs w/ feeding after prolonged starvation / malnutrition (eg ETOH abuse); MC on **Day 4** of re-feeding

Sudden shift from fat metabolism to carbohydrate metabolism results in ↓K^+, ↓Mg^{++}, and ↓PO_4^- (all move intracellular along w/ glucose)

Effects →

Encephalopathy (↓ PO_4^-)

Cardiac arrhythmias (↓K^+, ↓ Mg^{++})

Profound weakness (↓PO_4^- – lack of ATP)

CHF (↓PO_4^- - lack of ATP) – get *peripheral edema*

Failure to wean from ventilator or **respiratory difficulty (↓PO_4^- - lack of ATP)

Prevent this by starting feeds at a **low rate** (10–15 kcal/kg/day) and monitoring electrolytes w/ replacement

*Specific Deficiencies

*Cachexia – *anorexia, weight loss, wasting, *Mediated by TNF-alpha*

Kwashiorkor – protein deficiency

Marasmus – starvation

Vitamins required for normal bone growth *(CAD)* – ***Vit C, Vit A and **Vit D**

Vitamins important for wound healing *(CAZ)* – ***Vit C, Vit A and **Zinc**

Most Vit K produced by **bacteria** in the intestines

Vit K deficiency – coagulopathy (bleeding)

Steatorrhea - can occur w/ obstructive jaundice (lack of bile acids in bowel), terminal ileal resection (don't reabsorb bile acids), short-gut syndrome (bile acids not reabsorbed), chronic pancreatitis (lack of pancreatic enzymes) ****causes deficiency of **fat soluble vitamins** *(A, D, E, K)* and **essential fatty acids**

Trace element deficiencies associated w/ **long term TPN:

**Zinc - *poor healing, hair loss, diarrhea, skin lesions on extremities and peri-oral areas, body wasting.*

*Cx's after terminal ileum resection *(or from **severe terminal ileum disease** which has become non-functional for absorption)*

1) ↓ed **B-12** and **folate uptake** can result in **megaloblastic anemia**

2) ↓ed **bile salt uptake** causes osmotic **diarrhea** (bile salts) and **steatorrhea** (↓ fat uptake) in colon

3) ↓ed **bile salt uptake** can result in the formation of **gallstones**

4) ↓ed **oxalate binding to Ca** secondary to increased intra-luminal fat → oxalate then gets absorbed in colon → released in urine → **Ca-oxalate kidney stones** (hyperoxaluria)

Transferrin – transporter of iron; **Ferritin** – storage form of iron

Oncology

139. *All of the following are true except
    a. Ebstein Barr Virus (EBV) is associated w/ nasopharyngeal CA
    b. The src family of proto-oncogenes code for tyrosine kinases
    c. The ras family of proto-oncogenes code for G proteins
    d. p53 is primarily involved in angiogenesis

    Answer d. p53 is primarily involved in cell cycle regulation and apoptosis

140. *All of the following are true except
    a. The MC metastasis to the small bowel is lung CA
    b. The MC metastasis to an axillary node is lymphoma
    c. The most important prognostic factor for sarcomas devoid of metastases is tumor grade
    d. The most important prognostic factor for breast CA devoid of systemic mets is nodal status

    Answer a. *The MC metastasis to the **small bowel** is **melanoma**.*
    Notably, these metastases are most likely to cause bowel obstruction from **intussusception** (not tumor filling the lumen).
    The MC metastasis to an **axillary node is **lymphoma***
    The most important pre-op prognostic factor for **sarcoma is **tumor grade**. Sarcomas rarely go to lymph nodes.*
    The most important prognostic factor for **breast CA (devoid of mets) is **nodal status** (positive or negative, how many, IMA vs. axillary).*

141. *All of the following mechanisms are true except
    a. Taxol stabilizes microtubules
    b. 5-FU inhibits thymidylate synthetase
    c. Taxol can cause neuropathy
    d. Etoposide is an anti-metabolite

    Answer d. *Etoposide blocks DNA unwinding and replication by inhibiting topoisomerase.*

142. *All of the following toxicities are true except
    a. Cardiotoxicity at doses greater then 500 mg/m^2 is characteristic of Adriamycin (doxorubicin)
    b. Pulmonary fibrosis is characteristic of bleomycin
    c. Ototoxicity is characteristic of cisplatin
    d. Hemorrhagic cystitis is characteristic of etoposide

    Answer d. *Hemorrhagic cystitis is a side effect of cyclophosphamide.*
    This is prevented with the use of **mesna** during chemotherapy.

143. All of the following are true of directed immunotherapy for CA exceptt
    a. They take advantage of bodies adaptive immune system
    b. T Killer cells cannot be tumor specific
    c. Involves harvesting T cells
    d. IL-2 is added to T cells to form T killer cells (LAK cells)

    Answer b. **T killer cells** can be made to be tumor specific by adding tumor antigen. T-cells are harvested, **IL-2** is added as well as the tumor antigen to form tumor specific T killer cells. These cells attack the tumor. Has been used for melanoma with some success

144. *All of the following are true of XRT for tumor therapy except:
    a. Tumor cells are most sensitive to XRT during M stage of cell cycle
    b. The main target of XRT is DNA
    c. Damage is primarily due to formation of oxygen radicals
    d. Large sarcoma are generally considered extremely radio-sensitive

Answer d. Large sarcomas are considered radio-resistant (sarcomas considered radio-resistant, large tumors are radio-resistant due to lack of oxygen within the tumor).
*Tumor cells are most sensitive to XRT during the **M stage** of the cell cycle
*The main target of XRT is **DNA**
*Damage is primarily due to formation of **oxygen radicals**

145. *All of the following are true of PET scan except:
    a.   18-fluoro deoxyglucose is injected IV
    b.   PET detects fluorodeoxyglucose molecules (FDG-6-phosphate)
    c.   PET is good in detecting brain metastases
    d.   The test may not work well in diabetics

    Answer c. *Due to the high glucose metabolism in the brain, PET has not been very useful for the detection of metastases to the brain.
    *PET may <u>not</u> work well in **diabetics** or those w/ **hyper-insulinemia** (competes w/ glucose)
    *PET detects fluorodeoxyglucose molecules (**FDG-6-phosphate**)

146. *All of the following are true of sentinel lymph node biopsy except:
    a.   Lymph nodes staining blue after lymphazurin blue dye should be resected
    b.   The sentinel lymph node is the hypothetical first lymph node(s) reached by cancer cells from a tumor
    c.   lymph node with the highest gamma count should be resected
    d.   Lymph nodes within 10% of the highest gamma count should be resected
    e.   Pts w/ clinically positive nodes should undergo SLNB

    Answer d. *Pts w/ **clinically positive nodes** should undergo **formal lymph node dissection.**

147. *The genes involved in development of colon CA include the following except:
    a.   APC
    b.   p53
    c.   DCC
    d.   Ret

    Answer d. Ret is not routinely involved in the development of colon CA.

148. *A phase II clinical trial:
    a.   Evaluates whether or not a drug is safe and at what dose
    b.   Evaluates whether or not the drug is effective
    c.   Evaluates whether or not the drug is better than existing therapy
    d.   Involves implementation and marketing

    Answer b. *Phase II trials evaluate whether or not the drug is effective.

<u>Most commons</u> (MC)
   Cancer #2 cause of death in US (MC – heart disease)
   MC CA in women – breast CA
   MCC of CA death in women – lung CA
   MC CA in men – prostate CA
   MCC of CA death in men – lung CA

<u>Oncogenesis</u> (cancer transformation)
Retroviruses can contain **oncogenes**
> **Epstein-Barr** – Burkitt's lymphoma (8:14 translocation, B cell, mandible); Nasopharyngeal CA
>> Post-transplantation lymphoproliferative disease (PTLD)

> **HPV** – cervical CA
> **HepB, -C, -D** - hepatocellular CA

Tumor Suppressors – have 1 or both of the following functions
> 1) **Inhibit cell cycle**
> 2) **Induce apoptosis** (programmed cell death)

Generally need multiple oncogenic gene transformations and mutations in tumor suppressors to get cancer

<u>Proto-oncogenes</u>
Can be converted to oncogenes and promote CA
Growth factors (eg c-*sis* – PDGF)
Tyrosine Kinases (eg *src* family)
*****GTPase** (G proteins; eg *ras* family) – usually transmembrane
> **k-ras oncogene** – protein is a **GTPase** involved in signal transduction and cell cycle regulation; involved in colon CA

Transcription factors (eg *myc* family)

<u>Tumor suppressor genes</u>
*****APC** (adenomatous polyposis coli) - involved in *****cell cycle regulation** and **cell movement**
*****p53** - involved in **cell cycle regulation** and *****apoptosis** (normal gene induces cell cycle arrest and apoptosis; abnormal gene allows unrestrained cell growth)
BRCA 1 and **2** - proteins involved in **DNA damage repair** and **cell cycle regulation**
Bcl-2 - mitochondrial membrane permeabilization involved in *****apoptosis**

<u>Cancer Immunology</u>
Natural killer cells can independently attack tumor cells (attack cells w/ lack of MHC expression)
Cytotoxic T cells need MHC complex to attack tumor
> Tumor antigens are random unless viral-induced tumor

<u>Cancer spread</u>
Resection of a normal organ to prevent cancer
> **Breast** – BRCA I or II with strong family history
> **Thyroid** – RET proto-oncogene w/ family Hx of MEN or thyroid CA
> **Also** (although organ not totally normal)
>> **Undescended testicle in adults** (testicular CA)
>> **Colon** (FAP, long standing ulcerative colitis)
>> **Gallbladder [polyps** (esp w/ sclerosing cholangitis) or **porcelain gallbladder]** → gallbladder CA

****MC CA in suspicious axillary lymph node** (or any other nodal site) – **_lymphoma_**
Lymph nodes have poor barrier function
> → better to view them as signs of **probable systemic mets**

Sentinel lymph node biopsy – <u>no role for clinically palpable nodes</u>; you need formal lymphadenectomy
****MC met to small bowel** - <u>melanoma</u> *(causes intussusception)***
Krukenberg tumor – gastric CA mets to ovary (also colorectal CA)
Most successfully cured <u>isolated</u> mets w/ surgery (5-year survival)
> **Germ cell** (eg seminoma) to lung **75% 5-YS** *(best)*

Chemotherapy agents
Cell cycle–nonspecific agents (→ all DNA cross-linking + binding agents)
- Act at all phases of the cell cycle
- **Linear** response to cell killing (↑ dose → ↑ killing)
  - *Alkylating agents – add alkyl groups to DNA, covalent bond*
    - *Cisplatin (platinum)* – nephrotoxic, neurotoxic, **ototoxic**
    - *Carboplatin (platinum)* – **b**one (myelo-) suppression
    - **Oxaliplatin** (platinum) – nephrotoxic, neuropathy, ototoxic (all less than cisplatin), cold sensitivity; used for **colon CA**
    - *Cyclophosphamide – acrolein is active metabolite*
      - S/Es: *hemorrhagic cystitis*
      - **Mesna** can help w/ hemorrhagic cystitis.
    - *Busulfan* and *Bleomycin*: S/Es – pulmonary fibrosis
    - **Streptozocin** (nitrosurea) – used for **pancreatic islet cell tumors** 'Glucose mimic' to islet cells only → kills islet cells

Cell cycle–specific agents
- Act at specific stages of cell cycle (S or M); only cells <u>at that stage</u> affected; *exhibit plateau in cell-killing ability* (at certain point, ↑ dose→ killing doesn't change)

1) **S Phase** (interfere w/ DNA replication and synthesis)
   - *Methotrexate – inhibits <u>dihydrofolate reductase</u> (DHFR), which inhibits purine and DNA synthesis*
     - S/Es: renal toxicity, radiation recall
     - **Leucovorin rescue** (tetrahydro-folic acid) - reverses effects of methotrexate
   - *5-Fluorouracil (5FU) – inhibits <u>thymidylate synthase</u> (TS), which inhibits purine and DNA synthesis*
     - **Leucovorin** – ↑ toxicity of 5FU
   - *Topoisomerase Inhibitors (etoposide) – interferes w/ DNA replication by <u>*inhibiting topoisomerase</u>*
     - S/Es – bone marrow suppression
     - **Topoisomerase** normally unwinds DNA for DNA duplication
   - *Doxorubicin (Adriamycin) – <u>DNA intercalator</u>*
     - S/Es: **cardiomyopathy** (CHF) secondary to **O_2 radicals** at > 500 mg/m^2

2) **M** phase (<u>m</u>icrotubule <u>m</u>odulators – arrest <u>m</u>itosis)
   - **Alkaloids**
     - **Vincristine** (microtubule inhibitor) – **peripheral neuropathy**, neurotoxic
     - **Vin<u>b</u>lastine** (microtubule inhibitor) – **b**one (myelo) suppression
   - ****Taxanes** (docetaxel, paclitaxel, Taxol) – promote **microtubule formation** and **stabilization** that cannot be broken down; ****S/E- neuropathy**

Hormonal Therapy
- **Selective Estrogen Receptor Modulators** (SERMs)
  - *Tamoxifen* – Tx and prevention of <u>breast CA</u>
    - Preferred for **pre-menopausal:** 1) **prevention** and 2) **receptor positive breast CA** (or unknown status)
  - *Raloxifene* - preferred for **post-menopausal prevention** of **breast CA**; also decreases Fx's post-menopause
    - S/Es: DVT (1%), endometrial CA (0.1%) – less w/ Raloxifene
- *Aromatase Inhibitors* (anastrozole, letrozole)
  - Block conversion of androgens to estrogen
  - Preferred for **post-menopausal receptor positive breast CA** (or unknown receptor status)
  - S/Es: fractures (2x more common than SERMs)
- **GnRH analogues** (leuprolide): ↓s FSH + ↓s LH → ↓ testosterone; used for hormone sensitive <u>prostate CA</u>

Anti-androgens (flutamide, bicalutamide) – inhibit androgen
receptors (testosterone + DHT receptors); used in prostate CA
Monoclonal Antibody Therapy
Trastuzumab (Herceptin) – blocks **HER/neu receptor**, used for
breast CA; **HER/neu** - Human Epidermal Growth Factor
Receptor tyrosine kinase
Bevacizumab (Avastin)- blocks **VEGF receptor** and inhibits
angiogenesis; use in metastatic: 1) colorectal CA, 2) non-small
cell lung CA
Receptor Tyrosine Kinase Inhibitors (multi-RTKI)
Imatinib (Gleevec)
Binds **c-kit** (stem cell growth factor receptor)
Used for malignant GIST tumors (very effective)
S/Es: CHF (uncommon)
Immunotherapy
IL-2: metastatic melanoma or renal cell CA, can be used as single Tx
Vaccines to prevent CA – HepB vaccine, HPV vaccine (Gardasil)
Other
Mitotane (DDD) – cytolytic for adrenal cortex
Use - unresectable or metastatic adrenocortical CA
Octreotide – used for pancreatic islet cell tumors (including
gastrinoma) and carcinoid syndrome
Levamisole – **anti-helminthic drug** that ↑s immunity against CA
Important S/Es
****Bleomycin and busulfan** – can cause pulmonary fibrosis
Least myelosuppression – bleomycin, vincristine, busulfan, cisplatin
hormonal Tx, monoclonal antibody Tx

***Radiation therapy** *(XRT, ionizing radiation)*
*M phase – most vulnerable stage of cell cycle for XRT
*Most damage done by formation of **oxygen radicals**
→ maximal effect w/ **high oxygen levels**
Main target is DNA* – oxygen radicals **damage DNA, w/ damaged DNA,
the cell is **no longer able to divide** successfully
Higher-energy radiation has skin-preserving effect (maximal ionizing
potential not reached until deeper structures).
Very radio-sensitive tumors – seminomas, lymphomas
The more frequently the cells **divide**, the more **sensitive to XRT**
Very radio-resistant tumors – epithelial, sarcomas; **Large tumors* – *less
responsive to XRT due to *lack of oxygen in tumor*
Brachytherapy – source of radiation in or next to tumor (Au-198, I-128);
delivers high, concentrated doses of radiation
Gamma knife – high intensity **cobalt XRT** directed at brain tumors
XRT sensitizers – oxygen, chemo, hyperthermia
XRT can be used for **painful bony mets*
Half-lives – CEA: 18 days; PSA: 18 days; AFP: 5 days

Tumor lysis syndrome
Rapid **tumor lysis** following **chemo** leads to **acute metabolic disarray**
Destroyed cell releases of **purines** and **pyrimidines** (→ *uric acid*)
K^+ and PO_4^- also leaked from cell
Leads to: **acute renal failure** (uric acid nephropathy), **arrhythmias** (↑K^+)
RFs – lymphomas, leukemias
****Path: ↑ uric acid, ↑K^+, ↓Ca^{++}, ↑PO_4^-,**
Tx: aggressive **hydration, allopurinol** (↓ uric acid production),
rasburicase (converts uric acid to inert metabolite allantoin). PO_4^-
binding antacids before chemo, **loop diuretic**, HCO3⁻ (alkalinize
urine, prevent uric acid precipitation), **calcium, D50 + Insulin** for
hyperkalemia; **HD** if previous fail

*PET *(positron emission tomography)*

　　18-FDG (fluorodeoxyglucose) metabolized to **FDG-6-phosphate** by **hexokinase**

　　PET detects **FDG-6-phosphate** molecules

　　5-10% false positive rate (**inflammatory DZ** – histoplasmosis, TB)

　　5-10% false negative rate (**slow metabolizing tumors** – carcinoid, bronchoalveolar lung CA)

　　Accuracy for **brain low because of **increased glucose uptake in brain***

　　*Test may not work in ***diabetics** or ***hyper-insulinemia** (hyperglycemia competes w/ 18-FDG uptake; insulin promotes 18-FDG uptake into normal cells)

*SLNBx (sentinel lymph node biopsy)

　　Sentinel lymph node – hypothetical first lymph node(s) reached by cancer cells from a tumor

　　Lymphazurin blue dye and **technetium labeled sulfur colloid radiotracer** used; are injected around primary tumor area

　　　　Need 1-4 hrs for uptake → dye + radiotracer travel to sentinel node(s)

　　　　**Type I hypersensitivity reactions (1%) have been reported w/ lymphazurin blue dye

　　Usually find 1-3 nodes; send for permanent

　　All blue nodes and **nodes within 10%** of highest gamma count node should be taken

　　Can't find dye or gamma counts in OR → **formal lymph node dissection*

　　Tumor found in LN's along path → **formal lymph node dissection*

　　For a high gamma count outside area you were expecting (eg you are performing SLNB for breast CA and the supra-clavicular region lights up), you should sample lymph nodes in the area that has the high count if it is at least 10% of the highest count node

　　MC uses – breast CA and melanoma

Most impt prognostic factor of **breast CA** devoid of systemic mets – **nodal status

Most impt pre-op prognostic factor of **sarcoma** devoid of systemic mets – **tumor grade

*Ovarian CA – one of the few tumors for which **surgical debulking improves chemotherapy (not seen in other tumors, see Gynecology chp)

Colon CA

　　***Genes involved in development include **APC, p53, DCC, and K-ras**.*

　　*Colon CA does not usually go to bone

Curable solid tumors w/ chemo only – lymphoma

T-cell lymphomas – HTLV-1 (skin lesions), mycosis fungoides (Sezary cells)

Types of Tx

　　Induction – sole Tx; often used for advanced disease (eg metastatic lung CA) or when no other better treatment exists (eg lymphoma)

　　Primary (neo-adjuvant) – chemo given 1st, followed by another (secondary) therapy (XRT, surgery, or both)

　　Adjuvant – chemo given after another Tx is used (XRT, surgery, or both)

　　Salvage – for tumors that fail to respond to initial chemotherapy

Definitions

　　Hyperplasia – increased number of cells

　　*Metaplasia – replacement of one tissue with another (GERD w/ squamous epithelium in esophagus changed to columnar epithelium → Barrett's esophagus)

　　*Dysplasia – altered size, shape, and organization (Barrett's Dysplasia)

*Clinical trials

　　Phase I – is it safe and at what dose?

　　Phase II – is it effective?

　　Phase III – is it better than existing therapy?

　　Phase IV – implementation and marketing

Core needle biopsy (CNBx) – gives architecture

Fine needle aspiration (FNA) – gives cytology (just cells)

Trauma

149. **A 24 yo man is stabbed in the chest w/ an ice-pick just to the left of midline at the 5th intercostal space. The pts airway is intact, he is breathing spontaneously, and his blood pressure is 120/80 with a heart rate of 90. He has 2 large bore IVs placed. CXR shows a left pneumothorax so you place a chest tube. Which of the following is most appropriate next step in this patient's work-up:
    a. Careful observation only
    b. Pericardial window, esophagoscopy and bronchoscopy
    c. Median sternotomy and exploration
    d. Chest CT

    Answer b. **Pericardial window, esophagoscopy and bronchoscopy*

150. *A 21 yo woman shot in the left flank presents w/ a BP of 75 despite 2 L of crystalloid. You start giving blood. The most appropriate next step is
    a. FAST scan
    b. Abd CT
    c. Laparotomy
    d. Laparoscopy

    Answer c. *Penetrating abd injury in an unstable pt requires laparotomy.*

151. *A 26 yo woman is involved in a severe MVA. She is hypotensive (BP 80/40, HR 120), intubated, and has a distended abdomen. She also has a pelvic fracture. You give her 2 liters of lactated ringers and then start transfusing blood however she remains hypotensive. The most appropriate next step in management is:
    a. Abdomen and Pelvic CT
    b. Angiogram
    c. FAST scan
    d. Exploratory laparotomy

    Answer c. This is a very frequent occurrence in busy trauma centers. Put simply, in a hypotensive patient, you need to figure out if the bleeding is from the abdomen, pelvis, chest or extremities. The first test should be a FAST scan - **if positive**, go to OR.

    If FAST **is negative** (and you are reasonably sure the source of the bleed is not the chest - usually assessed by exam and CXR) place an external fixator in ED if ortho is standing there and waiting, but otherwise go to **angio** ASAP for embolization of pelvic vessels. Wrapping a sheet tightly around pelvis can be used to temporarily tamponade pelvic bleeding while waiting for angiography.

152. *You perform FAST on an unstable pt involved in a MVA which shows a large fluid collection in the peri-splenic space. The pt is hypotensive despite blood resuscitation. The pt has a blown pupil on the right. The most appropriate next step in management is:
    a. Head CT
    b. Abdominal CT
    c. Head and abdominal CT
    d. Go to OR

    Answer d. A positive FAST scan in a hypotensive patient means you go to the OR for laparotomy. In the ABC's scheme you need to take care of C (circulation) before assessing the head injury.

    While in the OR, you should place a **Burr hole** to decompress the side w/ blown pupil. This is placed 5 cm anterior and 5 superior to the external auditory canal (frontal bone).

153. **A 25 yo man involved in a motor vehicle accident will open his eyes only to painful stimuli, does not form words but mumbles, and withdraws to pain. All of the following are true except:
   a. Blunt injury carries a worse prognosis compared to penetrating injury give equal GCS scores
   b. His GCS is 8
   c. Motor score carries the most prognostic significance
   d. He should be intubated

   Answer a. **Penetrating injury** *carries a worse prognosis compared to blunt injury give equal GCS scores; Open eyes to painful stimuli is 2, incomprehensible sounds is 2, and withdrawals from pain is 4. 2 + 2+ 4 = 8*

   The **motor score *carries the most prognostic significance.*

154. **A 30 yo man involved in a MVA suffers an isolated closed head injury (CHI). After arriving at the ED, the pt starts making a copious amount of urine. All of the following are true of this patient except:
   a. This is most consistent with diabetes insipidus
   b. The urine specific gravity in this patient is likely low
   c. Serum sodium concentration is likely high
   d. This is most consistent with elevated anti-diuretic hormone (ADH)

   Answer d. *SIADH would result in fluid retention, not diuresis.*

155. **A 30 yo man involved in a MVA suffers an isolated closed head injury (CHI). He has low urine output and a sodium of 120. His CVP is 18. All of the following are true except:
   a. This is most consistent w/ SIADH
   b. The urine specific gravity is likely high
   c. Treatment mainstay for this problem is fluid restriction and diuresis
   d. He should receive aggressive fluid resuscitation

   Answer d. *Tx mainstay for SIADH is **fluid restriction** and **diuresis***

156. *A patient with a CHI is having difficulty maintaining his airway so you intubate him. Head CT shows loss of sulci and compression of cisterns and ventricles so you place an intra-cerebral pressure (ICP) catheter. All of the following are true of cerebral perfusion pressure (CPP) except:
   a. In general, a cerebral perfusion pressure of 60 or better is sufficient
   b. CPP = mean arterial pressure – intracranial pressure
   c. Mannitol can help lower intra-cranial pressure
   d. Hypoventilation benefits these patients

   Answer d. *Relative hyperventilation* for modest cerebral vasoconstriction (pCO_2 30–35) limits brain edema and lowers ICP.

157. All of the following are true except:
   a. Subdural hematomas are MC from torn bridging veins
   b. Loss of consciousness, then lucid interval, followed by neuro deterioration is classic for epidural hematoma
   c. A blown pupil with head injury is from compression of CN II
   d. Diffuse axonal injury indicates a poor prognosis

   Answer c. A blown pupil from head injury is due to compression of CN III.

   Subdural hematoma - *MC from torn **bridging veins** between the dura and arachnoid*
   Epidural hematoma – *MC from injury to the **middle meningeal artery***

158. **A 20 yo woman involved in a MVA is stable, complains of neck pain, and has a cervical spine X-ray which shows pre-vertebral soft swelling. You do not see any Fx's or dislocations. The most appropriate next step is:
   a. MRI
   b. CT scan
   c. Repeat cervical spine x-rays
   d. Close observation

   Answer a. **Pts w/ **pre-vertebral cervical soft tissue swelling** or w/ **neurologic deficits without bony injury** are at high risk for ligamentous injury or occult Fx. **The best study to check for this is an **MRI.**

159. *All of the following are true of maxillo-facial trauma except:
   a. The MCC of facial nerve injury is temporal bone fracture
   b. A Le Fort III fracture is across the orbital walls
   c. Malocclusion is the best indicator of mandibular injury
   d. Nasoethmoid fractures w/ CSF leak should undergo immediate repair

   Answer d. *Nasoethmoid Fx w/ CSF leak* is initially treated conservatively (epidural catheter to drain CSF – helps close leak).

160. *All of the following are true except:
   a. Zone II penetrating neck injuries are usually explored
   b. Aortic transection at the ligamentum arteriosum is best approached with median sternotomy
   c. Zone I innominate artery injury is best approached with median sternotomy
   d. Zone III extends from angle of the mandible to the base of the skull

   Answer b. *Left thoracotomy* is the approach for **aortic transection** at the ligamentum arteriosum (MC area for aortic transection)

   Zone I innominate artery injuries are approached w/ median sternotomy

161. **A 21 yo woman involved in a MVA sustains a direct blow to the neck. She is awake and asymptomatic. CT scan of her head, neck, chest and abdomen shows only a right carotid dissection. The most appropriate Tx for this injury is:
   a. Observation
   b. Open repair
   c. Stent placement
   d. Anticoagulation therapy

   Answer d. **The initial Tx of asymptomatic carotid artery dissections is **anti-coagulation** with heparin followed by Coumadin. This is done in an effort to prevent thrombotic and embolic events.

162. *A 21 yo patient has a persistent pneumothorax following a MVA despite 2 good chest tubes. Which of the following is the most appropriate next step:
   a. CT scan of chest
   b. Increase suction from 20 cm H20 to 40 cm H20
   c. Bronchoscopy
   d. Thoracotomy

   Answer c. Persistent pneumothorax despite 2 well placed chest tubes raises the suspicion of either a mucus plug (or foreign body) obstructing the airway or a tracheo-bronchial injury. **Bronchoscopy** is best for Dx.

163. A 23 yo involved in a MVA has a Grade V splenic laceration w/ active blush, an aortic transection, and a severe pulmonary contusion. The pt is hypotensive despite 4 units of packed RBCs. Which is most appropriate next step:

a. Splenectomy
b. Aortic transaction repair
c. ICU management
d. Abdominal CT

Answer a. *You should address other life-threatening injuries (bleeding spleen above) <u>before</u> the aortic transection.*

164. A 65 yo man involved in a MVA has 4 left sided rib fractures at 2 sites along each rib w/ paradoxical chest wall motion and poor oxygenation All of the following are true except;
    a. Mechanical impairment is the biggest factor for his poor oxygenation
    b. This patient may require intubation
    c. Para-vertebral block or epidural catheter reduces pain and improves oxygenation
    d. A PA catheter can help manage fluid status

    Answer a. *The underlying **pulmonary contusion** is the biggest impairment to respiratory status, <u>not</u> the **flail chest** itself.*

165. **All of the following are true of hemothorax except:
    a. Lung inflation generally worsens bleeding
    b. The most important RF for empyema after chest trauma is retained hemothorax
    c. Drainage of > 1500 cc of blood after initial chest tube placement is an indication for OR thoracotomy
    d. Unresolved hemothorax despite 2 well placed chest tubes requires VATS drainage when the pt is stable

    Answer a. Lung inflation generally decreases bleeding by compressing the bleeding area.

    Drainage of > 1500 cc *of blood after initial chest tube placement is an indication for OR thoracotomy*
    The most important RF for **empyema after chest trauma is retained hemothorax*
    Unresolved hemothorax *despite 2 well placed chest tubes requires **VATS drainage** when the pt is stable*

166. *All of the following are true of tracheo-bronchial injuries except:
    a. They are more common on the right
    b. Breathing may be worsened after chest tube placement
    c. Is one of the very few conditions in which clamping the chest tube may be beneficial
    d. Approach to the proximal left mainstem (< 1 cm from the carina) is best carried out through a left thoracotomy

    Answer d. Approach to the proximal left mainstem (< 1 cm from carina) is right thoracotomy *(**aorta is in the way on the left)*

167. *A 25 yo man comes to your office 3 months after a MVA with left chest pain. CXR shows air-fluid levels in the chest. The most appropriate next step is:
    a. Exploration through the abdomen
    b. Exploration through the chest
    c. Chest tube
    d. Percutaneous drain

    Answer b. The acute Tx of a **diaphragmatic injury** is to go through the **abdomen** for repair. **With **delayed presentation** (> 1 week), go through the **chest** because adhesions to the lung will have developed which you must take down through a chest incision.*

168. **All of the following are true of splenic injuries except:
    a. Hemodynamic instability is a contraindication to splenic salvage
    b. A large fluid collection 5 days following splenectomy that is high in amylase requires re-operation
    c. Immunizations should be given following a traumatic splenectomy
    d. Subcapsular hematomas should be left alone

    Answer b. **Pancreatic leak after splenectomy should be treated with percutaneous drainage (95% successful).*

169. **A 21 yo man has severe venous bleeding from an injury to the posterior portion of the liver following a MVA. You try the Pringle maneuver but this fails to control the bleeding. You try to get to the bleeding site but the blood wells up too fast. The most appropriate next step in management is:
    a. Liver resection
    b. Damage control
    c. Atrio-caval shunt
    d. Argon beam

    Answer b. This pt likely has an injury to hepatic veins where they enter the IVC or the IVC itself. These are hard to fix and are associated with high mortality. In general, if not easily fixed, go w/ *damage control peri-hepatic packing* and take pt to ICU. If packing fails to control the bleeding, place an **atrio-caval shunt** (32 fr chest tube) and repair injury.

170. **The above pt survives and the packs are removed the next day. The pt has a prolonged recovery period. On POD #21 he is noted to have abd pain and severe hematemesis. He has 2 large bore I.V.'s in place and you T and C for 6 units of blood. His Hct is 21 so you transfuse 2 units of blood. The most appropriate next step in this patient's management is:
    a. Exploratory laparotomy
    b. EGD
    c. Angiography
    d. TIPS procedure

    Answer b. **EGD is the best initial Dx test for pts with an upper GI bleed.*

171. **EGD in the above pt shows blood coming out of the Ampulla of Vater (hemobilia). The most appropriate next step in management is:
    a. Exploratory laparotomy
    b. ERCP w/ stent
    c. Angiography
    d. TIPS procedure

    Answer c. ***This pt has **hemobilia** from a **vascular to bile duct fistula** (usually hepatic artery to bile duct). Tx is **angio-embolization.***

172. *A 29 yo man is shot in the abdomen and you explore him. He has a severe anterior liver injury that you try to treat but blood keeps welling up out of the liver bed and you cannot control it. You perform a Pringle maneuver which is:
    a. Clamping of the portal triad
    b. Clamping the IVC
    c. Placing an atrio-caval shunt
    d. Packing off the area and heading to the ICU

    Answer a. ***The **Pringle maneuver** involves clamping the portal triad which is located in the hepato-duodenal ligament. The Pringle maneuver will not control bleeding from the hepatic veins or IVC (located posteriorly).*

The portal triad structures includes the **portal vein** (posterior), **common bile duct** (lateral) and the **proper hepatic artery** (medial). The portal triad enters the liver at **segments IV and V.**

173. A 22 yo woman was shot through the pancreas neck. She now has severe venous bleeding posterior to the pancreas which you cannot control. The most appropriate next step in this patient's management is:
    a. Portal vein ligation
    b. Whipple
    c. Transect the pancreas
    d. Splenectomy

    Answer c. Access to this portion of the **portal vein** is obtained by transecting the **pancreas neck** (need distal pancreatectomy w/ that move)

174. *A 22 yo man suffers a GSW to the right flank. During laparotomy, you notice bile stained fluid in the right upper quadrant. The most appropriate next step is:
    a. Endoscopy
    b. Gastrostomy
    c. Whipple
    d. Kocher maneuver

    Answer d. The most appropriate move is to perform a **Kocher maneuver** which entails mobilizing the duodenum (and colon hepatic flexure) and examining the duodenum, the portal triad, and the pancreas head.

    Findings requiring Kocher maneuver – para-duodenal (1st or 2nd) hematomas, bile staining, sucus drainage or fat necrosis.

175. **Concerning traumatic pancreatic injuries, all of the following are true except:
    a. The first concern is to figure out whether or not the duct is involved
    b. Edema, hematoma, fluid, and fat necrosis are worrisome for injury
    c. Trauma Whipples have an operative mortality similar to elective
    d. For pancreatic duct injury, the cut-off between distal pancreatectomy and Whipple is duct injury in relation to the superior mesenteric vein

    Answer c. Mortality is 50% for a trauma Whipple (trauma Whipple's should be <u>avoided</u> if at all possible).

    For pancreatic duct injury, the cut-off between distal pancreatectomy and Whipple is duct injury in relation to the **superior mesenteric vein.*

176. *A 15 yo old boy is struck in the abd when he goes over the handle bars on his bike. You get an abd CT w/ IV and oral contrast and you cannot identify any abnormality. The next day, you try to feed the child clears but he vomits twice. His abdomen also feels somewhat more distended compared to yesterday. The most appropriate next step in management is:
    a. Repeat abdominal CT
    b. Zofran (ondansetron)
    c. Phenergan (promethazine)
    d. Exploratory laparotomy

    Answer a. (see below)

177. *You repeat the child's CT scan with oral and IV contrast and identify a hematoma in the third portion of the duodenum. You do not see extravasation of contrast at the site. The most appropriate next step is:
    a. Exploratory laparotomy, evacuate the clot, close the duodenum
    b. Percutaneous evacuation of the clot
    c. NG tube suction and TPN
    d. Whipple

Answer c. The first lesson is that if a trauma pt has a change in clinical status or is failing to progress normally (eg N/V w/ clears), you need to repeat appropriate studies. Pancreatic injuries, small bowel tears, duodenal injuries and diaphragmatic injuries can present late.

Duodenal hematomas can occur as a delayed presentation in trauma. The 1st step is to make Dx. This is probably best done w/ an **UGI contrast study** (will show a "stacked coin" or a "coiled spring" appearance) although abd CT scan with oral and IV contrast can pick these injures up. *******Tx is NPO and TPN* for up to *3 weeks. The vast majority* of para-duodenal hematomas resolve w/ **conservative *Tx***.

If there were a contrast leak from the duodenal injury, open repair would be required.

178. ******A 25 yo man suffers a GSW to the lower abdomen. On exploration, the ureter above the pelvic brim is transected with a 1 cm segment missing. The most appropriate management of this injury is:
    a. Re-implantation into the bladder
    b. Trans uretero-ureterostomy
    c. Re-anastomosis
    d. Percutaneous drainage

    Answer c. (see below)

179. ******A 25 yo man suffers a GSW to the lower abdomen. On exploration, the ureter below the pelvic brim is transected with a 1 cm segment missing. The most appropriate management of this injury is:
    a. Re-implantation into the bladder
    b. Trans uretero-ureterostomy
    c. Re-anastomosis
    d. Percutaneous drainage

    Answer a. (see below)

180. ******A 25 yo man suffers a GSW wound to the lower abdomen. On exploration, the ureter above the pelvic brim is transected with a 2.5 cm segment missing. The most appropriate management of this injury is:
    a. Re-implantation into the bladder
    b. Trans uretero-ureterostomy
    c. Re-anastomosis
    d. Percutaneous drainage

    Answer d. Full transection ureteral injuries can be divided into **high/middle** (above pelvic brim) and **lower** injuries (below pelvic brim).

    Complete transections **below the pelvic brim (lower injuries) are always treated with **re-implantation into bladder** because a cysto-ureteral anastomosis has much higher success rate than a uretero-ureteral anastomosis (especially after trauma).

    Injuries **above the pelvic brim are handled in one of 2 ways:
    1) If there is just a short segment missing (< 2 cm), go ahead and mobilize as much ureter as you can without devascularizing it and perform re-anastomosis; place ureteral stent and leave drains

    2) If more than 2 cm is missing, place a percutaneous nephrostomy tube and tie off both ends of the ureter. At a later date, a urologist can perform a uretero-ureter anastomosis or an ileal conduit.

Partial ureteral injuries can be repaired over stent.
These injuries can occur w/ **pelvic tumor resections, LAR's** and **APR's**

181. *A 22 yo man suffers a severe pelvis fracture and has hematuria. You get a retrograde cystourethrogram and see an extra-peritoneal bladder rupture. The most appropriate therapy for this patient is:
    a. Foley drainage for 7 days
    b. Exploratory laparotomy
    c. Nothing
    d. Cystectomy

    Answer a. The most appropriate Tx for an **_extra_-peritoneal bladder rupture** is urinary catheter drainage for 7 days. The most appropriate Tx for an **_intra_-peritoneal bladder rupture** is laparotomy w/ surgical repair.

182. *You clamp the infra-diaphragmatic aorta in a trauma pt w/ a penetrating abd injury, perform a Mattox maneuver, and find the left renal vein is completely avulsed from its connection w/ the IVC. The most appropriate next step is:
    a. Oversew the renal vein and ligate IVC connection
    b. Perform primary repair
    c. Left nephrectomy
    d. Pack and go to the ICU

    Answer a. The ****_left renal vein_** has adrenal and gonadal vein collaterals making ligation at the IVC connection safe. The **right renal vein** has no collaterals and requires repair, or if ongoing shock w/ other severe injuries, nephrectomy.

183. **A stable 25 yo man involved in an MVA has fractured left posterior ribs and no left renal uptake of contrast. The most appropriate next step is:
    a. Chest tube
    b. Open repair
    c. Angiography
    d. Nephrectomy

    Answer c. ****This pt has an _intimal flap_** causing thrombosis and no flow to the left kidney. ****Immediate angiogram** should be performed w/ possible stenting of the left renal artery.

184. *A 25 yo man suffers a posterior knee dislocation with loss of pulse. You are able to get the knee back in place and a pulse is now present. The most appropriate next step in this patient's management is:
    a. Nothing else
    b. Heparin
    c. Exploration
    d. Angiogram

    Answer d. *Posterior knee dislocations* have a high incidence of popliteal artery injury. **Angiogram** is mandatory.

185. *Non-operative management is most appropriate for which of the following:
    a. Intimal flap in popliteal artery that is not flow limiting
    b. Cold foot after external fixation of femur fracture
    c. Traumatic large AV fistula
    d. Pulsatile bleeding from thigh stab wound

    Answer a. An intimal flap in the popliteal artery that is not flow limiting can be treated conservatively (Tx: ASA)

186. **All of the following are indications for angiogram of an extremity except:

a. Injury to anatomically related nerve
b. History of severe blood loss from the injury
c. Large hematoma
d. Obvious thrill and bruit

Answer d. ***Bruit or thrill is an indication for OR, not angiogram.*

187. *All of the following are true of hip dislocations except:
    a. Closed reduction with conscious sedation should be performed in the ED as soon as the patient is stable
    b. Anterior dislocations are associated with femoral artery injuries
    c. Posterior dislocations are associated with sciatic nerve injuries
    d. Bed rest and skeletal traction is the best Tx for hip dislocation

    Answer d. Hip dislocations are especially susceptible to **avascular necrosis**. **Closed reduction** should be performed in the ED as soon as the patient is stable.

188. **A stable, neurologically intact 35 yo man suffers a severe lower leg soft tissue crush injury and tibial plateau fracture after being pinned underneath a car. The pt initially does not have a pulse in the foot but after placing a traction splint, a pulse is restored. All of the following are true except
    a. He is at increased risk for popliteal artery injury
    b. This patient is at risk for compartment syndrome due to the crush injury and tibial plateau Fx
    c. Closed Fx reduction and re-assessment of pulse was the most appropriate step
    d. Concomitant venous and nerve injury do not increase his risk of amputation

    Answer d. Concomitant arterial, venous and nerve injury increase risk for amputation. ***This pt is at risk for **compartment syndrome** due to the **crush injury** and **tibial plateau Fx**. **Rhabdomyolysis** can occur from **crush injury** and from **compartment syndrome** resulting in **myoglobinuria** (Tx: volume, alkalinize urine), **hyperkalemia** (Tx; calcium gluconate, D50 + Insulin) and **metabolic acidosis** (Tx:HCO3-)*

189. *All of the following are true of electrical injuries except:
    a. Cataracts can occur
    b. Bone has the highest electrical resistance
    c. The MCC of early death is brain injury
    d. Compartment syndrome can occur in these patients

    Answer c. MCC of early death is cardiac arrest from ventricular fibrillation.

190. *All of the following are true except:
    a. Tx for Brown Recluse spider bites is Dapsone
    b. Thyroid hormone is released as part of the flight or fight response
    c. The MCC of airway obstruction is the tongue
    d. Head injury is the MCC of death after reaching the ED alive

    Answer b. **Thyroid hormone is NOT involved in fight or flight response*

Coding in ED
Need possible *ED thoracotomy* (loss of pulse or SBP < 60)
1) **Blunt trauma** - use only if pressure or pulse lost **while in ER**
   Consider reversible cause before thoracotomy (eg tension PTX)
2) **Penetrating trauma** - use only if pressure or pulse lost **on way to ER** or **in ER**
Penetrating right chest injury and pt codes – still do left thoracotomy
   Extend incision across sternum to explore right if needed (clamshell)

Penetrating Chest Injury
1) **Stable** patient

Chest in "box " → get CXR (if normal, repeat in 4-6 hrs)
Chest tube on side of injury (you are going to OR) + chest tube
on contra-lateral side if PTX or hemothorax on that side
OR for **pericardial window** (median sternotomy if blood
found), **esophagoscopy** and **bronch** (thoracotomy if
indicated)
Gastrografin swallow before commencing diet to R/O
esophageal injury (hard to find w/ esophagoscopy alone)
Esophageal injuries hardest to dx

Chest outside "box" → get CXR (if normal, repeat in 4-6 hrs)
Chest tube for PTX, hemothorax, or if going to OR for
something else

Injury **below nipples** requires **laparotomy** or **laparoscopy** to R/O
diaphragm injury and peritoneal penetration
"box" formed by nipples, sternal notch, and xyphoid process
Some use FAST instead of pericardial window to R/O
hemopericardium

2) **Unstable** patient (DDx:hemorrhage, tension PTX, cardiac tamponade)
Place chest tube(s) right away (diagnoses tension PTX and
hemorrhage; consider bilateral chest tubes right away):
→ If not much blood, go to OR for **pericardial window** and
laparotomy
→ If chest tube has **high output** (> 1000-1500) →
OR for **anterior-lateral thoracotomy** on **bleeding side**
(**clamshell incision** if you need to see whole heart
or contra-lateral side)
Keep pt **supine** for thoracotomy (anterior thoracotomy)
Clamp hilum if severe **lung injury** (then repair)
Clamp aorta if **aortic injury** (then repair)
Put finger in hole for **heart injury** (then repair)
Intercostal arteries and IMA can bleed significantly

Penetrating Abdominal injury (includes flank)
Unstable patient – laparotomy
Stable patient
1) **GSW to abdomen** – laparotomy **Tangential flank or low back –
laparotomy** is safest answer (can consider abd CT to confirm
trajectory)
2) **Low velocity penetrating abdominal injury** (eg stab wounds) –
need local **fascia exploration** in the ED
1) **Non-penetrating** – discharge home
2) **Penetrating** – **laparotomy or laparoscopy** (safest answer)

Blunt trauma
Stable → normal work-up
Unstable → (SBP ≤ 90 despite 2 L of LR) → **FAST scan** (or DPL)
If **positive** (bleeding from **abd source**) → OR (for laparotomy)
If **negative** → find source of bleeding:
Pelvic fx (exam, PXR)
Chest - hemorrhage, tension PTX, tamponade (exam, CXR)
Extremity bleeding – lacerations or femur fractures
Neurogenic shock (lateral c-spine) – R/O above 1st

Pelvic Fx's
Pelvic fixation will tamponade most pelvic *venous bleeding
Angio-embolization is required for most pelvic *arterial bleeding
All pts w/ significant pelvic fx's need **proctoscopy, RUG** (retrograde
urethrogram) and **cystogram** – these pts are at high risk for
genitourinary and **rectal injuries**

**Isolated anterior ring (ie pubic rami fx) w/ minimal sacro-iliac
displacement - Tx: weight bearing as tolerated*

FAST scan (focused abdominal sonography for trauma)
  U/S used to inspect heart and abdominal compartment (looks for blood in
  peri-hepatic fossa, peri-splenic fossa, pelvis, and **pericardium**)
  Morbid obesity can limit viewing
  May miss free fluid < 50 ml (eg hollow viscous injury)
  Need laparotomy (or median sternotomy/pericardial window if
  hemopericardium) if FAST is positive
  *FAST scan misses (false negatives) – retroperitoneal bleed, hollow
  viscous injury

Diagnostic peritoneal lavage (DPL)
  Used in **hypotensive pts** (SBP $\leq$ 90) with blunt trauma
  *Positive DPL (blunt): >10 cc blood, >100,000 RBCs/cc food particles,
  bile, bacteria, >500 WBC/cc
  Need **emergency laparotomy** if positive
  Perform **supra-umbilical DPL** if pelvic fracture present
  *DPL misses (false negatives) – retroperitoneal bleed, contained
  hematoma

*CT scan misses (false negatives) – hollow viscous injury, diaphragm injury

**Glasgow Coma Scale (GCS)
  Motor Function
      6 follows commands
      5 localizes to the pain site
      4 withdrawals from pain
      3 flexion with painful stimuli (decorticate)
      2 extension with painful stimuli (decerebrate)
      1 no response to painful stimuli
  Verbal Response
      5 oriented x 3
      4 confused but responds
      3 inappropriate words with speech
      2 incomprehensible sounds (grunting)
      1 no response verbally
  Eye opening
      4 spontaneous eye opening
      3 opens eyes to command
      2 opens eyes to pain
      1 no response to eye opening

  Most impt prognostic indicator of the GCS is the **motor score
  *Penetrating head injury has poorest survival of any head injuries given
  equal GCS scores
  Lowest score is **3**; intubated pts are given a verbal score of **1T**
  GCS score:
      $\leq$ 14   need head CT
      $\leq$ 10   need intubation
      $\leq$ 8   need ICP monitor

Diabetes Insipidus (decreased ADH)
  Sx's: copious **dilute urine output**
  Dx: ↑ serum Na; ↓ urine Na; ↓ urine specific gravity (nl 1.002-1.028)
  Tx: 1) **Replace free water** deficit w/ D5 water
          Correct Na < 0.7 mEq/L/h → avoid **brain swelling**
       2) **DDAVP** (desmopressin)

**SIADH (syndrome of inappropriate ADH; anti-diuresis)
> Sx's: **low urine output** and **fluid overload** *(no edema)*
>> ADH acts on distal tubules to reabsorb water (**cAMP** mediated)
>> ↓ serum Na; ↑ urine Na, ↑ urine specific gravity (concentrated)
> Tx: 1) ****Fluid restriction + diuresis** *(mainstay)*
>> Correct slowly (Na < 0.5 mEq/L/h) to ****avoid central pontine
>> myelinolysis**

*ICP monitors for:
> 1) **GCS ≤ 8**
> 2) **Suspected elevated ICP** based on CT scan
> 3) **Not able to follow neuro exam** w/ moderate to severe head injury (eg
>   in OR; paralyzed or sedated)

Cerebral perfusion pressure (CPP)
> **CPP** = Mean arterial pressure (MAP) *minus* intracranial pressure (ICP)
> **Elevated ICP findings on CT scan** - decrease in size of ventricles, loss of
>   sulci (flattening), loss of cisterns

*Supportive Tx for elevated ICP
> Normal ICP is 10; **ICP > 20** usually requires treatment
> Overall, want goal **cerebral perfusion pressure** (CPP) > 60
> **Sedate** and **paralyze**
> Raise **head of bed**
> **Relative hyperventilation** - want some cerebral vasoconstriction (keep
>   **pCO$_2$ 30–35**)
> **Keep sodium 140–150** - **normal saline** used for volume (draws edema
>   from brain and lowers ICP); also raises MAP
> **Volume + Pressors** (phenylephrine) to keep **MAP high**
> **Mannitol** - draws edema from brain and lowers ICP
> **Levetiracetam** (Keppra) or **Fos-phenytoin** - SZ prevention
>   *Do not need to check drug levels w/ these*
> **Barbiturate coma** - if refractory to above
> **Ventriculostomy** - removes **CSF fluid** which can help lower ICP
> **Craniotomy** - if refractory to all of the above (decompresses ICP)
> **Brain swelling**
>> ****Maximum brain swelling occurs *48-72 hours after trauma**
>>   *(peak ICP)*
>> **Symptoms** (Sx's) of ↑ ICP – stupor, headache, N/V, stiff neck
>> **Signs of ↑ ICP** – HTN, HR lability (high or low), slow RR
>> ***Intermittent bradycardia** is a sign of severely elevated ICP and
>>   impending herniation
>> **Cushing's triad** – HTN, bradycardia, and slow respiratory rate
>>   (signals impending herniation)
>> **Herniation** – shift of brain across skull structures; usually fatal

Subdural hematoma
> Greater incidence than epidural
> ***MCC** – *venous injury*; torn ****bridging veins** between dura and arachnoid
> **Head CT** – crescent-shaped deformity adjacent the skull
> Tx: Operate for significant **neuro degeneration** and **mass effect** (shift ≥
>   **10 mm** for subdural)
> **Chronic subdural hematomas**: MC - elderly after minor fall
>   Operation indications as above

Epidural hematoma
> ****MCC** – *arterial injury;* usually ****middle meningeal artery**
> **Head CT** – lenticular (lens-shaped) deformity adjacent the skull
> ***Typical pattern** – loss of consciousness (LOC) → then lucid interval →
>   then sudden deterioration (N/V, irritability, restless, LOC)
> Tx: Operate for significant **neuro degeneration** and **mass effect** (shift ≥ 5
>   **mm** for epidural).

Cerebral hematoma and **contusions** – MC in frontal lobe
  Coup or contra-coup (typically don't require operation)
Intra-ventricular hemorrhage – if hydrocephalus, place *ventriculostomy tube
Diffuse axonal injury (denotes very severe head injury)
  Dx: *MRI most sensitive*
  Tx: supportive care for elevated ICP, extremely poor prognosis
Dilated pupil (blown pupil)
  Possible ipsilateral temporal lobe pressure on *cranial nerve III*
   (**oculomotor**, can progress to **temporal uncal herniation**)
  Going to OR emergently for something else (and can't get head CT) →
   Burr hole on that side and on other side if that's negative 5 cm
    anterior and superior to external auditory canal
  In ER w/ blown pupil and pt stable → Get **Head CT** (could be baseline
   anisocoria; don't want Burr hole if pt had baseline pupil difference)

Cervical Spine

  Dens = odontoid process
  *MC location for spine injury** – cervical spine
  *MC cervical spine fx** – dens fx
  The higher the cervical spine fx, the higher the morbidity and mortality
  Best indication for **steroids** in spinal cord injury - worsening neuro deficit
  **Pts w/ neurologic signs of cord injury and negative CT scan* – get
   MRI to check for ligamentous injury

Thoracolumbar Spine

  Thoracolumbar spine contains 3 columns (anterior, middle, and posterior)
  If ≥ 2 columns are disrupted, spine considered **unstable:**
   Wedge Fx's usually **anterior** column only and considered **stable**
   Burst Fx's considered unstable (2 columns – anterior and middle)
    Tx: **spinal fusion**

Indications for emergent surgical spinal cord decompression - Open Fx,
  cord compression, progressive neuro dysfunction, Anterior Cord Syndrome

Upright fall – calcaneus, lumbar, and **wrist or forearm** fractures

Maxillofacial trauma

  Facial Fx's (Le Fort Fx's)
   Type I (- across maxilla)
   Type II (/ \ , lateral to nasal bone, underneath eyes, towards maxilla)
   Type III (- - , lateral to the orbital wall)
   Tx: **Maxillo-mandibular fixation** (MMF) for above ± miniplates
  Facial trauma at high risk for **cervical spine trauma**
  Facial nerve injury
   MCC facial nerve injury – temporal bone Fx (at **geniculate**
    ganglion; if severe nerve injury – repair)
   Iatrogenic injury – repair immediately
  Mandibular fx
   Malocclusion best indicator of injury
   Dx: thin slice CT w/ facial reconstruction
   Tx: external or internal fixation
  Nasoethmoid fx
   CSF leak in 70% (CSF has **tau protein + beta-transferrin**)
    Conservative Tx initially
    Can place *epidural catheter* to decrease CSF pressure
    Close dura if above fails (4-6 weeks of conservative Tx)
    If undergoing facial reconstruction, repair at that time
  Orbital fx (blowout fractures)
   Impaired gaze or diplopia requires repair
   Tx: restore orbital floor (bone fragments or graft)

Nosebleeds
- **Anterior** – Vaseline gauze packing
- ****Posterior** – Vaseline gauze deep packing; balloon tamponade if that fails (can use foley catheter); ***May require **angio-embolization** of **internal maxillary artery or **ethmoidal artery*

Tripod Fx (zygomatic bone) – internal fixation (just for cosmesis; not a functional problem)

Basal skull fx's - raccoon eyes (anterior fossa), Battle's sign (mastoid; middle fossa), hemotympanum, CSF rhinorrhea / otorrhea – most do basilar skull Fx's do <u>not</u> require surgery

*Operate on skull fx's if either:
1) Significantly **depressed** (≥ 1 cm, needs elevation) *or:*
2) **Contaminated** (dura penetration) *or:*
3) **Refractory CSF leak** (conservative Tx up to 6 weeks)
*Close dura w/ operation

Temporal skull fx's - injury to CN VII (facial) and VIII (vestibulocochlear)

**Zone I Neck (penetrating) – explore if symptomatic or significant finding
- Location – *clavicle to cricoid cartilage*
- W/U – angio, bronch, EGD and swallow (late), ± pericardial window
- Approach- median sternotomy (esp vascular injury; proximal control)

Zone II Neck (penetrating) – **explore all (if penetrating platysma muscle)
- Location – *cricoid cartilage to angle of mandible*
- Approach – **lateral neck incision** (trachea, esophagus, blood vessels)

**Zone III Neck (penetrating) – explore if symptomatic or significant finding
- Location – *angle of mandible to the skull base*
- W/U – angio and laryngoscopy
- Approach- jaw subluxation, digastric and sternocleidomastoid muscle release, ± mastoid sinus resection to reach vascular (ie carotid) injury

*Vascular injuries (thoracic)
In general get **proximal** and **distal control** before open repair (bypass graft usually used); endovascular repair being used for some injuries
- **Median sternotomy* for injuries to:
  - Ascending aorta
  - Innominate artery (may need cervical extension)
  - Proximal right subclavian artery (likely need cervical extension)
  - Proximal left or right common carotid artery
  - Proximal left subclavian artery (w/ **trap door** infra-clavicular incision)
  - Innominate vein
  - Superior vena cava (and intra-thoracic inferior vena cava)
- **Left thoracotomy* for injuries to:
  - Distal left subclavian artery
  - Descending thoracic aorta (eg aortic transection at ligamentum arteriosum)
- **Right mid-clavicular incision ± resection of medial clavicle**
  - Distal right subclavian artery

<u>Carotid artery</u>
Hemorrhage, pseudoaneurysm, or **AV fistula** (continual bruit)
- Tx: open **primary repair** or interposition graft
*Dissection (needs to be just carotid; not aortic dissection)
- **Asymptomatic* Tx: **anti-coagulate** (prevent thrombus formation)
- **Symptomatic* Tx: **carotid <u>stenting</u>** *(best);* open repair if that fails
Thrombosis
- **If antegrade flow is still present →**
  - Tx: open **primary repair** or interposition graft
- **No antegrade flow →** Tx: **anti-coagulate** to prevent thrombus extension and propagation
Carotid ligation – stroke in 20%

Thyroid gland injury – stop bleeding and place a drain (not thyroidectomy)
Recurrent laryngeal nerve injury- repair or re-implant in cricoarytenoid muscle

Persistent large PTX after chest tube

Make sure 1st chest tube has good placement and system working
Place 2nd chest tube anteriorly
*Still doesn't resolve → *bronch to look for tracheo-bronchial injury or mucus plug*

**Aortic transection

MC from rapid deceleration injury (MVAs); 90% of these pts die at scene
Address other life-threatening injuries 1st (eg severe solid organ laceration, pelvic fx w/ hemorrhage)→ repair aorta when pt stable
Mediastinal widening is MC from laceration of bridging veins and arteries (not leaking from aorta itself)
MC location for tear - ligamentum arteriosum
Dx: spiral chest CT (to screen; aortogram is the gold standard)
Repair options:
1) Left thoracotomy (posterolateral) w/ partial left heart bypass, place interposition graft (*Safest answer;* must be able to tolerate heparinization) *Significant cerebral hemorrhage is a contraindication to open repair (consider stent graft)*
2) Many being treated w/ stent grafts (off label indication)
**Important that you treat other life-threatening injuries 1st →*
Positive FAST or other life-threatening hemorrhage should be addressed *before* aortic transection

**Flail chest

≥ 2 consecutive ribs broken at ≥ 2 sites → paradoxical motion of chest wall
**Underlying pulmonary contusion biggest impairment to respiratory status (not the flail chest itself)*
Tx: may need intubation for underlying pulmonary impairment
Multiple rib fx's – thoracic *para-vertebral block* (or thoracic epidural) is best for pain relief; allows deep respiration (prevent hypoxemia)
**Hemothorax

Need to drain all blood from chest w/ chest tubes
Prevents fibrothorax and empyema, and to stop bleeding
Lung inflation compresses area (↓s bleeding)
*Most important RF for empyema after chest trauma is **retained hemothorax.*
**Unresolved hemothorax after two well-placed chest tubes*
*Tx: **VATS drainage (wait until pt stable from trauma)*
**Indications for OR thoracotomy after chest tube placement:*
1) > 1000-1500 cc after initial insertion
2) > 250 cc/hr for 3 hours
3) Unstable pt w/ significant bleeding
Lung injury bleeding

Perform tractotomy w/ GIA 45 stapler - place stapler in tract and fire to stop bleeding, resecting lung as you go (*no formal lobectomy)*
Clamp hilum if having trouble getting control
Cardiac contusion

*MCC death after heart contusion – *ventricular fibrillation (highest risk in 1st 24 hours)*
*MC arrhythmia after myocardial contusion – *SVT (supra-ventricular tachycardia)*
RFs – sternal Fx's, sternal contusion, no seatbelt
Dx: EKG (*best test)* - conduction abnormalities most significant finding
Anything other than NSR considered significant
Tx: need telemonitoring for 24 hours

Traumatic Cardiogenic Shock
1) ****Tension pneumothorax**
   Sx's: hypotension, ↓ breath sounds, bulging neck veins, tracheal
      shift away from injury, high airway pressures (if on ventilator)
      *Hypotension may worsen after being intubated
      Can see **bulging diaphragm** during laparotomy
   ****Cardiac compromise due to **decreased venous return to
      right atrium**
   Tx: chest tube
2) ****Cardiac tamponade**
   Sx's: hypotension, distended neck veins and muffled heart sounds
      (Beck's Triad)
   Dx: **FAST scan**
   If FAST scan shows **fluid** – pericardiocentesis or OR pericardial
      window to **decompress tamponade**
   Pericardial window or pericardiocentesis shows **blood** → need
      median sternotomy to find injury
   Pt coding → ED left anterior-lateral thoracotomy, open pericardium
   *1st ECHO sign of tamponade – right atrial diastolic compression
   **Mechanism of tamponade – _decreased ventricular filling_ due
      pericardial fluid (blood)

Tracheo-bronchial Injury
   Sx's: ***Worsening oxygenation** after chest tube placement (pt takes a
      deep breath in and goes out chest tube)
      Large **continuous air leak** after chest tube placement
      Large **pneumo-mediastinum** or severe **subcutaneous emphysema**
      Persistent PTX after chest tube placement
      MC after **blunt trauma**
   Dx: ***Bronchoscopy** (90% of injuries are within **1 cm of carina**)
      MC side – right (not as flexible as left side)
   Tx:

   Immediate tx - one of extremely few indications for **clamping a
      chest tube** (prevents the chest tube from sucking air out the
      injury and away from the lungs)
   Indications for repair:
      1) Respiratory compromise
      2) Persistent air-leak (1-2 weeks)
      3) Can't get lung up
      4) Injuries > 1/3 the tracheal or bronchial lumen
   Surgery
      *Mainstem intubate unaffected side w/ long ***single lumen
         tube** (double lumen tube too large, can **worsen tear**)
      *Right thoracotomy - for _right mainstem, trachea, and
         proximal left mainstem in_juries (avoiding the aorta on the
         right which is in the way for repair)
      *Left thoracotomy - for _distal left mainstem injuries_
   Note - you rarely ever want to clamp a chest tube in trauma because of the
      risk of tension pneumothorax

<u>Diaphragm Injury</u>
   MC on **left side** (liver protects the right side); MC after **blunt trauma**
   Dx: **CXR** or **CT scan** (can be hard to Dx)
      Air-fluid level in chest from **stomach herniation** through hole
      NGT in chest
   Tx: ***Trans-abdominal approach** if < 1 week (look for other injuries)
      *Chest approach if > 1 week (adhesions in chest prevent safe trans-
         abdominal approach)
      May need **PTFE mesh** to repair hole in diaphragm

Spleen trauma

MCC – blunt injury (MC organ injured w/ blunt trauma); heals in **6 weeks**

Threshold for splenectomy in **children** is high – unusual for children to undergo splenectomy

**Subcapsular splenic hematomas – _leave_

*Contraindications to splenic salvage – unstable, DIC, grade IV (hilar injury) or higher, other serious injuries (eg head injury, liver injury → don't want spleen to be a confounding issue), penetrating injury

Transfusion rate increased w/ splenic salvage

**Pancreatic leak after splenectomy

Presents as ****fluid collection** (*high amylase*) after splenectomy

Can injure the **tail of the pancreas** w/ splenectomy

Tx: ***percutaneous drain _only_** (*cures > 95%*)

Can also present as late fluid collection after conservative Tx for splenic trauma (fracture in tail of pancreas); same Tx

Post-splenectomy issues:

Give **immunizations** (Pneumococcus, Meningococcus, H. influenza)

ASA for platelet count > $1-1.5 \times 10^6$

Prophylactic Augmentin for 6 mos in children < 10 (give every day)

Liver trauma

MCC – blunt trauma

Lobectomy almost _never_ necessary

Leave drains w/ liver injuries

Intra-op hepatic bleeding (both penetrating and blunt):

**Pringle maneuver

For **severe hepatic bleeding**

Consists of intermittent clamping of ****portal triad** in the hepato-duodenal ligament (leave clamp on for 20 miin intervals while you perform repair, 5 min of reperfusion)

**Does _not_ stop bleeding from hepatic veins or IVC

Effective for portal venous or hepatic artery bleeding

**Hepatocytes most sensitive to ischemia – central lobar (acinar zone III)

*Damage Control Peri-hepatic packing

For **severe hepatic bleeding**

Pack severe liver injuries if pt becomes unstable (or severely coagulopathic) in OR and you are not able to easily fix problem. Go to ICU and get pt **warmed, stabilized, correct coags**, transfuse **blood**; remove packs next day

Place **sterile covering** (instead of closing abdomen) to prevent compartment syndrome if hard to get abdominal contents back in abdomen (occurs w/ massive resuscitation)

Severe retro-hepatic venous bleeding (from **hepatic veins** or **IVC**)

Tx – **Pack** (*best option*) hard to fix these injuries; damage control peri-hepatic packing and see if its **controlled**:

a. If **bleeding controlled** → go to ICU and follow damage control peri-hepatic packing pathway above

b. If **bleeding not controlled** → **Atrio-caval shunt** (32 Fr chest tube, allows blood diversion) and **repair**

**Subcapsular hepatic hematomas – _leave alone_

*Portal triad hematomas – open (both blunt and penetrating)

Common bile duct injury

< 50% of circumference – **primary repair** over stent

> 50% of circumference or complex injury- **choledocho-jejunostomy**

Kocher maneuver and dissect out the portal triad to find these injuries

Late cx's – biliary stricture at site of repair

Portal vein injury or SMV injury

Need to repair (ligation has 50% mortality)

*May need to transect neck of pancreas to get to injury

Need to perform ***distal pancreatectomy** with that move

Place **side-biting clamp** (allows blood flow while you repair) and
perform *lateral venorraphy*

**Hemobilia
Sx's: **abd pain, jaundice and hematemesis* (± melena) <u>late</u> after
trauma (*classic*; mean **4 weeks**; can also follow hepatic
surgery, percutaneous intervention to liver, trauma)
MCC – <u>iatrogenic</u> (eg PTC tubes, laparoscopic liver Bx)
**MC situation - hepatic artery to biliary duct fistula
Dx: **EGD** - will see **blood coming out of the Ampulla of Vater**
**Tx: **angio embolization; surgical ligation if that is unsuccessful
*Mesenteric artery injury (eg celiac, SMA) w/ blush, pseudoaneurysm or
large hemoperitoneum – <u>*no angio-embolization*</u>, go to OR for repair

Pancreatic trauma
MCC – penetrating trauma (80%)
Blunt trauma can cause perpendicular **pancreatic duct fractures**
Intra-op **pancreatic hematoma** – open (both penetrating and blunt)
Intra-op Assessment of Pancreas
Kocher maneuver and open **lesser sac** through omentum to
evaluate pancreas
Need to evaluate **duodenum** w/ pancreatic injuries
80% of pancreatic injuries discovered in OR are treated w/ just
drains (ie pancreatic duct <u>not</u> involved)
*Intra-op, the primary concern is to figure out if the **duct is injured:**
If **pancreatic duct not involved** (eg contusion) → just leave **drains**
If **pancreatic duct involved** →
Distal pancreatic duct injury
Tx: **Distal pancreatectomy** (can take 80% of gland)
*Splenic vein is directly posterior to pancreas
*Splenic artery is superior and posterior
Place **drains**
Pancreatic head duct injury (ie ampulla blown out) - Tx:
Place **drains** initially, usually **delayed Whipple** (mortality
too high w/ trauma Whipple → 50%)
***Whipple vs. distal pancreatectomy - based on duct injury in
relation to* **SMV**
**Late Dx of pancreatic injury (eg abd pain or rising amylase)
Will have **large fluid collection* around pancreas (necrosis, edema)
Dx: Abd CT usual
Tx: ***percutaneous drain* (cures 95%)

Duodenal trauma
Path
MCC – blunt trauma (crush or tears from deceleration injury)
*MC location for <u>tears</u> – 2nd portion (near Ampulla of Vater)
Can also get tears near ligament of Treitz
*MC location for <u>hematoma</u> – 3rd portion (overlying spine)
25% mortality w/ **blunt duodenal injuries** due to associated **shock**
Fistulas – major source of morbidity w/ duodenal injuries
Debridement and either: 1) **primary repair** or 2) **primary anastomosis**
treats 85% of all duodenal injuries requiring operation
Used when there is a **leak** or **loss of integrity** of bowel wall
If circumference of wall is reduced by > 50%, can't use primary repair
Segmental resection w/ **primary anastomosis** is possible w/ all
portions of duodenum <u>except</u> **2nd portion** (can do **primary
repair** to most 2nd portion injuries)
Dx of suspected duodenal injury
CT scan findings - bowel wall **thickening, hematoma, air,** contrast
leak, retroperitoneal **fluid/air**
UGI (best test for Dx of duodenal injury)
Leak → OR, **No leak →** conservative tx

Para-duodenal hematomas on **CT scan
> **MC location** – 3rd portion of the duodenum overlying the spine
> Sx's: ****high small bowel obstruction** 12–72 hrs after injury (eg N/V)
> Dx: ****UGI study** (best test) → 'stacked coins' or 'coiled spring'
> > appearance, R/O leak w/ this study as well
> Tx: **Conservative Tx 1st , ****TPN + NGT** resolves 95% of these within
> > **3 weeks** (hematoma gets reabsorbed)

Para-duodenal hematomas in **OR** (> 2 cm) – need to explore these
> **Kocher maneuver** and open **lesser sac through omentum**

Kocher – peritoneum to right of duodenum incised; duodenum and
> pancreas reflected towards midline (inspects 2nd and 3rd portions of
> duodenum and pancreatic head); assess duodenal wall, pancreas,
> portal triad, surrounding areas

Kocher maneuver indicated for:
> 1) **Bile staining** (biliary system or duodenal injury)
> 2) **RUQ sucus drainage** (duodenal injury)
> 3) **Fat necrosis** (pancreatic injury – pancreatic enzyme release)
> 4) **Para-duodenal hematomas** discovered intra-op

Colon trauma

Penetrating colon trauma – **primary repair** without ostomy is effective for
> the majority of penetrating injuries to the ascending, transverse or
> descending colon; use of an ostomy does not influence infection rate

*Indications for ostomy
> 1) *Pt in **shock** (a leak might kill the patient) or:
> 2) *Extensive **local damage** [eg devastating left colon injury w/
> > significant fecal spillage and prolonged (> 6 hrs) time to repair]
> **Ileostomy** w/ colo-colonic anastomosis for most (exception would
> > be pt in **shock** – just place colostomy and *avoid* anastomosis)

**Ureteral trauma

MCC – penetrating injury

**Hematuria NOT reliable sx

Blood supply is **medial** to upper 2/3 of ureter and **lateral** to lower 1/3 of
> ureter

Dx: **Multiple shot IVPs** (best test, looking for leak)
> Get this for penetrating wounds to lower quadrants (or worried about
> ureteral injury); identifies injury and 2 functional kidney's

Tx: **Cattel or Mattox** maneuver or exposure

1) ****If large ureteral segment is missing** (>2 cm; cannot perform re-
> anastomosis):
> **Upper 1/3** and **middle 1/3 injuries** won't reach bladder (injuries
> > above pelvic brim)
> > → temporize with ****percutaneous nephrostomy**, tie off both
> > > ends of ureter; go with **ileal interposition** or **trans-**
> > > **uretero-ureterostomy** later
> **Lower 1/3 injuries** → ****Re-implant in bladder**; may need **bladder**
> > (psoas) **hitch** procedure so that ureter can reach

2) ****If small ureteral segment is missing** (<2 cm):
> **Upper 1/3 or middle 1/3 area**
> > → ****primary repair** (spatulate ends, 6-0 PDS sutures, use
> > > absorbable suture); Repair over a ureteral stent
> **For lower 1/3** → ****Still re-implant in bladder** (ureter to bladder
> > anastomosis more durable than ureter-ureter anastomosis)
3) **Partial transections** can be repaired over stent

**Renal trauma
MCC – blunt trauma
95% of renal injuries are treated **non-operatively (esp. blunt trauma)*
*Hematuria – *best indicator of renal trauma; requires a **CT scan**
Anatomy
Gerota's Fascia covers kidney
**Anterior to posterior renal hilum structures (VAP) - renal vein,
renal artery, renal pelvis
*Right renal artery is posterior to IVC (MC)
*Left renal vein is MC anterior to aorta - need to watch for
retro-aortic left renal vein when placing aortic clamp for
open AAA repair
**Left renal vein
**Can be ligated near IVC in emergency situation (has
adrenal vein and **gonadal vein** collaterals)
Right does not have these collaterals (plugs directly into IVC) –
need repair or nephrectomy (**only if life saving**)
**Flank trauma *(eg fractured ribs) and* **pre-op IVP or CT scan has no
renal uptake** *on that side (ie no blood flow to kidney)* → *Dx + Tx:*
**immediate angio; *can stent if intimal flap*
Urine extravasation on CT scan – vast majority do *not* require operation
Indications for operation w/ blunt renal trauma:
1) **Acute ongoing renal hemorrhage in unstable patient**
2) **After acute phase:** severe collecting system disruption or
massive hematuria
Intra-op
1) **Expanding peri-renal hematomas or free hemorrhage** (blunt or
penetrating injury) → **Exploration**
2) **Non-expanding, stable, peri-renal hematomas** (blunt or
penetrating injury) → **Get IVP**
If vascular injury, open and repair, o/w leave
Penetrating more likely requires exploration than blunt
**Persistent shock despite ongoing fluid resuscitation with severe
vascular kidney injury and other concomitant major injuries –
need* **nephrectomy** *(feel for contra-lateral kidney 1st)*
Exploration
Left side → Mattox maneuver; **Right side** → Cattel maneuver
Get control of **vascular hilum 1st**
Can use SVG (saphenous vein graft) if not enough length for renal
artery or renal vein repair
*Kidney cortical injuries (> 95% non-operative) – when you do have
to repair these, just perform **primary closure**; place **drains**
Mattox maneuver – left colon, spleen, and pancreas brought up
Good for retroperitoneal exposure of aorta, left iliac, left renal
Cattel maneuver – right colon and duodenum brought up
Good for retroperitoneal exposure of IVC, right iliac, right renal

Bladder trauma
Hematuria – *best indicator of bladder trauma* (although not specific)
MC associated injury – pelvic fx (95%)
Sx's: hematuria, meatus blood, sacral or scrotal hematoma
Dx: **cystogram** *(best)*
*Extra-peritoneal bladder rupture – MC with pelvic fractures
Cystogram – **starbursts*; Tx: urinary catheter 1-2 weeks
*Intra-peritoneal bladder rupture
Cystogram – **leak*; Tx: OR for repair

Urethral and Genital trauma
  Sx's: **hematuria** or **blood at meatus** *(best indicator)*, free-floating prostate
  MC associated injury – pelvic fx, increased in males
  No Foley if urethral injury suspected (membranous portion of urethra at risk for dissection)
  Dx: **RUG** (retrograde urethrogram) - *best test for urethral injury*
  Tx:
      1) ***Significant tears** (**most injuries treated this way);*
          ****Supra-pubic cystostomy** tube and **repair in 2–3 months**
              (delayed repair); There is a **high stricture** and
              impotence rate if repaired early
      2) Small, partial tears Tx: bridging urethral catheter across tear for 3
          weeks (usually definitive)

Vascular Trauma
  ****Major (hard) signs of vascular injury:**
      Active hemorrhage is present
      Pulse deficit
      Expanding or pulsatile hematoma
      Distal ischemia
      Bruit or thrill is present
      Tx: For any of the above, go emergently to OR for exploration (get
          proximal and distal control 1st)
  ****Moderate (soft) signs of vascular injury:**
      History of hemorrhage at the scene
      Anatomically related nerve deficit
      A large stable hematoma
      Injury close to major artery (eg GSW to the medial thigh)
      ABI < 0.9
      Unequal pulses
      Dx: For any of above, get angiogram (some groups get **CT angio**)

      **All posterior knee dislocations require angio*

  Small injuries that are <u>not</u> flow limiting (small intimal flaps, small
      segmental stenosis, small pseudoaneurysms, small focal narrowings,
      small dissections) - Tx: **observation,** consider **heparin** (prevents
      thrombus formation)
  Injuries w/ flow limitation → Tx: operate w/ primary repair or covered
      stent

  Special issues:
      Vein injuries that require repair – femoral, popliteal, innominate,
          subclavian, axillary, superior mesenteric vein, portal vein
      ****Single artery transection in calf** in o/w healthy patient → ligate
      Consider **prophylactic fasciotomy** if ischemia >4-6 hours –
          prevents compartment syndrome
  Exposure for lower leg:
      1) **Above knee** popliteal - posterolateral retraction of **sartorius**
      2) **Below knee** popliteal - posterolateral retraction of **gastrocnemius**
          (medial head)

Orthopaedic Trauma
  Can loose 2 L of blood w/ a femur fx (class IV shock)
  Long bone fx or **dislocations w/ loss of pulse** (or weak pulse)
      1) *Immediate reduction* of Fx or dislocation, **re-assess pulse, ABI**
          a. If **pulse does not return** → OR for vascular bypass or repair
          b. If **pulse is weak** or **ABI < 0.9** → angiogram
      2) ****All knee dislocations** → angio after reduction (unless pulse is
          absent, in which case you would just go to OR)

Orthopaedic Trauma and Associated Injuries
Upper Extremity

Anterior Humerus dislocation	**Axillary nerve**
Posterior Humerus dislocation	Axillary artery
Proximal Humerus Fx	Axillary nerve
Mid-shaft Humerus Fx (spiral Fx)	**Radial nerve**
Distal (supra-condylar) Humeral Fx	Brachial artery
Elbow (Ulnar) dislocation	Brachial artery
Distal Radial Fx	Median nerve

Lower Extremity

Anterior Femur (hip) dislocation	Femoral artery
Posterior Femur (hip) dislocation	**Sciatic nerve**
Distal Femur (supra-condylar) Fx	Popliteal artery
Posterior (MC) Knee dislocation	Popliteal artery
Fibula neck Fx	Common peroneal nerve

Avascular Necrosis – femoral neck Fx's at high risk: Tx: hip replacement

Compartment syndrome
MC in leg **anterior compartment** (get foot-drop from dead muscle)
High risk fx's – supracondylar humeral fx (Volkmann's contracture), tibial
   plateau fx, elbow dislocations; also with **crush injuries**
Any injury resulting in interruption and then restoration of blood flow
Is a reperfusion injury mediated by PMNs
Can occur in any muscle compartment (compartment pressure exceeds
   capillary filling pressure)

Sx's: **Classic scenario:** fx w/ loss of blood flow → repair (> 4-6 hours later)
         → **pain** and **swelling** soon post-op
     1st finding – pain w/ passive motion
         Others – swelling, paresthesias → anesthesia → paralysis →
             poikiothermia → pulselessness (late finding)
         Distal pulses can be present w/ compartment syndrome → last
             thing to go

Dx: Based on **clinical suspicion** (if suspected → fasciotomy)
     Pressure **> 20 mmHg** abnormal
     Undiagnosed compartment syndrome can present as **renal failure**
         (*myoglobin* release from injured muscle)
     **The rhabdomyolysis also results in hyperkalemia, acidemia, and
         hyperphosphatemia**
     **Crush injury can also cause reperfusion injury, rhabdomyolysis
         and possibly compartment syndrome**

Tx: **Fasciotomy**, after 5-10 days place skin grafts
     With fasciotomy, you are through the fascia when the **muscle bulges**
     Incise the **total length of compartment** (eg the length of the leg)
     Remove all dead tissue (myoglobinuria if you don't resect)
     Myoglobinuria Tx: normal saline **volume** (most important) and
         alkalinize urine (HCO3 – drip)
     Watch for **hyperkalemia** (Tx: calcium gluconate, D50 + insulin) and
         metabolic acidosis (Tx HCO3-)
     **Nerve most at risk for lower leg fasciotomy – superficial
         peroneal nerve (goes to lateral compartment, can't evert foot)**

<u>Hematomas</u> (Intra-op; > **2 cm** considered significant)

Location	Penetrating	Blunt
Pelvic	explore	leave
Para-duodenal	explore	explore
Portal triad	explore	explore
Retro-hepatic	leave if stable	leave
Midline^	explore	explore
Peri-colonic	explore	explore
Peri-renal	explore *	leave†

^Explore both supra-mesocolic and infra-mesocolic
*Unless preoperative CT scan or IVP shows no injury and hematoma
    is not expanding.
†Unless preoperative CT scan or IVP shows vascular injury or there
    is an expanding hematoma

Retroperitoneal Hematomas
   Zone I Central Hematoma (medial to psoas) → open (potential for great
       vessel injury); If more to the **right** → Cattel; If more to **left** → Mattox
   Zone II Lateral Hematomas (lateral to psoas) → open (safest answer);
       potential for colon, duodenal, kidney injury
       If blunt trauma w/ no obvious colon or duodenum injury, IVP is OK
           and hematoma not expanding → observe
       If on right → Cattel; If on left → Mattox
   Zone III Pelvic Hematoma → leave if blunt; usually open if penetrating
       w/ penetrating - can pack pelvis w/ angio-embolization if
           uncontrollable

Placental abruption after trauma
   MCC – *shock* (mechanical disruption is #2)
   Placental lining separates from the uterus; 50% fetal demise
   Sx's: vaginal bleed, uterine tenderness, contractions, fetal HR <120
   ***Kleihauer-Betke test** – detects and measures fetal blood in maternal
       circulation → **sign of placental abruption**

Electrical Injuries
   These pt's are at risk for **rhabdomyolysis** and **compartment syndrome**
   Do not put IV's into affected limbs
   All need significant **volume resuscitation** (cell necrosis inside body)
   Other injuries – quadriplegia, organ necrosis, intestinal or GB perforation,
       ***cataracts**
   Evaluate for **compartment syndrome** → would need fasciotomy
       All extremities susceptible
   EKG and **telemetry** for 24 hours if having arrhythmias
   Electrical burns to mouth in children (electrical cord) – wait 6-9 months
       before repair unless child cannot eat
   MCC immediate death from electrical injury – cardiac arrest from
       ventricular fibrillation
   Highest resistance – bone

Extreme Hypothermia (temp < 27 C) Tx: <u>cardiopulmonary bypass</u> (highest rate
   of heat transfer)
DO <u>not</u> stop CPR until warm and dead

Shock
   Respiratory rate progressively ↑s w/ shock
   ***Shock = inadequate tissue oxygenation*
   1st response to hemorrhagic shock- ↑ diastolic pressure (vasoconstriction)

Trauma Statistics

Trauma deaths

1st **peak** (0 to 30 min) – most deaths due to **hemorrhage** (MC, lacerations of heart, aorta) and brain; can't save these pts

2nd **peak** (30 min to 4 hrs) – deaths due to **head injury** (MC) and **hemorrhage** pts you can <u>save</u> w/ rapid assessment golden hr

3rd **peak** (days to weeks) – deaths due to **MSOF** and **sepsis**

1) **Hemorrhage** – MCC of death in 1st hour
2) **Head injury** – MCC death after reaching the ER alive
3) **Infection** – MCC death long term

Blunt injury – 80% of all trauma
Penetrating injury – **small bowel** MC injured
Blunt Injury – **spleen** MC injured (some say liver)
Tongue – MCC of upper airway obstruction → perform jaw thrust
Seat belts – small bowel perforations, lumbar spine Fx, sternal Fx
Catecholamines – *peak 24-48 hours after injury*
ADH, ACTH, and glucagon – also ↑ after trauma (fight or flight response)
Thyroid hormone <u>not</u> involved in flight or flight

Critical Care

191. **All of the following are true except:
    a. Coronary sinus blood has the lowest venous oxygen tension
    b. Renal vein blood has the highest venous oxygen tension in the body
    c. The most important determinant of myocardial oxygen consumption and energy expenditure is wall tension
    d. Arterial pressure is equal to heart rate x systemic vascular resistance

    Answer d. Arterial pressure is equal to cardiac output x systemic vascular resistance.

    > **The heart consumes a lot of oxygen and the **coronary sinus** has the **lowest oxygen saturation** in the body (30%).
    > **The kidney receives 25% of C.O. for clearing solutes and regulating body water. This does not require a large amount of oxygen. The **renal vein** therefore has the **highest venous oxygen saturation** (80%)
    > **The most important determinant of **myocardial oxygen consumption** and energy expenditure is **wall tension** (others – HR, contractility)

192. *All of the following are most often associated with a decrease in SVO2 (mixed venous oxygen saturation) except:
    a. Myocardial infarction
    b. Cardiac tamponade
    c. Hemorrhagic shock
    d. Septic shock

    Answer d. A **decrease in SVO2** is caused by either decreased delivery of oxygen to the periphery or increased consumption. Delivery problems can be the result of a low cardiac output (MI, tamponade), decreased oxygen carrying capacity (low Hct, hemorrhage), or a low oxygen saturation.

    An **increase in SVO2** can occur with anything that causes a left to right shunt or that causes a decreased oxygen consumption in the periphery. A left to right cardiac defect (at the atrial level), cirrhosis, and septic shock all result in left to right shunt. Cyanide toxicity would result in decreased peripheral oxygen consumption and an elevated SVO2.

193. **All of following shift the oxygen dissociation curve to the **left** (**decreased p50**) except:
    a. Decreased CO2
    b. Low temperature
    c. High pH
    d. 2-3 DPG

    Answer d. **Items that cause a **left shift** (oxygen becomes more bound to hemoglobin) include decreased CO2, decreased temp, and high pH. Items that cause a right shift include low pH, increased CO2, 2-3 DPG, and ATP.

194. **Which if the following equations determines myocardial oxygen consumption:
    a. $= C.O. \times (CaO_2 - CvO_2)$
    b. $= C.O. \times (CvO_2 - CaO_2)$
    c. $= C.O. - (CaO_2 - CvO_2)$
    d. $= C.O. - (CvO_2 - CaO_2)$

    Answer a. **O_2 consumption** (VO_2; Fick equation) = C.O. x ($CaO_2 - CvO_2$)
    CvO_2 = venous O_2 content (mmHg) or *coronary sinus O_2 content for above
    CaO_2 = arterial O_2 content
    O_2 content = Hgb x 1.34 x O_2 saturation (%)

195. **A 67 yo woman develops urosepsis following a LAR for adenocarcinoma. She has been started on broad spectrum antibiotics. She is intubated, has a wedge pressure of 18, a HR of 120, a blood pressure of 70/50, and a C.O. of 8. The most appropriate next step in this patient's management is:
    a. Norepinephrine
    b. Dobutamine
    c. Dopamine
    d. Epinephrine

    Answer a. **Levophed (norepinephrine) is primarily an alpha agent and decreases vasodilatation associated w/ septic shock. This is the initial pressor of choice for septic shock despite fluid resuscitation.*

196. **A 50 yo man 6 hours out from a 5 vessel CABG has a cardiac index of 1.4 with a wedge pressure of 20 and a systemic pressure of 90/50. His HR is 90 and his SVR is 1400. The most appropriate initial step for this patient is:
    a.   Phenylephrine
    b.   ACE inhibitor
    c.   Nitroglycerin
    d.   Dobutamine

    Answer d. **Initial Tx for **cardiogenic shock is w/ an **inotrope** (eg dobutamine).*

197. *You place a swan ganz catheter in a 70 kg man through the left subclavian vein and get a wedge pressure. The approximate distance into the patient should be:
    a.   45 cm
    b.   50 cm
    c.   55 cm
    d.   60 cm

    Answer c. The approximate swan distance to wedge from the left subclavian vein is 55 cm. If you place a swan-ganz catheter and wedge it but the distance is significantly longer than expected (8 cm or greater), you likely have a loop or your catheter is in the wrong place.

198. **All of the following concerning pulmonary artery catheters are true except:
    a.   If possible, they should be avoided in pts w/ left bundle branch blocks
    b.   Excessive PEEP can artificially decrease wedge pressure
    c.   Zone III of the lung is the optimal site of placement
    d.   Pulmonary vascular resistance (PVR) can only be measured using a PA catheter (ECHO does not measure PVR)

    Answer b. Excessive PEEP can artificially increase wedge pressures. The optimal site of placement of the PA catheter is in *lung zone III (bases usually) to avoid the effects of airway pressures on wedge pressures. Wedge pressure measurement is taken at *end expiration.

    ***Pulmonary vascular resistance** (PVR) can only be measured using a PA catheter (ECHO does not measure PVR).*

199. **A critical care pt s/p thoracoabdominal aortic aneurysm repair has the following pulmonary artery catheter values: cardiac index 1.8, systemic vascular resistance 3000, and wedge pressure of 5. This is most consistent with:
    a.   Septic shock
    b.   Hypovolemic shock
    c.   Cardiogenic shock
    d.   Neurogenic shock

    Answer b. Poor cardiac index, poor filling pressures and a high SVR suggests **hypovolemic shock**.

200. **A critical care patient has the following pulmonary artery catheter values: cardiac index 5.0, systemic vascular resistance 500, and wedge pressure of 7. This is most consistent with:
   a. Septic shock
   b. Hypovolemic shock
   c. Cardiogenic shock
   d. Neurogenic shock

   Answer a. An elevated cardiac index of 5, a low SVR of 500, and a wedge pressure of 7 suggests **septic shock**.

201. **A critical care patient has the following pulmonary artery catheter values: cardiac index 2.0, systemic vascular resistance 500, and wedge pressure of 5. This is most consistent with:
   a. Septic shock (early)
   b. Hypovolemic shock
   c. Cardiogenic shock
   d. Neurogenic shock

   Answer d. A cardiac index of 2.0, SVR of 500, and wedge pressure of 5 is most consistent with **neurogenic shock**. (note that late, end stage septic shock could present like this as the heart starts to give out but the answer above states early septic shock).

202. **A 38 yo woman in the ICU 2 weeks after a severe episode of hemorrhagic pancreatitis w/ pancreatic abscess requiring open debridement is now septic and suffering ARDS. Despite fluid resuscitation (CVP 18) and pressors (Levophed and vasopressin) her SBP remain in the 80's. Her electrolytes show a Na of 130 K of 5.3, Ca of 8 and Hgb 8. The most appropriate next step in management is:
   a. Dexamethasone
   b. Add another pressor
   c. Calcium
   d. Blood transfusion

   Answer a. **The pt is likely suffering from relative *acute adrenal insufficiency* based on the clinical scenario. Dexamethasone is indicated while a corticotropin stimulation test is performed.*

203. **The most sensitive test for adrenal insufficiency is:
   a. ACTH stimulation test
   b. 24 urine cortisol
   c. Random serum cortisol
   d. Serum ACTH level

   Answer a. ***The most sensitive test for adrenal insufficiency is the corticotropin (ACTH) stimulation test.*

204. *Each of the following drugs causes stimulation of adenylate cyclase except:
   a. Dopamine
   b. Dobutamine
   c. Epinephrine
   d. Milrinone

   Answer d. *Milrinone works by inhibiting **cAMP phosphodiesterase** (which increases cAMP).* Milrinone is not subject to receptor down-regulation with prolonged use. Dopamine, epinephrine, and dobutamine are all beta-agonists and stimulate **adenylate cyclase** to increase cAMP and are subject to receptor down-regulation.

205. **All of the following are true of nitric oxide except:
    a.   Increases cAMP
    b.   The precursor is arginine
    c.   It is primarily released from vascular endothelium
    d.   Inducible nitric oxide synthetase is involved in hypotension w/ sepsis

Answer a. *Arginine* is the precursor to **nitric oxide**. NO acts on *guanylate cyclase* to increase **cGMP** and cause **vasodilatation**. **Inducible nitric oxide synthetase* is involved in **hypotension w/ sepsis**

206. *All of the following are true of intra-aortic balloon pumps (IABPs) except:
    a.   The tip should be placed 2-3 cm below the aortic arch
    b.   Inflation occurs with T wave and deflation on P wave
    c.   Improvement in coronary blood flow is primarily due to diastolic augmentation
    d.   The IABP is inflated during systole

Answer d. The IABP is *deflated* during systole to help reduce afterload. Coronary perfusion to the heart occurs primarily during diastole. During diastole, the IABP inflates and improves perfusion to the coronaries.

207. Which of the following is most renal protective for patient's with renal insufficiency receiving a dye load:
    a.   ASA
    b.   Pre-dye load hydration
    c.   HCO3-
    d.   N-acetylcysteine

Answer b. *Pre-dye **hydration** has been shown to be the most renal protective measure in pts w/ an elevated creatnine receiving a dye load.* **HCO3-** and **N-acetylcysteine** are also effective protective agents.

208. **All of the following are true except::
    a.   The MCC of acute renal failure (or oliguria refractory to fluid challenge) post-op (eg following AAA repair) is hypotension intra-op.
    b.   Renin converts angiotensinogen to angiotensin I
    c.   Angiotensin converting enzyme (ACE) converts angiotensin I to angiotensin II
    d.   The highest concentration of ACE is in the liver

Answer d. The highest concentration of ACE is in the **lung**. **The MCC of acute renal failure (or oliguria refractory to fluid challenge) post-op is hypotension intra-op.* **Renin* converts angiotensinogen to angiotensin I

209. All of the following are true of aldosterone except:
    a.   Causes reabsorption of Na
    b.   Causes excretion of H and K ions
    c.   Acts at the distal convoluted tubule
    d.   Primarily acts on protein kinase C

Answer d. Aldosterone causes the resorption of Na and excretion of H and K at the distal convoluted tubule by stimulating the **transcription** of Na/K ATPase and Na/H ATPase. This causes **water reabsorption**.

210. *A patient stops making urine after surgery. All of the following values are consistent with pre-renal renal failure except:
    a.   Urine Na 5
    b.   BUN/Cr ratio 35
    c.   FeNa = 0.1%
    d.   Urine osmolality 200 mOsm

Answer d. Urine osmolality > 500 mOsm consistent w/ pre-renal Azotemia *FeNa is the most sensitive test for acute renal failure.*

211. *FeNa is:
    a. [(Urine creatnine/Plasma creatnine) / (Urine sodium/Plasma sodium)]
    b. [(Urine sodium/Plasma sodium) / (Urine creatnine/Plasma creatnine)]
    c. [(Plasma sodium/Urine sodium) / (Urine creatnine/Plasma creatnine)]
    d. [(Urine sodium/Plasma sodium) / (Plasma creatnine/Urine creatnine)]

    Answer b. This is the formula for FeNa.

212. *The mechanism of activated protein C in the treatment of patients with multi-system organ failure and sepsis is:
    a. Activation of the clotting cascade
    b. Platelet inhibition
    c. Platelet activation
    d. Fibrinolysis

    Answer d. Activated protein C increases **fibrinolysis**.

213. *While trying to treat a pt with severe ARDS, you increase the PEEP to improve oxygenation. After doing this, you notice a decrease in urine output. The mechanism of decreased urine output with increased PEEP is:
    a. Compartment syndrome
    b. Decreased cardiac output (C.O.)
    c. Reduced oxygenation
    d. Retained CO_2

    Answer b. *Progressively increasing **PEEP** will compress the SVC and IVC, leading to decreased right atrial filling and **decreased C.O.***

214. **PEEP improves oxygenation by:
    a. Increasing functional residual capacity
    b. Increasing tidal volumes
    c. Increasing respiratory rate
    d. Increasing residual volume

    Answer a. Positive end expiratory pressure **(PEEP)** improves oxygenation by improving **functional residual capacity** (FRC). This effectively keeps alveoli open at the end of the breath so oxygen exchange can continue.

215. *All of the following are true of lung dead space except:
    a. Refers mostly to the conductance portion of the airway
    b. Is about 150 ml in most adults
    c. Refers to areas that are ventilated and not perfused
    d. Refers to areas that are perfused but not ventilated

    Answer d. Dead space is the area of lung that is ventilated but not perfused. In normal individuals, this is about 150 cc and refers mostly to the conduction portion of the airways (everything proximal to the respiratory bronchioles). Pathology which can increase dead space includes excessive PEEP (collapses the alveolar capillaries), PE, ARDS, and pulmonary hypertension. Increased dead space can lead to *CO_2 build-up.*

216. **All of the following are true except:
    a. Vital capacity is the maximal amount of air exhaled after a normal inhalation.
    b. Residual volume is the volume of air left in the lung after maximal exhalation.

c. Tidal volume is the volume of air exhaled with normal inspiration and exhalation.
d. Functional residual capacity is the volume of air left in the lung after a normal exhalation

Answer a. **Vital capacity** *is the maximal amount of air exhaled after a maximal inhalation.*

*****Residual volume** *is the volume of air left in the lung after maximal exhalation.*
*****Tidal volume** *is the volume of air exhaled with normal inspiration and exhalation.*
*****Functional residual capacity** *is the volume of air left in the lung after a normal exhalation*

217. *Post-op day 1 after a right upper lobectomy, your pt has a fever to 102.0. The most likely source of the fever is:
    a. PMNs
    b. Platelets
    c. Macrophages
    d. Lymphocytes

Answer c. *Alveolar macrophages* *are activated w/ atelectasis and release of IL-1, which acts on the hypothalamus to cause* **fever**.

218. **A patient with severe pancreatitis develops diffuse pulmonary infiltrates, hypoxemia, and eventually requires intubation. All of the following are true of the patients condition except:
    a. High plateau pressures improve patient outcome.
    b. Diffuse bilateral pulmonary infiltrates versus uni-lateral infiltrate suggests ARDS over pneumonia
    c. Diffuse bilateral pulmonary infiltrates with <u>low filling pressures</u> suggests ARDS over cardiogenic pulmonary edema
    d. Reducing barotrauma by lowering tidal volumes and allowing permissive hypercapnea has improved the outcome for ARDS

Answer a. Acute Respiratory Distress Syndrome **(ARDS)** can result from various issues (eg pancreatitis, shock, sepsis, etc.).

ARDS is characterized by impaired gas exchange leading to hypoxemia and diffuse infiltrates on CXR. **Maintaining low plateau pressures *w/* **permissive hypercapnea** *is a key principle for ARDS tx.*

**Diffuse bilateral pulmonary infiltrates versus uni-lateral infiltrate suggests ARDS over pneumonia.

**Diffuse bilateral pulmonary infiltrates with <u>low filling pressures</u> suggests ARDS over cardiogenic pulmonary edema.

******Reducing barotrauma** *by lowering tidal volumes and allowing* **permissive hypercapnea** *has improved the outcome for ARDS.*

219. **A 35 yo woman undergoing routine laparoscopic bilateral tubal ligation develops severe hypotension, tachycardia, and a drop in end-tidal CO2. The pt still has bilateral breath sounds. The most likely Dx is:
    a. A disconnection between the patient and the ventilator
    b. The patient has developed atelectasis
    c. Myocardial infarction
    d. CO2 embolus

Answer d. End tidal CO2 specifically reflects the exchange of CO_2 from blood to the alveolus. A gradual rise in ET-CO2 usually reflects impaired exchange from lung collapse or atelectasis.

A sudden drop in ETCO2 can be from something simple like disconnection from the ventilator or something more serious such as an embolus. The abrupt drop in ETCO2 following an embolus is from the interruption of CO_2 exchange at the alveolar level. Because of the hypotension associated with a drop in ETCO2 in the above pt, the most likely Dx is CO_2 embolus.

220. **Tx of the above problem involves removing the abdominal insufflation and:
    a.   Emergent TPA therapy
    b.   Coronary catheterization
    c.   Bilateral chest tubes
    d.   Trendelenburg, left side down, and 100% oxygen

Answer d. **Tx of CO2 embolus involves stopping insufflation** (1st step), placing pt in **trendelenburg** position w/ **left side down** (prevents any more propagation of CO2 into lungs) and then **ventilating w/ 100% oxygen**.

221. *A 50 yo woman undergoing laparoscopic tubal ligation has a sudden drop in her end-tidal CO2. The anesthesiologist states he cannot hear any breath sounds. Her blood pressure is 120/60 and her HR is 70. The most likely diagnosis is:
    a.   A disconnection between the patient and the ventilator
    b.   The patient has developed atelectasis
    c.   Myocardial infarction
    d.   CO2 embolus

Answer a. Because this patient is totally stable, the most likely cause of the decreased ETCO2 is **disconnection from the ventilator**.

222. *A 50 yo woman undergoing routine laparoscopic bilateral tubal ligation has a sudden rise in end-tidal CO2. The anesthesiologist states that the pts breath sounds are present but are decreased in both the bases. Her blood pressure is 120/60 and her HR is 70. The most likely diagnosis is:
    a.   A disconnection between the patient and the ventilator
    b.   The patient has developed atelectasis
    c.   Myocardial infarction
    d.   CO2 embolus

Answer b. The most likely cause of the rise in ETCO2 is **atelectasis**. The patient needs larger tidal volumes.

223. *All of the following are true except:
    a.   Presence of deep tendon reflexes precludes diagnosis of brain death
    b.   A positive test for apnea is consistent with brain death
    c.   Absent oculocephalic reflex is consistent with brain death
    d.   Fixed and dilated pupils is consistent with brain death

Answer a. *You can still have **brain death** w/ intact deep tendon reflexes

224. *A 27 yo man is in the ICU 6 hours after splenectomy following a MVA. The pt had a prolonged transport time and received 10 units of blood prior to arrival and 5 liters of crystalloid. You are having trouble ventilating the pt. Currently, his peak airway pressures are 70 (plateaus 50), his abdomen is distended, he is not making any urine, and his bladder pressure is 40. His CVP is 15 and his BP is 85/40. The most appropriate maneuver in this patient is:
    a.   Increase PEEP
    b.   Volume resuscitation
    c.   Decompressive laparotomy
    d.   CT scan

Answer c. This patient has classic signs of **abdominal compartment syndrome**. Tx - <u>decompressive laparotomy</u>

225. *A 25 yo woman involved in a MVA has a severe posterior hepatic laceration that you are trying to treat with damage control. You pack the area off and head to the ICU. She has received 20 units of blood, 10 FFP, and 10 platelets but remains hypotensive (BP 80/40). Her hematocrit is stable at 30. The most likely cause of her persistent hypotension is:
   a. Cardiac tamponade
   b. Sepsis
   c. Low calcium
   d. Low magnesium

   Answer c. Low calcium can occur after massive transfusion. This in turn can cause hypotension.

226. **All of the following are true except:
   a. A hyperechogenic focus w/ posterior shadowing on U/S is consistent w/ a gallstone
   b. Respiratory acidosis w/ laparoscopy can be reduced by decreasing pneumoperitoneum pressure and by increasing minute ventilation
   c. Pneumoperitoneum will increase renin production
   d. Reperfusion injury is mediated primarily by lymphocytes

   Answer d. Reperfusion injury is mediated primarily by **PMNs**.
   Respiratory acidosis w/ laparoscopy can be reduced by **decreasing pneumoperitoneum pressure** and by **increasing minute ventilation**
   Pneumoperitoneum compresses the IVC, decreases venous return to the heart, lowers C.O. and BP which is sensed by the kidney, and results in increased **renin** production

227. *All of the following are true except:
   a. Tx for nipride toxicity is amyl nitrate, then sodium nitrite
   b. Tx for methemoglobinemia is methylene blue
   c. Tx for carbon monoxide poisoning is primarily amyl nitrate
   d. Methemoglobinemia results in a right shift

   Answer c. *The Tx for **CO poisoning** is **intubation w/ 100% oxygen***

Hemodynamics
Mean arterial pressure = C.O. x SVR
Cardiac output (CO) = HR x stroke volume
Cardiac index (C.I.) = CO / BSA
Systemic vascular resistance (SVR) = 80 x [(MAP – CVP) / CO]
Cardiac Output - <u>Kidney</u> gets 25%, <u>Brain</u> gets 15%, <u>Heart</u> gets 5%
Preload – pressure stretching the ventricle of the heart
    Linearly related to left ventricular end-diastolic **volume** (**L**VEDV)
    Wedge pressure – used as a measurement of preload
    Starling's Law – the greater volume of blood entering the heart (LVEDV), the greater the ejection (stroke volume or ejection fraction); termed **right shift along curve** – at some point along the curve, increased volume no longer increases ejection and can worsen it (<u>over-distension</u> → **extreme right shift on Starling curve**)
Afterload – tension produced by the heart in order to contract
    Related to the resistance (ie SVR) against the ventricle contracting
    High SVR – hard for the ventricle to contract
    Low SVR – easier for the ventricle to contract
Stroke volume = LVEDV – LVESV
    Is determined by LVEDV, contractility and afterload

LVEDV – determined by preload and distensibility of ventricle
LVESV (LV end-systolic volume) – determined by contractility and afterload
Ejection fraction = stroke volume / LVEDV

Oxygen delivery and consumption

*O_2 delivery
  = C.O. x arterial O_2 content (CaO_2) x 10
  = C.O. x [Hgb x 1.34 x O_2 saturation + (pO_2 x 0.003)] x 10
**O_2 consumption (VO_2; Fick equation)* -
  = C.O. x ($CaO_2 - CvO_2$); CvO_2 = venous O_2 content (mmHg)
Normal O_2 delivery to O_2 consumption ratio is 4:1 (25% utilized; **SvO_2 75%**)
  Thus there is 4 x more oxygen delivered then used
  C.O. will increase to keep ratio constant
  O_2 consumption is normally **supply independent**
Most impt determinant of myocardial O_2 consumption (energy expenditure) – **wall tension** (followed by heart rate, contractility)
Oxygen-Hgb dissociation curve
  1) **Right Shift** (decreased O_2 affinity, p50 increases) – ↑ CO_2 (Bohr effect), ↑ temp, ATP, 2,3-DPG, ↓ pH, methemoglobinemia
  2) **Left shift** (increased O_2 affinity, p50 decreases) – opposite above, fetal Hgb, carbon monoxide poisoning
  Normal p50 (O_2 tension w/ 50% of O_2 receptors saturated) = 27mmHg
*Mixed Venous Saturation (SvO_2 pulmonary artery catheter)
  Oxygen saturation of mixed venous blood (nl 75% ± 5), measurement taken in pulmonary artery (allows mixing), assesses tissue oxygenation
  1) **Elevated SvO_2** – shunting of blood or decreased O_2 extraction (eg septic shock, cirrhosis, cyanide toxicity, hypothermia, paralysis, coma, sedation)
  2) **Decreased SvO_2** – occurs with:
     Increased O_2 extraction (eg malignant hyperthermia) or;
     Decreased O_2 delivery (eg hypoxia, cardiogenic shock, low Hct)
Bronchial blood flow becomes unsaturated after delivery to bronchus and lung tissue, then empties into pulmonary veins; thus, left ventricle blood pO_2 is 5 mmHg lower than pulmonary capillaries
Coronary sinus blood (ie coronary venous blood) – has lowest venous oxygen saturation in body (**30%**)
Renal veins – have highest venous oxygen saturation in body (**80%**); receives 25% of C.O. but does not have high oxygen expenditure
Pulse oximeter – reads Hgb-O2 as **red** and unbound Hgb as **infrared** (Red / Red + Infrared) x 100 = % sat
  Pulse oximeter **miss-reads** - nail polish, dark skin, low cardiac output, ambient light, low Hct, hypothermia, carbon monoxide
During hypoxia, blood is shunted to the heart and brain
*Shock = inadequate tissue oxygenation (most basic definition)

Pulmonary artery catheters (PA catheter)
Inaccurate measurements can be caused by:
  1) PA catheter **not in lung zone III** (lower lobes)
  2) **Wedge pressure > LA pressure** (mediastinal fibrosis, pulmonary vein obstruction, pulmonary HTN, high PEEP – compresses pulmonary veins)
  3) **LA pressure > LV end diastolic pressure** (mitral regurgitation, mitral stenosis)
*PA catheter distances to wedge (apx):
  *R SCV   45 cm
  R IJ   50 cm
  L SCV   55 cm
  L IJ   60 cm

If distance much longer/shorter than expected (ie 8 cm) → in wrong
place or have loop
Optimal lung placement for PA catheter – **zone III** *(lower lobes)*
Has **less respiratory influence** *on measurements*
Wedge measurements are taken at *end-expiration*
Contraindications
> **Absolute** – right sided endocarditis or thrombus, right mechanical
> heart valve
> **Relative** – coagulopathy (reverse), recent pacemaker (use fluoro),
> left bundle branch block (can cause complete heart block)

High PEEP:
> 1) Can affect wedge measurements
>> Subtract 1/2 the PEEP from wedge value if PEEP > 10
> 2) Can cause **decreased C.O.** from **decreased *right atrium* filling**
>> (main mechanism); **high PEEP causes poor UOP due to
>> decreased C.O.** *(will also increase* **renin**)

Pulmonary vascular resistance *(PVR) can be measured* only *using a
PA catheter (*not *measured w/ ECHO)*
Diabetics – have increased SVR from arteriopathy

	Swan Numbers (normal)
Cardiac output (C.O.)	4–8 L/min
Cardiac index (C.I.)	2.5–4 L/min
Systemic vascular resistance (SVR)	800-1400 (**1100**)
Pulmonary capillary wedge pressure (wedge)	7-**11**
Central venous pressure (CVP)	**7**
Mixed venous oxygen saturation (SvO$_2$)	**75%** ± 5

Types of Shock	CVP and wedge	C.I.	SVR	SvO$_2$
1) Hemorrhagic	↓	↓	↑	↓
2) Septic (hyperdynamic)	↓ (MC)	↑	↓	↑
3) Cardiogenic (eg MI)	↑	↓	↑	↓
4) Cardiac Tamponade	↑	↓	↑	↓
5) Neurogenic	↓	↓	↓	↑
6) Adrenal Insufficiency	↓ (MC)	↓	↓	↓
7) Pulmonary Embolus	↑	↓	↑	↓

1) **Hemorrhagic** *shock* – initial response is an increase in diastolic
pressure; Tx: volume (LR, then blood in trauma pts)
2) **Septic shock**
> Sx's: Initial sepsis (early) - **mental status changes** *(eg confusion)*
> **hyperventilation** *(resp alkalosis)* + **hypotension** *(classic triad)*
>> **Hyperglycemia** – common early sign before clinical sepsis
>>> **Early** sepsis – ↓ insulin, ↑ glucose (impaired utilization)
>>> **Late** sepsis – ↑ insulin, ↑ glucose (insulin resistance)
> Tx: **abx's**, **volume**, **Levophed** (NE, **best pressor Tx** for septic
> shock); **Vasopressin** 2nd line agent; **Consider testing for
> adrenal insufficiency** *if refractory to volume and pressors;
> consider* **activated protein C** *(Xigris) if severe sepsis w/ MSOF
> (causes* **fibrinolysis; cx's** *- bleeding)*

3) **Cardiogenic shock (eg large acute MI, CHF exacerbation)
   Sx's: pulmonary edema (SOB), low C.O.
       Heart can't contract effectively → pulmonary congestion
       Heart also becomes over-distended → worsens contractility
   Tx: **inotrope (best Tx, Dobutamine); morphine, NTG
       Intra-aortic balloon pump if necessary to stabilize (see below)
4) *Cardiac tamponade
   Fluid around heart causes **decreased ventricular filling in
       diastole (mechanism) → results in hypotension
   Sx's: hypotension, jugular venous distention, and muffled heart
       sounds (Beck's triad, complete triad present in minority of pts)
   Dx: Initial ECHO sign of early cardiac tamponade (1st sign) →
       impaired diastolic filling of right atrium (from compression)
   Tx: Drain pericardial fluid (eg pericardiocentesis or pericardial
       window); fluid resuscitation to temporize until fluid drained;
       pericardiocentesis blood does not form clot
5) *Neurogenic shock
   Neuro injury results in loss of sympathetic tone and decreased SVR
   Sx's: low HR, low BP, warm extremities (loss of autonomic tone)
   Tx: Volume 1st , phenylephrine after resuscitated to raise SVR
6) **Acute Adrenal Insufficiency
   Sx's: fever, N/V, abd pain and hypotension (unresponsive to fluid and
       pressors); Causes – withdrawal of exogenous steroids (MCC),
       bilateral adrenal hemorrhage (MC related to sepsis, eg
       Waterhouse-Friderichsen syndrome), adrenalectomy
       **Relative adrenal insufficiency can occur in severely ill critical care
           pts (**hypotension refractory to fluid and pressors)
   Dx: increased ACTH and decreased cortisol (↓ed Na and ↑ed K
       due to low aldosterone)
       Corticotropin stimulation test (best test, ACTH given, cortisol
           measured)
       Baseline cortisol < 15 or change < 9 ug/dl after stimulation
           test = adrenal insufficiency
   Tx: **Dexamethasone (2 mg IV Q 6) + fludrocortisone (50 ug/d)
       *Give prior to corticotropin stimulation test (dexamethasone
           does NOT interfere w/ test)
   Relative potency of steroids
       1 x – cortisone, hydrocortisone
       5 x – prednisone, prednisolone, methyl-prednisolone
       30 x – dexamethasone
7) Pulmonary Embolism (PE)
   Sx's:tachypnea, chest pain; **hypoxia + hypocarbia; ↓ BP + ↑ HR
       MC EKG finding – *SVT
       *Respiratory alkalosis from hyper-ventilation
       Intubated pt – decreased ET-CO2 initial finding
           (sudden decrease in ET-CO2 + hypotension, classic)
       Blood can't get to left side of heart due to PE
   *MC source - *ilio-femoral DVT
   Dx: chest CT angio (99% sensitive); 1/3 have negative LE duplex
       **ECHO - distended right ventricle, under-filled left ventricle
   Tx: volume, inotropes, pressors, heparin; for refractory
       hypotension despite inotropes and pressors, consider suction
       catheter embolectomy or open removal on cardiopulmonary bypass

Receptors
   *Inotropes that directly ↑cAMP – Dopamine, Dobutamine, Epinephrine
       (mostly an inotrope, some pressor activity), Isoproterenol
   *Inotropes that inhibit cAMP phosphodiesterase (indirectly ↑ cAMP)
       Milrinone
   Inotropes that inhibit Na/K transporter - Digoxin

Inotropes (↑ cardiac output)
1) **Dopamine** (1-20 μg/kg/min)
    Low (1-5)   **DA receptors**
    Moderate (6-10)   **Beta-1** and **Beta-2** (↑ contractility + HR)
    High (>10)   **Alpha-1** (vasoconstriction, ↑ MAP)
2) **Dobutamine** (1-20 μg/kg/min); **Beta-1** (contractility)
    some beta-2 (vasodilation) at higher doses (> 15)
3) **Milrinone**
    cAMP phosphodiesterase inhibitor (results in ↑ed cAMP)
    Ca^{++} influx ↑s myocardial **contractility**
    Also a **pulmonary vasodilator** (relaxes vascular smooth muscle)
    **Not** subject to **beta-receptor down-regulation like other
        inotropes** (good for long-term use; eg pts awaiting heart TXP)
        Other drugs lose potency w/ time
4) **Isoproterenol**
    Beta-1 (↑ HR and contractility) and **Beta-2** (vasodilates)
    S/Es: arrhythmogenic; increases heart metabolic demand (rarely
        used); may actually ↓ BP (beta-2)

Pressors (↑SVR and ↑MAP; NE and Epi also inotropic)
1) **Phenylephrine** - **Alpha-1** (vasoconstriction)
2) **Norepinephrine** (NE, Levophed; 1-40 μg/min)
    Predominantly **Alpha-1** and **Alpha-2** (vasoconstriction); some Beta-1
    Acts as a potent **splanchnic vasoconstrictor**
3) **Epinephrine** (1-20 μg/min)
    Low Dose (1-5)   **Beta-1** and **Beta-2**
    High Dose (> 5)   **Alpha-1** and **Alpha-2**
    Can _lower_ blood pressure at low doses (Beta-2 > Beta-1)
4) **Vasopressin** (0.01 - 0.1 U/min); **AVPR-1** receptor; arterial
    vasoconstriction

Vasodilators
1) **Nipride** - NO mediated; predominantly arterial dilatation
    S/E - Cyanide toxicity (at risk if >3 μg/kg/min for 72 hours)
        Check for **metabolic acidosis** and **thiocyanate** level
        Cyanide binds to cytochrome c in mitochondria and **disrupts
            electron transport chain**; cell cannot use O_2 so you get
            a left to right shunt (↑ SvO_2)
        Tx: **amyl nitrite** 1st, then **sodium nitrite; hydroxy-cobalamin**
2) **Nitroglycerin** - NO mediated; predominantly venodilation, coronary
    artery dilator, decreases **ventricle wall tension** by decreasing pre-
    load
3) **ACE inhibitors** - **decreases angiotensin II** (predominantly results in
    vasodilation and ↓ed aldosterone)
    1) reduce mortality post-MI and 2) prevent CHF post-MI
    Absolute contraindications – previous angioedema, renal artery
        stenosis
    Relative contraindications – impaired renal function, hypovolemia,
        aortic stenosis
    S/Es – cough, angioedema
5) _Inhaled_ **NO** - pulmonary vasodilator (soluble guanylate cyclase receptor)
    Also called **endothelium-derived relaxing factor** (EDRF)
6) **Sildenafil** (Viagra) – pulmonary vasodilator (NO mediated)

*_Intra-aortic balloon pump_ (IABP)
    Sequence:
        Inflation – on **T wave** (diastole)
        Deflation – on **P wave** or start of **Q wave** (systole)
    Tip should be just distal to left subclavian (2 cm below top of arch)
    Effects:
        Improves MAP (inflation w/ ventricular diastole)

Improves diastolic coronary perfusion (coronaries fill in diastole and ↑ed diastolic MAP improves coronary perfusion)
Decreases afterload (deflation w/ ventricular systole)
IABP Indications:
1) **Cardiogenic shock** post-MI
2) **Ventricular septal rupture** (VSR) post-MI
3) **Acute mitral regurgitation** (MR, eg ruptured papillary muscle either spontaneously or post-MI)
4) **Unstable angina** (improves coronary flow)
5) Pre-op before high risk cardiac surgery (eg pts w/ low EF)
Has increased survival following 1) VSR and 2) acute MR
Absolute contraindications – aortic regurgitation, aortic dissection, severe aorto-iliac occlusive DZ
Relative contraindications – vascular grafts in aorta; aortic aneurysms

Atrial fibrillation is the MCC of delayed discharge after cardiac surgery
Magnesium is used to Tx **torsades de pointes** (a type of ventricular tachycardia)

Kidneys *(renal system)*
   *Renin-Angiotensin System
       Glomerular filtration rate (GFR) is controlled by the **efferent limb**
       Renin *(*released from **kidney***)
           Release caused by:
               ↓ed **pressure** sensed by **juxta-glomerular apparatus**
               ↑ed **sodium** concentration sensed by **macula densa**
               Additional releasing factors - Beta-2 receptor, ↑ed K^+
           Inhibition of release – ↓ed K^+
           ***Renin* converts **angiotensinogen** *(synthesized in **liver**) to angiotensin I*
       Angiotensin converting enzyme (ACE, *in **lung***)
           Converts angiotensin I to angiotensin II
           ACE inhibitors work here; ACE also breaks down **bradykinin**
       Angiotensin II effects (binds AG II receptor):
           Primary effect – *release of **aldosterone** from **adrenal cortex***
           Secondary effects:
               1) **Vasoconstrictor** (potent, ↓s renal blood flow), ↑s BP
               2) ↑ed **sympathetic tone** (↑ed HR and contractility)
               3) **Release of ADH** (vasopressin, posterior pituitary)
       Aldosterone (steroid hormone)
           Upregulates Na^+/K^+ **ATPase** in *distal convoluted tubule* (cell membrane)→ Na^+ and **water reabsorption**; K^+ **excretion**
           Also upregulates Na^+/H^+ **exchanger**→ H^+ excretion (can get metabolic alkalosis)
           Hyperkalemia can also stimulate aldosterone release
   Anti-diuretic hormone (ADH; vasopressin)
       Released by posterior pituitary gland when **osmolality** is high
       Acts on *collecting ducts* for **water resorption**
       Also a **vasoconstrictor**
   Renal Toxic Drugs
       *NSAIDs - inhibit prostaglandin synthesis**, causes renal arteriole vasoconstriction
       *Aminoglycosides, contrast dyes** and myoglobin – direct injury to renal tubules
   Electrolyte abnormalities w/ renal failure - volume overload, ↓ed Na^+ + Ca^{++}; ↑ed K^+, urea, Mg^{++} + $PO4^-$, *Avoid* Mg antacids / laxatives
   Indications for dialysis: 1) fluid overload, 2)↑ed K^+, Mg^{++}, $PO4^-$
       3) metabolic acidosis, 4) uremic encephalopathy (really high BUN), 5) uremic coagulopathy, 6) poisoning
   Hemodialysis – can cause **hypotension** from large volume shifts
       Hct increases 5–8 for each liter taken off

CVVH – slower then HD, good for pts that cannot tolerate volume shifts
Elevated creatinine in pt needing contrast dye (eg CT scan or
    angiogram)
    1) **Pre-op hydration** – *most renal protective measure*
    2) **HCO3⁻ drip** (next best Tx), **N-acetylcysteine**
    Note - gadolinium for MRI can cause **contrast nephropathy and*
            nephrogenic systemic fibrosis** in pts w/ **renal insufficiency
    Can use **CO_2 angiogram** (contrast not as good, less renal toxic)
Myoglobinuria
    Released from muscle after trauma (eg crush injury) or compartment
        syndrome
    Myoglobin converted to **ferrihemate** in acid environment (renal toxic)
    Tx: **fluids** *(best)* + **HCO3⁻** to alkalinize urine (prevents conversion)

**Poor urine output post-op (oliguria, rising Cr; acute renal failure)
    Try fluid challenge (1-2 L LR or NS) and/or **lasix challenge
    *Dx studies:
        FeNa – fractional excretion of Na
            **Best test for acute renal failure (azotemia)
        FeNa = (urine Na/Cr) / (plasma Na/Cr)
            Pre-renal: FeNa < 1%, urine Na < 20, BUN/Cr ratio > 20
                Urine osmolality > 500 mOsm (concentrated)
            Renal (ie ATN): FeNa > 2% and opposite above
        ARF (acute renal failure, ↑ Cr ≥ 0.5); 70% of renal mass must be
            damaged before ↑ Cr and BUN
    Use above to figure out cause:
        1) **Pre-renal** oliguria / ARF - Tx: Optimize **volume**
        2) **Renal** oliguria / ARF (ATN, acute tubular necrosis)
            *****MCC renal ATN** – hypotension intra-op*
            Tx: **Diuretic** trial (Lasix and Mannitol); try to make **non-oliguric**
        3) **Post-renal** oliguria / ARF (ureteral obstruction)
            Renal U/S shows **hydronephrosis**; Tx: **relieve obstruction**

    **MCC post-op poor UOP – *hypovolemia*
    **MCC post-op ARF – *hypotension (MC intra-op), resulting in ATN (eg s/p*
    open AAA repair now w/ oliguria despite fluid resuscitation)

<u>Pulmonary Function Tests</u> (PFTs)
    Lung Measurements
        Total lung capacity (TLC)
            Lung volume after maximal inspiration
            TLC = VC + RV
        *****Vital capacity** (VC)*
            Volume of air w/ maximal exhalation after maximal inhalation
        *Residual volume (RV)
            Lung volume after maximal expiration (comprises 20% of TLC)
        *Tidal volume (TV)
            Volume of air w/ a normal inspiration and expiration
        *****Functional residual capacity** (FRC)*
            Lung volume after normal exhalation
            FRC = ERV + RV
            Surgery (atelectasis), sepsis (ARDS), and trauma (contusion,
                atelectasis, ARDS) – *all ↓ FRC*
            **PEEP increases FRC
        Expiratory reserve volume (ERV)
            Volume of air forcefully expired after normal expiration
        Inspiratory capacity
            Maximum amount of air breathed in after normal exhalation
        FEV_1 – forced expiratory volume in 1 sec (after maximal inhalation)
        Minute ventilation = tidal volume x resp rate
        *Compliance = (change in lung volume) / (change in lung pressure)

High compliance - lungs easy to ventilate (eg COPD)
Low compliance - lungs hard to ventilate (eg ARDS, fibrotic lung diseases, reperfusion injury, pulmonary edema)
Ventilation to perfusion ratio (V/Q ratio)
Normally highest in upper lobes, lowest in lower lobes
Dead space
Part of lung that is ventilated but <u>not</u> perfused
Normally, dead space is the airway to level of the bronchiole (comprises 150 ml; conductive airways)
Causes of increased dead space – ↓ed C.O. (capillary collapse), PE, pulmonary HTN, ARDS (edema compresses capillaries), excessive PEEP (capillary compression)
Increased dead space leads to **increased pCO_2**
V/Q mismatch (poor ventilation but good perfusion)
MCC – atelectasis; others – ARDS

Pulmonary vasodilators – prostacyclin, nitric oxide
Pulmonary vasoconstrictors – **hypoxia** (very potent), acidosis
Pulmonary shunting can be caused by – nipride, nitroglycerin, nifedipine
Manifests as **hypoxia**

<u>Ventilator</u>
Improving Oxygenation →
↑ PEEP – improves **functional residual capacity** (FRC; *best initial method to ↑ pO_2*); causes alveolar recruitment
↑ FIO_2 – NOT as effective as ↑ed PEEP
Excessive PEEP Cx's:
↓ed **right atrial filling** → ↓ed C.O. → ↓ renal blood flow→ ↓ **UOP** (***main mechanism of ↓ed UOP w/ ↑ed PEEP is low C.O.*); also results in increased **renin**
↑ed **pulmonary vascular resistance** (pulmonary capillary compression)
↑s **wedge pressure**
Improving Ventilation (removing CO_2)
↑ respiratory rate
↑ tidal volume
Pressure support – decreases work of breathing (inspiratory pressure held constant until minimum tidal volume is achieved)
Barotrauma – prevent by keeping *plateau pressures* **< 30** (most important) and peaks < 50
*Increasing inspiratory time (**inverse ratio ventilation**) can result in significant *auto-PEEP* because lungs are not given enough time to exhale (stacking breaths, results in barotrauma or decreased C.O. from decreased right atrial filling)
Normal inspiration to expiration time ratio (I:E ratio) is **1 : 3**

<u>Atelectasis</u> (from alveolar hypoventilation)
Bronchial obstruction and ↓ed respiratory effort main causes
MCC of fever in 1st 48 hours *after abdominal or lung* **surgery**
Sx's: fever, tachycardia; *Fever caused by release of **IL-1** (acts at hypothalamus) from *alveolar macrophages*
Tx: incentive spirometer, pain control

<u>ARDS</u> (Acute Respiratory Distress Syndrome)
Direct causes – **pneumonia** (MCC overall, 40%), aspiration (15%),
Indirect causes – sepsis (25%), shock, DIC, pancreatitis, trauma
Criteria *(see below)*
Impaired gas exchange + inflammatory mediator release causes **MSOF**
***PMN's** have a prominent role in ARDS w/ **inflammation** of lung parenchyma

Reducing barotrauma by using **permissive hypercapnea and low tidal
volumes has **improved outcome for ARDS**

Permissive hypercapnea - increases **inspiratory time** (to improve
oxygenation at the expense of expiratory time (causes pCO2 to rise)

Correct pH to > 7.30 (give HCO3⁻, may be able to ↑ RR)

Avoid FiO₂ > 60% for > 24 hrs - causes **O2 radical induced lung injury

**DDx: ARDS vs VAP vs PE vs CHF

Ventilator Associated Pneumonia Criteria (VAP)
1) New unilateral infiltrate
2) Fever
3) Purulent sputum (consider bronchoalveolar lavage)
4) > 48 hours on ventilator

Pulmonary Embolus Findings
1) Normal CXR (sometimes have wedge shaped infarct)
2) Hypoxemia *and* hypocarbia
3) Sudden onset
4) Predisposing condition

ARDS
1) Acute onset
2) Bilateral diffuse patchy air space disease (CXR)
3) ***Absence of heart failure* (Wedge < 18, normal PA pressures)
4) PO2/FiO2 < 300

CHF
1) bilateral pulmonary edema, cardiomegaly
2) ***elevated filling pressures* (wedge > 18)

**SIRS (Systemic Inflammatory Response Syndrome)
MC etiology – infection (eg bacteremia, PNA)

Non-infectious etiologies – severe trauma, shock (any form),
anaphylaxis, burns, acute pancreatitis

***All mediated by massive **TNF-alpha** and **IL-1** cytokine release*

***Most potent stimulant for SIRS* (TNF-alpha release) – **GNR endotoxin**
(lipopolysaccharide – lipid A portion)

Criteria for SIRS (need ≥ 2):

Temp	> 38°C or <36°C
HR	> 90 (or on pressors)
RR	> 20 (or requiring intubation)
pCO₂	< 32 mmHg
WBC	> 12 or < 4

Can lead to **hypotension, shock, MSOF** (eg ARDS, ARF, liver failure,
cardiac failure) and **death**

Tx: **Identify** and **treat underlying cause; ICU care**

**Sepsis = SIRS + infection
Hyperglycemia – often occurs *just before* clinical sepsis

***Optimal glucose level in septic pts** – 80-120

Sepsis causes inflammation, hypercoaguability, and decreased
fibrinolysis

SIRS + infection + hypotension = **septic shock**

****Hypotension** w/ septic shock related to up-regulation of **inducible nitric
oxide synthase** (iNOS)

**Air embolus (CO₂ embolus similar)
MC occurs w/ sucking air through **central line or central line site**

CO₂ embolus can occur w/ **laparoscopic** procedures (eg laparoscopic
cholecystectomy)

Sx's: **sudden ↓ in ET-CO2, hypotension** and **tachycardia** (*classic*)
May have 'mill wheel' murmur

Can lodge in RA, RV, and/or pulmonary arteries causing **air lock,**
which **prevents venous return**

**Tx:
 1st step – *Stop insufflation* if laparoscopic procedure
 Trendelenburg (head down)
 Left lateral decubitus position (keeps air in RA and RV)
 Give **100% oxygen** (comes into equilibrium w/ embolus and is
  reabsorbed faster) – *stop nitrous oxide (doesn't diffuse quickly)*
 Hyperventilation (↑ minute ventilation, RR x TV)
  ↓s blood pCO2, which ↑s gradient for CO2 or air to diffuse
 Prolonged CPR if needed to allow embolus to be absorbed
 Aspirate central line if present (gets air out of RA)
 Intubate if necessary; **fluid, pressors** and **inotropes** to maintain BP

****Brain death**
EEG – should show electrical silence
MRA or angiogram, not necessary; but should show no brain blood flow
Apnea test - Pt is **disconnected from ventilator** after pre-oxygenation
 (FiO2 100%) and monitored:
 → pCO_2 > 60 mmHg or ↑in CO_2 by 20 is a **positive test for apnea**
 → If arterial pressure drops to < 60 or pt desaturates, test is
  terminated (**negative test for apnea**)
**Can still have deep tendon reflexes (DTRs) w/ brain death

****Abdominal compartment syndrome**
Sx's:
 1) *Distended abdomen*
 2) *Low UOP* (*decreased C.O.* from IVC compression biggest factor,
  also renal vein compression)
 3) *Increased airway pressures* (upward displacement of diaphragm)
Occurs w/ **hypotension** and **massive blood / fluid resuscitation** due to
 trauma (esp w/ prolonged transport time) and abd surgery →
 abdominal contents become swollen and compress IVC
**IVC compression (leading to decreased venous return) is the final
 common pathway for ****decreased C.O.**
Dx: ****bladder pressure > 20** (hook foley up to CVP monitor)
Cx's: gut malperfusion, poor ventilation
Tx: *decompressive laparotomy*, sterile cover for abdominal contents
Can't get abdomen closed after operation because of swollen bowel
 → cut sterile IV bag and sew to skin; Ioban drape over that; bring
  back in 48 hrs and close abdomen when visceral swelling goes down

*Tx for **nipride toxicity** (cyanide toxicity) is amyl nitrite, followed by sodium
 nitrite; **hydroxy-cobalamine**
*Tx for **methemoglobinemia** is methylene blue
*Tx for **carbon monoxide poisoning** is intubation with 100% oxygen

****CO_2 pneumoperitoneum** (normal 10-15)
Cardiopulmonary dysfunction can occur w/ intra-abdominal pressure **> 20**
Pneumoperitoneum *increases*: pulmonary artery pressure, pulmonary
 vascular resistance, HR, systemic vascular resistance, central
 venous pressure, mean and peak airway pressure, renin, CO_2
**Pneumoperitoneum *decreases*: pH, venous return (IVC compression,
 leads to decreased cardiac output), renal flow (primarily due to
 decreased cardiac output, some from renal vein compression, ****will
 increase renin production**)
Hypovolemia lowers pressure necessary to cause compromise
CO_2 can ↓ in **myocardial contractility**
**Can minimize respiratory acidosis from CO2 pneumoperitoneum by
 decreasing pneumoperitoneum pressure and **increasing minute
 ventilation** (RR or TV)

Surgical technologies
Harmonic scalpel
- Cost-effective for **medium vessels** (short gastric arteries)
- Disrupts **protein hydrogen bonds**, causes **coagulation** of vessels

Ultrasound
- **B-mode** (MC used, B = brightness; assesses relative density of structures); forms 2 dimensional structure
  - *Shadowing – dark area posterior to object indicates mass (eg gallstone, breast fibroadenoma)
  - *Enhancement – brighter area posterior to object, indicates fluid-filled cyst or structure (eg gallbladder, breast cyst)
  - *Lower frequencies – good for deep structures, less resolution
  - **Higher frequencies** – good for superficial structures, more resolution
- **Duplex ultrasound** combines **B mode** and **doppler**; looks at how sound waves bounce off moving objects like blood; gives colored visual description of blood flow (can see velocity, stenosis and direction)

*Acute Gout Flare
- Due to **uric acid** buildup (end product of purine metabolism)
- Sx's: painful arthritis, esp MTP of great toe (podagra), warm, tense
- Dx: needle shaped *negatively bi-refringent crystals*, ↑ WBCs in joint
- Tx: **Acute attacks** – **indomethacin**, **colchicines** (*microtubule inhibitor*, prevents WBC migration), steroids
  - **Allopurinol** (xanthine oxidase inhibitor) – inhibits uric acid synthesis
  - **Probenecid** – inhibits renal reabsorption of uric acid

**Carbon monoxide poisoning (CO)
- **MCC fatal poisoning** (from suicide)
- Binds Hgb and creates **carboxy-hemoglobin** → O_2 can't bind anymore
- **Carbon monoxide has as a greater affinity for Hgb than oxygen (250 x)**
- **Results in a left shift in the oxygen dissociation curve**
  - Hgb will not let go of bound O_2
  - Additionally O_2 has to compete w/ CO for binding sites
- Sx's: ↑ HR, HTN, mental status changes (headache, seizures)
- Dx: **Falsely elevates oxygen saturation reading** on pulse oximeter
  - Abnormal carboxy-hemoglobin
    - **Non-smokers** > 10%
    - **Smokers** > 20%
- **Tx: 100% oxygen on ventilator (best Tx, displaces CO)**

**Methemoglobinemia
- Oxygen carrying ferrous ion (Fe^{2+}) of heme group is oxidized to ferric ion (Fe^{3+}) → forming methemoglobin **which cannot bind oxygen**
- **Results in a right shift is oxygen dissociation curve**
- **Causes** – topical anesthetics for EGD [benzocaine (Hurricaine spray)], dapsone, fertilizers (nitrates) – **all act as oxidizing drugs**
- Sx's: ↑ RR, dyspnea; metabolic lactic acidosis (anaerobic metabolism)
  - **O_2 saturation reads 85%**
- **Tx: oxygen + methylene blue**

Reperfusion injury - Critical role of **PMNs

Burns

228. Each of the following are true of 1st and superficial 2nd degree burns except:
     - a. Epithelialization occurs primarily from hair follicles
     - b. Epithelialization can occur from the edges of the wound
     - c. These usually require skin grafts
     - d. A sunburn is an example of a 1st degree burn

     Answer c. 1st and superficial 2nd degree burns do not require skin grafts.

229. *The primary fuel used in burn wound infections is:
     - a. Protein
     - b. Fatty acids
     - c. Glucose
     - d. Glutamine

     Answer c. Although protein is extremely important for repair of burn wounds, it is the structural component, not the fuel used by the cells. Burn wounds use **glucose** in an obligatory fashion.

230. *A 54 yo man involved in a house fire was trapped in an enclosed space. As you evaluate him, he spits up a fair amount of carbonaceous sputum. You notice upper airway stridor and his throat feels tight. All the following are true except:
     - a. This patient should be intubated
     - b. Lung / tracheal injury is caused by carbonaceous sputum, not heat
     - c. Burn wound infection is the MC infection w severe burns (>30% BSA)
     - d. ETOH is a risk factor for inhalational injury

     Answer c. *Pneumonia* is the MC infection in pts w/ significant burn wounds. In some series, 70% of all pts w/ large burns get pneumonia.

231. *A 28 yo man suffers severe 2nd and 3rd degree burns over 60% of total body surface area. He is intubated and currently undergoing appropriate fluid resuscitation. The patient has 3rd degree burns across his entire chest extending to his back. The patient also has a circumferential burn to his right arm with decreased perfusion to his right hand. The next appropriate step is:
     - a. Escharotomy
     - b. Arm elevation
     - c. Thrombectomy of the right brachial artery
     - d. TPA

     Answer a. Patients with circumferential 2nd and 3rd degree burns and poor distal perfusion should undergo **escharotomy** to that extremity.

     Occasionally for deep burns, escharotomy is not enough because the muscle compartment is involved in the burn and fasciotomy is required. For the arm, opening the dorsal and ventral compartments is required.

     Pts with severe burns **across the chest** can have trouble with ventilation due to decreased chest wall compliance (from both the burn and from edema with subsequent fluid resuscitation). Tx chest escharotomy

     Pts w/ severe burns to the **fingers** and decreased perfusion require **mid-axial incisions** (not lateral – the nerves travel here)P

232. **All of the following are true of fluid resuscitation for burn wounds except:
     - a. Lactated ringers is the fluid of choice
     - b. Aggressive fluid resuscitation is indicated for $\geq$ 2 degree burns over $\geq$ 20% of BSA
     - c. CVP is the best measure of fluid resuscitation
     - d. ½ the volume should be give in the 1st 8 hours

124

Answer c. **Adequate urine output** is the best measure of successful resuscitation (<u>Adults</u> - 0.5 cc/kg/hr, <u>Child</u> - 1 cc/kg/hr.

**Lactated ringers *is the fluid of choice for resuscitation in severe burns.*

**Parkland formula: 4 cc/kg x % burn over 24 hours
Give **1/2 volume in 1st 8 hours,** next **1/2 over 16 hours**
Calculate only for $\geq 2^{nd}$ degree burns that are $\geq 20\%$ BSA

233. *Treatment of patients with severe burn injuries and myoglobinuria consists of:
    a. Broad spectrum antibiotics
    b. Aggressive inotropic support
    c. Fluid resuscitation and HCO3- drip
    d. CVVH to clear the myoglobin

    Answer c. The best Tx for patients with burn injuries and myoglobinuria is fluid resuscitation and HCO3- to prevent precipitation of the myoglobin.

234. *The best way to diagnose burn wound sepsis is:
    a. Culture swab of the wound
    b. Biopsy of the wound
    c. Blood cultures
    d. Examination

    Answer b. The best way to Dx burn wound infection is wound biopsy.

235. *You are getting ready to place a skin graft on a burn area. A burn wound biopsy shows 10^4 staph epidermidis/gram of tissue. The next appropriate step in management is:
    a. Nothing
    b. Broad spectrum antibiotics
    c. Vancomycin
    d. Proceed with auto-grafting

    Answer d. The diagnosis of a burn wound infection requires $> 10^5$ organisms/gram of tissue, otherwise it is considered colonization. The best way to diagnose a burn wound infection is with a burn wound biopsy (avoids contaminates from just swabbing it)

    If there was an **infection present** in the burn wound, in addition to starting antibiotics, going ahead with excising the burn wound (and the infection) and placing a temporary porcine allograft is a reasonable option. *You would <u>not</u> want to place an autograft in this situation.*

236. *The most common organism involved in burn wound infection is:
    a. Staph epidermidis
    b. Pseudomonas
    c. Strep viridans
    d. Klebsiella

    Answer b. Pseudomonas is the MC organism in burn wound sepsis (some recent studies state staph aureus is the MC organism, but pseudomonas has been the classic answer)

237. **All of the following are true except:
    a. Silvadene can result in neutropenia and thrombocytopenia
    b. Silver nitrate can result in methemoglobinemia
    c. Mafenide sulfate can result in metabolic alkalosis
    d. Topical abx's result in decreased burn wound infections

Answer c. ***Sulfamylon (mafenide sulfate) can result in **metabolic acidosis** through inhibition of carbonic anhydrase.*

238. **Skin grafts survive in the 1st 48 hours primary by:
     a. Neovascularization
     b. Reliance on stored glycogen
     c. Gluconeogenesis
     d. Imbibition

     Answer d. ***Skin grafts survive by **imbibition** (osmotic exchange of nutrients) for the 1st 48 hours. After that, neovascularization takes over.*

239. **In comparison of split thickness skin grafts (STSG) to full thickness skin grafts (FTSG), all of the following are true except:
     a. STSG are more likely to survive
     b. FTSG have less wound contraction
     c. FTSG are good for palmar burns
     d. The most common reason for skin graft loss is infection

     Answer d. ***STSG are more likely to survive compared to FTSG because they are thinner and more likely to survive **imbibition** and early neovascularization periods (harder for imbibition to work with thicker grafts).*

     ***The MCC of **skin graft loss** is **seroma** (or hematoma) formation underneath skin graft, which raises it and prevents neovascularization. Make sure skin graft is compressed down w/ xeroform gauze to prevent.*

     ***Donor sites for STSGs heal in **3 weeks** and can be used again*
     ***STSGs are apx 0.15 mm (includes **epidermis** and **part of dermis**)*
     ***FTSGs include the **epidermis** and all of the **dermis** (requires primary closure)*

240. **You bring an intubated 30 yo man with a 60% total body surface burn back to the OR for his 3rd debridement in 3 days and the anesthesiologist gives him succinylcholine. Shortly after this, his EKG shows T wave abnormalities, then a widened QRS, and then asystole. You cannot feel a pulse so you start CPR. The 1st drug you should give for this problem is:
     a. Dantrolene
     b. Calcium chloride
     c. Methylene blue
     d. Atropine

     Answer b. Burn patients are at increased risk for **hyperkalemia** because of myonecrosis and leaking of potassium into the blood stream. This, combined with succinylcholine which causes potassium release when it depolarizes the cell membrane, results in hyperkalemia. ***The 1st Tx of choice for **hyperkalemia** with arrhythmias is **calcium.***

241. **All of the following are true except:
     a. Seizures following burn wounds are MC due to infection
     b. Ectopia is best treated w/ surgical release
     c. Hydrofluoric acid burns are best treated w/ calcium (topical, intra-arterial)
     d. Steroids are contraindicated in Toxic Epidermal Necrolysis

     Answer a. Seizures following burn wounds are MC due to **hyponatremia** related to fluid resuscitation

     *****Hydrofluoric acid** burns best Tx - **calcium** (topical, intra-arterial)*
     Steroids are <u>contraindicated</u> in **Toxic Epidermal Necrolysis

*Burns Wounds
    1st degree - sunburn (epidermis)
    2nd degree
        Superficial dermis (papillary) - painful; blebs and blisters; hair follicles
            intact; blanches to touch (heals in 2 weeks)
        Deep dermis (reticular) - decreased sensation; loss of hair follicles,
            slow to blanch, *(need skin grafts)*
    3rd degree - leathery; down to subcutaneous fat (sub-dermal)
        (need skin grafts)
    4th degree - down to bone, adipose, tendon or muscle

1st and superficial 2nd degree burns heal by **epithelialization**
    Epithelial cells come from hair follicles (primary site) and edges of wound

*Escharotomy indications (perform within 4–6 hours to prevent myonecrosis)
    1) **Circumferential** burns w/ *decreased* temp, pulse, capillary refill, pain
        sensation and/or neurologic function in extremity
    2) **Problems ventilating** with significant chest torso burns
    May also need **fasciotomy** if compartment syndrome suspected
    Escharotomy (fasciotomy) **types:**
        1) ***Medial and lateral sides of limbs** (*except* fingers, see 3 below)
        2) **Dorsum of hand** (*avoid* palm)
        3) ****Fingers** – mid-axial incision (*avoid lateral incisions → nerves there*)
        4) **Chest** – lateral chest wall, sub-clavicular and above costal margin

**Inhalational injury
    Important prognostic factor for **mortality** after burn
    Most of injury from **carbonaceous materials** *and* **smoke**, *NOT* heat
    RFs – ETOH, trauma, closed space, age > 10 or < 50, delayed extrication
    Sx's (possible injury)- stridor, facial burn, wheezing, carbonaceous sputum
    Cx's of inhalational injury: pneumonia, upper airway obstruction,
        bronchospasm, atelectasis, carbon monoxide poisoning
    Dx: **fiberoptic bronchoscopy** *(best test)* – look for soot, edema, erythema
    Intubation criteria – upper airway stridor or obstruction, worsening
        hypoxemia, massive volume resuscitation (often w/ very large burns)
    MC infection in pts w/ significant burns (> 30% BSA) → **pneumonia
        RFs – **inhalation injury (#1),** fluid resuscitation w/ pulmonary edema
    **MCC death after significant burn – *infection (#1 pneumonia)*

**Carbon monoxide poisoning (carboxy-hemoglobin levels)

Normal level	10%
Normal level in smokers	20%
Coma	50%
Death	70%

    Tx: **intubate w/ 100% O2** *(best Tx)*

**Volume resuscitation
    **Parkland formula: 4 cc/kg x % burn over 24 hours
        Give **1/2 volume in 1st 8 hours**, next **1/2 over 16 hours**
        Calculate only for ≥ 2nd degree burns that are ≥ 20% BSA
    **Use lactated Ringer's (LR) in 1st 24 hrs (switch to D5 1/2 NS after 24
        hrs)
    **UOP best measure of resuscitation: Adults - 0.5 cc/kg/hr
        Child - 1 cc/kg/hr, Infant (< 6 mos) - 2 cc/kg/hr
    Parkland can grossly underestimate requirements w/ inhalational injury,
        ETOH, electrical injury or post-escharotomy
    Children need **Ca++** and **glucose** in 1st 24 hours
    Albumin *avoided* in resuscitation (increases **pneumonia**)

*Renal issues w/ severe burns:
> **Hyperkalemia** (released from dead tissue)
> **Myoglobinuria** (from dead muscle; **Tx:** fluid resuscitation *(best Tx)* + HCO3⁻ to alkalinize urine
> **Renal failure** (from volume loss, myoglobinuria)

*Burn wound infections
> <u>No</u> role for prophylactic IV antibiotics
> **Sx's of burn wound infection** - rapid eschar <u>separation</u>, <u>edema</u>, 2nd to 3rd degree <u>conversion</u> (partial thickness → full thickness), <u>hemorrhage</u> in wound, <u>erythema gangrenosum</u>, <u>green</u> discoloration of fat (or other color changes), <u>black</u> skin around the wound, <u>pseudomonas</u> smell
> ****Dx burn wound infection** *(differentiate from colonization)* →
> ***biopsy* of burn wound** (best method; > 10⁵ organisms = infection)
> Path **MC organism** in burn wound infection – <u>pseudomonas</u> (some say staph aureus); **MC fungal infection** – Candida
> **MCC burn wound sepsis** – pseudomonas (some say staph aureus)
> The larger the burn, the greater risk of infection
> **Cell mediated immunity** is decreased in burn wound due to decreased granulocyte chemotaxis
> Tx: **Burn wound excision w/ allograft** *(best Tx)* + **systemic abx's**
> *Do <u>not</u> use autograft when excising infected burn wounds*
> If just cellulitis around burn wound → systemic and topical abx's
> ****Prevention** - Topical abx's decrease incidence of burn wound infections
> (Candida infections have ↑ed as a consequence)
> **Silvadene** (silver sulfadiazine)
>> Limited eschar penetration (bacteriostatic)
>> Contraindicated w/ **sulfa allergy**
>> S/Es: **neutropenia** and **thrombocytopenia**
> **Silver nitrate**
>> Limited eschar penetration
>> S/Es: **Electrolyte imbalances** (↓Na⁺, ↓Cl⁻, ↓Ca⁺⁺, ↓K⁺)
>>> **Methemoglobinemia** → contraindicated w/ G6PD deficiency; discoloration
> ****Sulfamylon** (mafenide sodium)
>> **Painful** application
>> Good **eschar penetration**, good for **cartilage**
>> Good for **pseudomonas**
>> S/Es: ****Metabolic acidosis** due to carbonic anhydrase inhibition

1st week: need to 1) **excise burned areas** and 2) **start nutrition**
> **Early excision of burned areas** (48-72 hours after burn)
>> Use **dermatome** for deep 2nd degree and 3rd degree wounds
>> **Residual skin viability** based on **color, texture,** and ****punctate bleeding** after eschar removal
> **Infected areas**
>> 1) excise, 2) place allograft, 3) then re-excise later (don't use autograft for infected areas); **Biopsy** suspected burn wound infections *(best method of Dx)*
>> ****Autografts** contraindicated if culture positive for **beta-hemolytic strep** or ** bacteria >10⁵**
> Skin grafts need to be **compressed** w/ xeroform gauze / cotton balls - don't want seroma or hematoma to form which prevents graft from attaching *(MCC of skin graft failure)*
> **For each burn wound excision session:**
>> < 1 L blood loss
>> < 20% of skin excised
>> < 2 hours in OR
>> Blood loss is to be expected
>> Pts can get extremely sick if too much time spent in OR

Types of Grafts
- **Autografts** [split-thickness (STSG) or full-thickness (FTSG)] *best overall*
    - ****STSG**
        - ****more likely to survive** compared to FTSG (graft not as thick; ****easier imbibition**, subsequent re-vascularization)
        - **STSG** - 0.015 cm, includes **epidermis** and part of **dermis**
        - **Meshed grafts** for large area (eg back, trunk, arms, legs)
    - ****FTSG**
        - ****less wound contraction** than STSG
        - Not as many donor sites
        - Can get better skin color match
        - **Donor site must be closed primarily*
        - Good for face, palms back of hands, genitals
        - <u>Not</u> good for large areas
        - **FTSG** can be harvested from **behind ear**, above **clavicle**, or **groin** (loose skin areas – **primary closure**)
    - **Homografts** (**allografts** - cadaveric skin; **xenografts** - porcine)
        - Not as beneficial as autografts
        - Good temporizing material (lasts 2 weeks); may be good for infected burn wounds
        - ***Eventually allografts become **vascularized, undergo rejection, thrombosis,** and then **require removal***
- **STSG donor site**
    - **Hemostasis w/ epinephrine soaked gauzes**
    - Covered w/ Op-site (*semi-occlusive dressing*) - heals in **3 wks*
    - Can use as a **donor site** *again* (w/ STSG, epithelium migrates primarily from **hair follicles**, also from wound edges; these are termed **epithelial appendages**)
    - Donor site healing time *inversely* proportional to **thickness of graft** harvested
- **FTSG donor site** – need primary closure
- ****Graft survival:**
    - ****Imbibition** (days 0-3) – osmotic nutrient and oxygen supply to graft for 1st 3 days
    - **Neovascularization** (day 3+) new blood vessel growth to graft
    - **Areas w/ poor vascular supply will likely NOT support skin grafting → tendons, bone w/o periosteum, radiated skin*
    - **Unusual areas that can support grafts – omentum, bowel wall, bone w/ periosteum intact*
- ****MCC skin graft loss → seroma or hematoma formation under graft**
- **Nutrition**
    - ***Burn wounds must use <u>**glucose**</u> in an obligatory fashion*
    - **Caloric need** – 25 kcal/kg/day + (30 kcal/d x % burn) – *don't exceed* 3000 kcal/d
    - **Protein need** – 1 g/kg/day + (3 g/d x % burn)
    - **Glucose** – best source for calories (non-protein) w/ burns

2nd week
- **Hands, feet, face,** and **genital areas treated**
- **Allograft replaced w/ autograft**
- **Face** – topical abx 1 week, FTSG (*non-meshed*) for unhealed areas
- **Hands** – immobilize in functional position
    - Abx's for 1 week, then FTSG and immobilize in functional position for another week, then physical therapy
    - May need wire fixation of joints if unstable or open.
- **Palms** - **preserve** specialized **palmar aponeurosis** (**<u>avoid</u> palmar fasciotomy or escharotomy* – go on dorsal surface)
    - ***Splint hand in **extension for 1 week; FTSG in 2nd week*
- **Genitals** – topical abx's for 1 week; FTSG in 2nd week

Admission criteria

1) **2nd and 3rd degree burns**
> **> 10% BSA** in pts aged < 10 or > 50 years
> **> 20% BSA** in all other pts
> Significant portions of **special areas** (hands, face, feet, genitalia, perineum, or skin overlying major joints)

2) 3rd degree burns > 5% (any age group)

3) **Electrical and chemical burns**

4) Concomitant **inhalational** injury, mechanical **trauma** or medical co-morbidities

5) Pts w/ special needs (social, emotional or long-term rehabilitation)

6) **Child abuse** (or suspected; accounts for 15% of burns in children)

Rule of 9's – assessing % of body surface burned
> Head = 9, arms = 18, chest = 18, back = 18, legs = 36, perineum = 1
> **Patient's palm** = 1% BSA (can use to measure size of burn)

Highest deaths – children and elderly (can't get away)

MC burn – scald burn (eg stove)

MC burn to present to ED and be admitted – flame burn (eg fire)

Items that suggest child abuse

Delayed care	Lack of splash marks
Conflicting histories	Stocking or glove pattern
Previous burns or injuries	Flexor area sparing
Sharp demarcation	Dorsal area of hands
Uniform depth of burn	Deep and localized

Complications after burns

Seizures – MC iatrogenic (related to **Na^+ concentration** and resuscitation)

Ectopia –contraction of burned adnexae and can't see out of eye.
> Tx: surgical eyelid release

Eyes – fluorescein staining to Dx injury; Tx: fluoroquinolone ointment

Corneal abrasion – Tx: topical fluoroquinolones ointment

Symblepharon – eyelid stuck to underlying conjunctiva
> Tx: release with glass rod and amniotic tissue transplantation

Curling's ulcer – duodenal ulcer w/ burns

Marjolin's ulcer – highly malignant, ulcerative, **squamous cell CA** in chronic non-healing burn wounds or in chronic healing unstable scars (osteomyelitis, venous ulcers, post-XRT → latency period 30 years)

Acalculous cholecystitis

Hypertrophic scar (does not go beyond original border of scar like keloids)
> Usually occurs 3 - 4 months after injury
> Secondary to increased **neovascularity**
> MC w/ deep thermal injuries that take > 3 weeks to heal, heal by contraction and epithelial spread, or heal across flexor surfaces
> Tx: steroids, silicone injection, compression
> If disfiguring - scar excision, primary closure, then steroid injections

Special burns

Acid and alkali burns
> Need vigorous water irrigation (30-60 min)
> **Alkalis** deeper than acid due to **liquefaction necrosis**
> **Acid burns** result in **coagulation necrosis**

Hydrofluoric acid burns – topical **calcium gluconate** spread over wound (neutralizes burn); can also inject calcium around site or give **intra-arterial calcium**

Powder burns – wipe off before irrigation

Tar burns – cool, wipe off w/ lipophilic solvent (eg **glycerol**)

Phenol burns – are not water soluble; use lipophilic solvent (eg **glycerol**)

Erythema multiforme and Variants

All involve **detachment of epidermis from dermis
Erythema Multiforme - least severe form (self-limited, target lesions)
Stevens-Johnson Syndrome (more serious), < 10% BSA
Toxic Epidermal Necrolysis (TEN)
> Most severe form of erythema multiforme major
> Drugs MCC (phenytoin, bactrim, PCN); viruses
> > 30% BSA
> Mouth, lungs and GI tract can be involved

Staph Scalded Skin Syndrome (caused by staph aureus)
Tx:
> Remove offending agent if drug related
> **Topical antimicrobial** (<u>no</u> silvadene if thought to be sulfa related)
> **Topical Allografts** to prevent wound desiccation and super-infection
> **Wrap area w/ Telfa gauze**
> **Fluid resuscitation** (weeping wounds)
> **Abx's** if due to staph aureus
> ***NO steroids*
> May need future skin grafts

Frostbite

Rapid re-warming of part in circulating warm water 40-42°
Pain control, Tetanus shot, Silvadene over blistered areas
May need amputation or skin graft later

Head and Neck

242. *All of the following are true except:
    a. Torus palatine is generally resected
    b. The inferior thyroid artery is a branch of the thyrocervical trunk
    c. The facial nerve provides motor function to the face
    d. The phrenic nerve is located along the anterior scalene muscle

    Answer a. Torus palatine (benign congenital bony mass on upper palate of mouth) is left alone.

243. **A 65 yo man presents to your office with a left sided 2 cm neck mass just below his jaw on the anterior border of the sternocleidomastoid muscle. The mass has been present for about 3 months. He denies fevers or other sx's. The mass is not tender. PMHx significant for a 30 pack-year smoking and alcohol abuse. On exam, the mass is mobile and you do not feel any adenopathy. The most appropriate next step for this patient is:
    a. Perform excisional biopsy
    b. FNA in the office
    c. Radiation therapy
    d. I-131

    Answer b. **FNA** (w/ U/S if possible) is the next appropriate step. FNA can make a definitive Dx in 90% of the time.

244. **FNA in the above pt shows squamous cell CA in a lymph node. In addition to physical exam, the test most likely to identify this patient's primary lesion is:
    a. MRI
    b. Pan endoscopy with random biopsies
    c. CT scan
    d. PET scan

    Answer b. You are trying to find the primary tumor at this point. It would be premature to go with just excisional biopsy. Although CT scan will be needed in the work-up, **physical exam** and **pan-endoscopy** detects 80% of head and neck tumors of unknown origin.

245. **Instead of the above, the FNA is negative despite 3 attempts. Pan-endoscopy with random biopsies and chest/abd CT are negative except for the 2 cm lesion. The lesion is non-cystic and does not appear to be invading any other structures. The most appropriate next step in this patients management is:
    a. Excisional Biopsy
    b. Modified radical neck dissection
    c. Radiation therapy
    d. I-131

    Answer a. Perform excisional biopsy is the most appropriate next step. You have performed an appropriate W/U to find primary tumor and the patient does not have diffuse adenopathy suggestive of lymphoma. One should always be prepared to perform a modified radical neck dissection when biopsying an anterior neck mass in case multiple nodes are found but this should not be the initial step.

246. **The excisional biopsy for the above pt comes back as a lymph node with squamous cell carcinoma. The most likely source for the primary tumor is:
    a. Palate
    b. Tonsil
    c. Tongue
    d. Pharynx

    Answer b. MC location for head / neck CA of unknown origin is **tonsils.**

247. **For the above pt, which of the following is the most appropriate next step:
    a. Selective neck dissection
    b. Induction chemo w/ 5-FU and cisplatin
    c. XRT only
    d. Modified radical neck dissection

    Answer d. **Metastatic squamous cell CA** w/ occult primary is treated w/ **ipsilateral MRND, ipsilateral tonsillectomy** and post-op **bilateral neck XRT.**

248. **Instead of the above (question 246), the biopsy comes back as thyroid tissue (pathology reports it as **lateral aberrant thyroid tissue**). All of the following are true except:
    a. The patient should undergo total thyroidectomy
    b. The patient should undergo MRND
    c. The patient should receive post-op XRT
    d. The patient should be treated w/ I-131

    Answer c. **Occult thyroid papillary carcinoma** can present in this fashion (the papillary CA has spread to a cervical node). Post op XRT is indicated for papillary (and follicular) CA only if it is not responsive to I-131.

249. **A 50 yo man w/ a long history of chewing tobacco presents w/ a 2 cm ulcer on his inner cheek. You get a core needle biopsy which shows a verrucous (buccal squamous cell) CA. The most appropriate management of this patient is:
    a. Pre-op chemo-XRT followed by resection
    b. Chemo-XRT only
    c. Full cheek resection with flap
    d. Full cheek resection with modified radical neck dissection

    Answer c. **Verrucous ulcer CA** (buccal squamous cell CA) is not aggressive and can undergo full cheek resection +/- a flap w/ 0.5 cm margins. No chemo or XRT is indicated. Lymph node dissection is not indicated either.

250. **All of the following are true of oral cavity squamous cell CA except:
    a. The lower lip is more commonly involved than the upper lip
    b. Nasopharyngeal SCCA is associated w/ human papilloma virus
    c. Nasopharyngeal SCCA is treated primarily w/ XRT
    d. Flaps are needed if more than 1/3 of the lip is removed

    Answer b. **Nasopharyngeal CA** is associated w/ **Ebstein Barr Virus**
    Nasopharyngeal SCCA is treated primarily w/ **XRT** (very sensitive)
    Flaps are needed if **more than 1/3** of the lip is removed

251. *A 50 yo man has a mass 1 cm anterior to the ear. The mass causes him pain and he has a facial droop. CT of the head shows the tumor is involved in both the deep and superficial portions of the gland. This most likely represents:
    a. Mucoepidermoid carcinoma
    b. Adenoid cystic carcinoma
    c. Pleomorphic adenoma
    d. Warthin's Tumor

    Answer a. There are 2 features of this presentation that make the parotid tumor almost certainly malignant. The first is that it invades both the superficial and deep glands (unusual for benign tumors) and the second is that the **facial nerve** is affected (facial droop). Given that this tumor is almost certainly malignant, you have to go with the MC malignant tumor of the parotid, which is mucoepidermoid carcinoma.**The **facial nerve** courses through the **parotid gland** and controls **motor function to face**.

252. *The nerve most likely injured with submandibular resection is:
    a.   Vagus
    b.   Hypoglossal
    c.   Auriculo-temporal
    d.   Marginal mandibular

    Answer d. The nerve most commonly injured with resection of the submandibular gland is the *marginal mandibular nerve* (inferior alveolar branch). *This nerve supplies **motor function** to the **lower lip and chin**.

253. *A 55 yo man with a pre-auricular mass undergoes head, neck and chest CT which shows a parotid tumor involving both lobes with no additional lesions or adenopathy. EGD and bronch are also negative. The patient has a normal neurologic exam. At resection, a mucoepidermoid carcinoma is completely encasing the facial nerve. Which of the following is the appropriate next step:
    a.   Superficial parotidectomy
    b.   Total parotidectomy and stripping the tumor off the facial nerve
    c.   Total parotidectomy and resection of the facial nerve
    d.   Close and give XRT

    Answer b. Due to morbidity associated with resection of the facial nerve, an attempt should be made to preserve it, even if you have to peal the tumor off. This area should receive post-op XRT after surgery.

254. *A 55 yo woman with a pre-auricular mass undergoes head, neck and chest MRI which show a diffusely infiltrative parotid tumor extending to and encasing the carotid sheath and vagus nerve. The external carotid artery is narrowed from compression. Bx shows adenoid cystic CA. The most appropriate next step is:
    a.   Total parotidectomy with carotid reconstruction
    b.   Total parotidectomy and stripping the tumor off the carotid artery
    c.   XRT
    d.   chemo

    Answer c. Adenoid cystic CA can be extensively infiltrative, with a propensity to invade nerve roots. Additionally, it is very sensitive to XRT and typically has a long indolent course. Given the diffuse DZ in this pt, *XRT* is indicated as sole therapy.

255. **All of the following are true except:
    a.   The most common benign parotid tumor is pleomorphic adenoma
    b.   The tumor most likely to involve bilateral parotid glands at time of Dx is Warthin's Tumor
    c.   Tx of most benign parotid tumors involves enucleation
    d.   Following a parotidectomy, gustatory sweating is most likely caused by cross-innervation of the auriculo-temporal nerve and sympathetic nerves to the skin

    Answer c. **Tx of most **benign parotid tumors** involves **superficial parotidectomy**. Enucleation is <u>contra-indicated</u> due to high recurrence.

    The MC benign parotid tumor is **pleomorphic adenoma
    ***Post-op gustatory sweating** (Frey's syndrome) is caused by cross-innervation of auriculo-temporal nerve and skin sympathetic nerves
    The tumor most likely to involve **bilateral parotid glands at time of Dx is **Warthin's Tumor**

256. *A 35 yo woman comes in with the chief complaints of unsteadiness, tinnitus and hearing loss. You order a head MRI and there is a tumor at the cerebello-pontine angle. The most likely diagnosis is:

a. Glioma
b. Glioma multiforme
c. Neuroma
d. Medulloblastoma

Answer c. *Unsteadiness, tinnitus, and hearing loss are the classic symptoms of an **acoustic neuroma**. A tumor at the cerebello-pontine angle almost ensures the diagnosis.*

257. *A 10 yo boy presents with a cyst and a cyst tract near the angle of his mandible. This cyst has had recurrent infections in it. This cyst most likely connects to the:
    a. External auditory canal
    b. The tonsilar pillar
    c. The nasal septum
    d. Thoracic duct

Answer a. **Type I** *branchial cleft cysts extend from the angle of the mandible to the* **external auditory canal**.
Type II *(MC Type) goes from anterior SCM muscle to the* **tonsilar pillar**
Type III *goes from the deep SCM muscle to the* **pyriform sinus**
Tx for all of these cysts is resection

258. **A 5 yo girl presents with a midline anterior neck mass that moves with tongue protrusion and swallowing. This most likely represents:
    a. Thyroid cancer
    b. Branchial cleft cyst Type I
    c. Branchial cleft cyst Type II
    d. Thyroglossal duct cyst

Answer d. *A midline anterior neck mass in a child that moves with tongue protrusion and swallowing is classic for a **thyroglossal duct cyst**. Thyroid CA would appear more lateral as would branchial cleft cysts.*

Tx: *excision of entire* **cyst, tract,** *and* **central portion of** <u>hyoid</u> *bone (midportion) through lateral neck incision (Sistrunk procedure)*

259. *A 1 yo girl has a fluctuant multi-loculated mass on the lower lateral neck (posterior to the SCM) that has repeated infections. This most likely represents:
    a. Branchial cleft cyst Type I
    b. Branchial cleft cyst Type II
    c. Thyroglossal duct cyst
    d. Cystic hygroma

Answer d. *Cystic hygroma. Tx is **resection***

260. *All of the following are true except:
    a. The MC childhood aural CA is rhabdomyosarcoma
    b. Pinna lacerations should be repaired with full thickness sutures including cartilage
    c. The most effective surgery for obstructive sleep apnea is uvulopalatopharyngoplasty
    d. Sepsis from suppurative parotitis requires parotidectomy

Answer d. *Sepsis (MC from staph aureus) from suppurative parotitis requires **incision and drainage***

The most effective surgery for obstructive sleep apnea is **uvulopalatopharyngoplasty**

Anatomy

Phrenic nerve – on anterior scalene muscle, controls diaphragm

Trigeminal nerve – ophthalmic, maxillary, mandibular branches
> Sensation for most of face
> Mandibular branch – taste anterior ⅔ of tongue and floor of mouth

Facial nerve – temporal, zygomatic, buccal, marginal mandibular, and cervical branches; motor to face; runs through the parotid gland

Glossopharyngeal nerve
> Sensory to posterior 1/3 tongue; motor to pharynx
> Injury – trouble swallowing

Hypoglossal nerve
> Motor to all of tongue except palatoglossus
> Tongue deviates to **ipsilateral side** w/ injury

Thyrocervical trunk – "**STAT**":
> **S**uprascapular artery
> **T**ransverse cervical artery
> **A**scending cervical artery
> Inferior **T**hyroid artery

Trapezius muscle flap (spinal accessory nerve, allows shoulder shrug) – flap based on **transverse cervical artery**

Pectoralis major muscle flap – flap based on **thoracoacromial artery**

Torus palatini – benign congenital bony mass on upper palate of mouth
> Tx: nothing

Torus mandibular – as above but on anterior lingual surface of mandible

Neck mass (Enlarged lymph node)

Dx (for lymph node):
> If **inflammatory** (tender, URI sx's), can tx w/ **abx's, F/U in 2 weeks**
> > Make sure getting **smaller**
> *1st* – **FNA** *(best initial Dx test)* + CXR (in office, that day)
> > If it shows CA, base w/u on type of cells
> > If work-up and biopsy indeterminate, go to 2nd below
> *2nd* – Bronch / EGD (w/ random Bx's if no lesion found)
> > **Neck/chest/abd CT** (neck CT picks up carotid body tumor)
> > **Mammogram** in women
> > All above looking for *primary lesion*
> *3rd* – still can't figure it out → **perform excisional biopsy** → send FS
> > Need to be prepared for MRND

Squamous cell CA (ie epidermoid CA) found in **cervical node <u>without</u> known primary** (cant' find primary despite work-up) **Tx: ipsilateral MRND, ipsilateral tonsillectomy** (25% of occult primaries eventually found here), **bilateral neck XRT** (to nodal region + potential head and neck primary sites)

Enlarged lateral neck lymph node w/ normal thyroid tissue (**lateral aberrant thyroid tissue) = **papillary thyroid CA** w/ lymphatic spread, Tx: **total thyroidectomy, ipsilateral MRND,** and post-op [131]I

Verrucous ulcer (**buccal** squamous cell CA) - often presents as **leukoplakia** on cheek; associated w/ **chewing tobacco**
> Very **low grade,** well-differentiated squamous cell CA
> Locally aggressive but **very rare nodal or systemic mets**
> Often on **inner cheek** but can be anywhere in mouth
> **Tx: full cheek resection ± flap; **<u>No</u> lymph node dissection**

Oral cavity cancer (oro-pharyngeal, above larynx)
> **MC site for oral cavity CA** - lower lip (lip considered anterior oral cavity)
> **RFs** – ETOH and tobacco
> **MC type** – vast majority **squamous cell CA** (ie epidermoid)

CA risk – **erythroplakia** worse than leukoplakia
Division of anterior oral cavity and **posterior oral cavity** marked by:
> Tonsilar pillars
> Junction between the hard and soft palates
> Tongue papilla

Lip CA and **Tonsilar CA** considered anterior oral cavity CA

Anterior oral cavity CA→ submental + submandibular chain 1st
> *Exception* **Tongue CA** goes to cervical chain nodes (early)

Posterior oral cavity CA → cervical chain nodes 1st
> 1) ****Nasopharyngeal SCCA**: Sx's – epistaxis or obstruction
> > EBV associated; Chinese
> > ****_Very_ responsive to XRT** (do _not_ resect these tumors)
> 2) **Oropharyngeal SCCA**; Sx's – neck mass, sore throat
> 3) **Hypopharyngeal SCCA**; Sx's – hoarseness **(early LN spread)**

*Location w/ lowest survival rate – *hard palate (hard to resect)
Need **1 cm margin** for all _except_ tongue (2 cm margin required)
Tx:
> **Stage I + II anterior tumors** (< 4 cm, no nodal or bone invasion) →
> > **Resection**
> **Stage I + II posterior tumors** (< 4 cm, no nodal or bone invasion) →
> > **XRT _only_** (include neck nodes) hard to resect these tumors
> > ***Nasopharyngeal SCCA very sensitive to XRT*
> **Stage III anterior or posterior** (> 4 cm _or_; nodal or bone invasion)
> > All get: 1) *Resection*, 2) *node dissection*, and 3) postop **chemoXRT**
> > *Exception – **nasopharyngeal CA** → get **chemo-XRT** only (no
> > > resection; include neck nodes in XRT field)
> **Stage IV** (mets) - palliative chemo-XRT (5-FU + cisplatin)

Special Issues
> ****Lip CA**
> > **Lower lip** CA MC than upper due to sun exposure
> > Lesions at **commissure** (angle of mouth) are **most aggressive**
> > Needs to involve **mucosa** or its _not_ lip CA (would the Tx like skin CA)
> > ****Flaps needed** if more than 1/3 of lip is removed
> **Tongue CA** – jaw invasion still operable; **early nodal invasion** (cervical chain)
> > Commando procedure – removes portion of the mandible
> **Maxillary sinus CA Tx:** maxillectomy
> **Tonsil CA:** Sx's – asymptomatic until large; **RFs** - ETOH, tobacco
> > **MC type** – SCCA
> > Considered **anterior oral cavity CA**
> > 80% have **lymph node spread** at time of dx
> > Tx: **tonsillectomy** (best way to get Dx + Tx lesion)
> > > Therapy then same as above for anterior tumors
> > **_Parotid tumors can invade oral cavity and deviate the ipsilateral tonsil_**
> **Other nasopharynx tumors**
> > **MC benign tumor of nasopharynx* – papilloma
> > **MC tumor of nasopharynx in children* – lymphoma Tx: chemo
> > **Nasopharyngeal angiofibroma* - benign, **extremely vascular**
> > > Males < 20 years (obstruction or epistaxis)
> > > Tx: **angio-embolization** (MC internal maxillary artery), then
> > > > resection; XRT for inaccessible tumors

Salivary gland cancers
> Parotid, submandibular, sublingual, and minor salivary glands
> **Mass in large salivary gland** → MC benign
> **Mass in small salivary gland** → MC malignant
> > Although parotid gland is MC site for a malignant tumor
> **MC salivary gland tumor in children** – hemangiomas

Parotid Mass

Pre-auricular mass just above angle of mandible, anterior to ear
  All are parotid tumors until proved otherwise
  Dx usually made after **superficial parotidectomy**
Sx's: painless mass; **pain or facial nerve paralysis** suggests CA
Dx: *NO FNA* if parotid mass is mobile, discrete and confined to superficial
        lobe (perform **superficial parotidectomy** – this is your biopsy)
     If mass is in deep parotid gland, the pt is poor surgery risk, or the
        mass is felt to be metastatic (eg melanoma), then FNA useful

Path
  80% of all salivary tumors in parotid
  80% of parotid tumors benign (MC - pleomorphic adenomas)
  Malignant parotid tumors metastasize to **lung**

*Malignant parotid tumors
  Mucoepidermoid CA – MC malignant tumor of salivary glands
  Adenoid cystic CA – #2 malignant tumor of salivary glands
     Long, indolent course → propensity to **invade *nerve roots***
     Very sensitive to XRT *(can just give XRT if extensive)*
  Tx:
     Total parotidectomy + prophylactic MRND + post-op XRT
     Only exception is low grade mucoepidermoid CA → just total
        parotidectomy (no MRND or XRT)
     Try to preserve facial nerve branches, even if you have to
        peel tumor off (unless already out on **pre-op exam**)
        XRT to that **area post-op**
  Melanoma and SCCA skin CA can metastasize to parotid gland (see
     Skin and Soft tissue section)

*Benign parotid tumors
  Pleomorphic adenoma *(mixed tumor)*
     **MC benign tumor of salivary glands
     Malignant degeneration in 5%
  Warthin's tumor (papillary cystadenoma lymphomatosum)
     #2 benign tumor of salivary glands; **bilateral** in 10%
     Enucleation NOT performed due to high recurrence rate
  Tx: **superficial parotidectomy** (total parotidectomy if deep gland
     involved)

Technical considerations
  MC injured nerve w/ parotid surgery – greater auricular nerve
     (numbness over lower portion of ear auricle)
  MC injured nerve w/ submandibular gland resection – marginal
     mandibular nerve (inferior alveolar nerve branch; motor to lower
     lip and chin)
  Deep parotid tumor extending to **para-pharyngeal space** (ie –
     pushing tonsil towards midline); Tx – **median
     mandibulotomy** for exposure (need mandibulectomy if bone
     involved)

Frey's syndrome – cross innervation of the **auriculo-temporal nerve** w/
  sympathetic fibers in skin sweat glands following parotidectomy
  Sx's: **gustatory sweating** (sweating on cheek while eating)
  Tx: usually self limiting (use roll-on anti-perspirants) → If refractory, can
     place *alloderm skin graft* between skin flap and nerve

Modified radical neck dissection (MRND)
  Takes omohyoid, submandibular gland, sensory nerves C2–C5, cervical
     branch of facial nerve, and cervical chain LN's
  No real mortality difference compared to RND

Radical neck dissection (not really used anymore)
Same as MRND _plus:_ **accessory nerve (CN XII), sternocleidomastoid,**
and **internal jugular**
*Most morbidity w/ *accessory nerve* resection (muscles of neck including
sternocleidomastoid; trapezius)*

*Acoustic neuroma (vestibular schwannoma, CN VIII, vestibulocochlear)
Benign, slow growth; associated w/ neurofibromatosis (von
Recklinghausen's DZ)
Sx's: Tinnitus, hearing loss, unsteadiness, vertigo, N/V
Dx: **MRI** *(best test)* – classically at the *cerebello-pontine angle*
Tx: Craniotomy and resection including superior/inferior vestibular nerves;
facial nerve at risk w/ surgery; XRT is alternative

*Branchial cleft cysts – can lead to sinus tracts, fistulas, and infection
1st Branchial Cleft Cyst – **angle of mandible**
Can connect with *external auditory canal*
Very often associated w/ facial nerve
2nd Branchial Cleft Cyst *(**MC location)* – **anterior border of SCM muscle;**
goes through **carotid** bifurcation and into *tonsillar pillar*
3rd Branchial Cleft Cyst – deep in SCM, emerges in *pyriform sinus*
Tx for all cysts: resection

**Thyroglossal duct cyst
From descent of thyroid from **foramen cecum**
Possible that this is only thyroid tissue the pt has
Goes through **hyoid bone**
Risk of **infection**; 1% **malignancy** risk (MC papillary thyroid CA)
Sx's: **Midline cervical mass**; MC between hyoid and thyroid isthmus
Classically **moves upward with swallowing
May cause dysphagia, susceptible to infection
Tx: excision of entire **cyst, tract, and **central portion of _hyoid_ bone**
(midportion) through lateral neck incision (Sistrunk procedure)

Lingual thyroid
Thyroid tissue that persists in area of foramen cecum at **base of tongue**
The only thyroid tissue in 70% of pts who have it
1% malignancy risk
Sx's: dysphagia, dyspnea, dysphonia
Tx: **Thyroxine** suppression for sx's; abolish w/ **I-131** or **resection** if it does
not shrink after thyroxine; resection if worried about CA

**Cystic hygroma
Classically found in **lateral posterior neck triangle (posterior to SCM)
Fluctuant, multi-loculated area under skin
Form sinuses and get infected; is a macrocytic **lymphatic malformation**
Tx: resection

Ear Disorders (ear = pinna)
Cauliflower ear (ie boxers ear, UFC fighters) – un-drained hematomas that
organize and calcify; Tx: drain hematomas to avoid this
Cholesteatoma - epidermal inclusion cyst of ear
Slow growing but erode as they grow - damage middle ear bones
(malleus, incus and stapes) and/or mastoid
Sx's: hearing loss and brown/yellow/bloody drainage from ear
Tx: **surgical excision** ± mastoidectomy
Pinna lacerations (ear) –need full thickness sutures through involved
cartilage
Ear Infections need to be treated promptly to avoid **cartilage necrosis**
MC childhood aural CA – rhabdomyosarcoma of middle or external ear

<u>Laryngeal Cancer</u> (vocal cord and surrounding structures)

Sx's: Hoarseness, aspiration, dyspnea, dysphagia

Tx **XRT** (vocal cord only) or **chemo-XRT** (beyond vocal cord)

*Surgery is not the primary Tx; Try to **preserve larynx***

XRT – spread field to get **ipsilateral neck nodes** (cervical chain);
If tumor **crosses midline** → **bilateral neck XRT**

Stage III (positive nodes)→ need above + MRND (take **ipsilateral thyroid**)

MC benign tumor of larynx – papilloma

*Stenson's duct (ie parotid duct)

Opens into vestibule of mouth opposite upper 2nd molar

***Primary repair** of lacerations over catheter stent*

Ligation causes painful parotid atrophy and facial asymmetry

*Suppurative parotitis

MC in elderly patients w/ dehydration; **MC organism** – staph

Tx: fluids, salivation, abx's; ***incision and drainage if abscess develops***
or pt not improving; can be a life-threatening problem

*Sialoadenitis

Acute inflammation of salivary gland related to **stone** in duct

Most calculi near orifice

80% involves submandibular or sublingual glands

Tx: ***Incise duct and remove stone**; gland excision for recurrent DZ*

*Paraganglioma

MC ENT site – carotid body (**carotid body tumor**, at bifurcation)

Can secrete **norepinephrine** (↑ HR + HTN; palpations, HA's)

Sx's: ***neck mass w/ bruit**; Dx: angio; highly vascular*

Tx: surgical excision

*Sleep apnea

Pt rarely aware of problem (spouse brings them in)

Pauses in breathing w/ sleep

Cx's: cor pulmonale, MI's, arrhythmias, and death

Tx: ***CPAP** (continuous positive airway pressure at night (best Tx)*
***Uvulopalatopharyngoplasty** (UPP, best surgical option)*

Prolonged oral intubation – can lead to **sub-glottic stenosis**

Tx: tracheal resection and reconstruction *(best Tx)*; can dilate temporarily

Tracheostomy – consider if pt requires intubation for > 7–14 days

Benefits – ↓ secretions, easier ventilation, ↓ PNA risk

Median rhomboid glossitis – failure of fusion of the tongue. Tx: none required

*Cleft lip (primary palate)

Highest prevalence – Native Americans

Failure of fusion of **maxillary** and **medial nasal processes**

Involves lip, alveolus, or both structures; may have poor feeding

*Repair at **10 weeks** of age, **10 pounds**, and a **Hgb 10***

Tx: **Millard procedure** (Z plasty); repair nasal deformities at same time

*Cleft palate (secondary palate)

Two plates of hard palate are not completely joined; also involves soft palate

Hole in roof of mouth connects directly w/ **nasal cavity**

Affect **speech** and **swallowing** if not closed soon enough; can affect
maxillofacial growth if closed too early → ***repair at 12 months***

Palatal obturator used to temporarily close hole before surgery

Hemangioma – MC benign head and neck tumor in adults

MC tumor overall of childhood

Mastoiditis

Infection of the mastoid cells; can destroy bone; rare

From untreated **acute supportive otitis media**

MC organism – strep pneumoniae

Ear is pushed forward

Tx: **abx's;** if condition does not improve quickly insert **tympanostomy tube**
to drain pus from middle ear; possible emergency ***mastoidectomy** if
abx's and drainage fails

Adrenal

261. All of the following are true except:
    a. The right adrenal vein drains into the right renal vein
    b. Cortisol level generally peaks between 4-6 am
    c. Adult excess androgen or estrogen secretion from an adrenal source is almost always CA
    d. Glucocorticoid and mineralocorticoid Tx after adrenalectomy prevents Addison's Disease and Nelson's Syndrome

    Answer a. The right renal vein drains into the inferior vena cava.

262. **During a negative trauma workup, you discover an adrenal tumor. All of the following are appropriate in this pt's management except:
    a. Urine catecholamines and metabolites should be checked
    b. > 5 cm is an indication for resection
    c. Bloody cyst fluid requires resection
    d. Angiomyolipomas require adrenalectomy

    Answer d. **Angiomyolipomas are benign and can be observed**

    **Urine catecholamines and metabolites should be checked*
    ***> 5 cm* is an indication for resection*
    ***Bloody** cyst fluid requires resection*

263. *All of the following are true of pheochromocytomas except:
    a. The MC location for extra-adrenal pheochromocytomas is the aortic bifurcation
    b. Alpha blockers should be given before beta-blockers to avoid hypertensive crisis
    c. The most sensitive test for pheochromocytoma localization is MIBG
    d. Adrenal venous sampling is the best method for localizing adrenal pheochromocytomas

    Answer d. Adrenal venous sampling should be _avoided_ to prevent hypertensive crisis.

264. **A 25 yo women presents to the hospital w/ HTN, polydipsia, and polyuria. She has a serum sodium of 150 and a serum potassium of 2.9. She has been off diuretics for some time. All of the following are true except:
    a. This patient likely has a plasma aldosterone to renin ratio > 20
    b. A 24 urine aldosterone > 14 mcg after a 3 day salt loading (salt suppression test) helps confirm diagnosis
    c. Adrenal venous sampling helps differentiate unilateral vs. bilateral DZ
    d. The MCC of this syndrome is adrenal hyperplasia.

    Answer d. **The MCC of **hyperaldosteronism** is **aldosterone adenoma****

    This patient likely has a **plasma aldosterone to renin ratio > 20*
    ***A 24 urine **aldosterone > 14 mcg** after a 3 day salt loading (salt suppression test) helps confirm Dx of hyper-aldosteronism*
    ***Adrenal venous sampling** helps differentiate unilateral vs. bilateral DZ*

265. **All of the following are true except:
    a. Adrenal adenoma is the MCC of Cushing's Syndrome
    b. At least 50% of adrenocortical CA's are functional tumors
    c. High ACTH and a high dose dexamethasone test that does not suppress cortisol production suggests an ectopic ACTH producer
    d. Mitotane is used for unresectable adrenocortical CA

    Answer a. Pituitary adenoma is the MCC of Cushing's Syndrome.

Adrenal blood supply
Superior adrenal artery – off inferior phrenic artery
Middle adrenal artery – off aorta
Inferior adrenal artery – off renal artery

Left adrenal vein – goes to **left renal vein**
Right adrenal vein – goes to **IVC**
Lymphatics – drain to sub-diaphragmatic and renal lymph nodes

Hypothalamic-pituitary-adrenal axis
Hypothalamus releases **CRH** (corticotrophin releasing hormone), which goes to anterior pituitary gland
Anterior pituitary gland then releases **ACTH** which goes to adrenal cortex
Adrenal cortex then releases **cortisol**
Diurnal (high am, low pm) peak at 4-6 a.m.; also increased w/ **stress**
Cortisol effects – proteolysis, lipolysis, gluconeogenesis, hyperglycemia (partly from insulin resistance) inotropic, vascular tone

Adrenal Medulla
Produces **catecholamines** (norepinephrine + epinephrine)
Tyrosine hydroxylase - rate-limiting step for catecholamines
Phenylethanolamine N-methyltransferase (PNMT), converts norepinephrine (NE) → epinephrine (EPI, enzyme _only_ found in **adrenal medulla** (exclusive producer of endogenous EPI)
Only adrenal pheochromocytomas produce EPI
Monoamine oxidase (MAO) – breakdowns NE and EPI to normetanephrine and metanephrine; *__Vanillylmandelic acid__ (VMA) produced from these*

After bilateral adrenalectomy → need glucocorticoids and mineralocorticoids
1) prevents **Addison's Disease** (adrenal insufficiency)
2) prevents **Nelson's Syndrome** (pituitary enlargement compresses optic nerve); from chronic CRH stimulation of pituitary adenoma

**_Asymptomatic adrenal mass_ (incidentaloma, > 1 cm)
1% of CT scans show incidentalomas in adrenal gland (increase w/ age)
MC adrenal tumor (also MC malignant adrenal tumor) - met from another primary (lung-MC, breast, melanoma)
MC adrenal tumor _without_ previous history of CA (also MC primary adrenal tumor) – non-functional adrenal adenoma (50%)
Dx (*need to R/O functional tumors*):
Pheochromocytoma - 24 hour urine (Epi, NE, VMA, metanephrines nor-metanephrines) – *do this _before_ any biopsy*
Cushing's Syndrome – overnight **urine cortisol + serum ACTH**
Aldosteronoma – serum aldosterone, renin, K and Na
Adrenocortical CA – CT/MRI findings generally suggests diagnosis
**_FNA_ indicated for:
1) **> 10 Hounsfield units** or has **poor contrast washout** (< 50% at 10 min) on CT (both indicative of malignancy)
2) **Previous CA** or if you think it is a **met from a separate primary**
**_Surgery_ (resection) indicated for:
1) **≥ 5 cm**
2) **Ominous characteristics** (complex, hemorrhagic areas, irregular margins, heterogeneous, dense, vascular appearance)
3) **Functional tumor**
4) Is **enlarging**
5) Significant **FNA finding** (eg adrenocortical CA,)
If going to follow – repeat abd CT every 3 months for 1 year, then yearly
Adrenal cysts → aspirate;
Clear fluid → follow, resection if recurs; **Bloody** fluid → resection
Angiomyolipomas (on biopsy) – benign, leave

*Pheochromocytoma

Chromaffin cells, usually slow growing, from **sympathetic ganglia** or ectopic **neural crest cells**

MC location – adrenal gland (MC **right** side; **adrenal medulla**)

10% rule – malignant, bilateral, in children, familial, extra-adrenal, MEN

Extra-adrenal tumors more likely **malignant** (25%) and *do not produce epinephrine*; only adrenal pheochromocytomas produce epinephrine from norepinephrine (have **PNMT enzyme**)

Sx's: HTN (episodic, eg weight-lifting), HA, diaphoresis, palpitations,

Dx:

> ***24 hour urine** (best test for Dx, highest specificity, 98%) – *VMA (most specific),* Epi, NE, metanephrines, nor-metanephrines
>
> **CT scan** (or MRI) to localize tumors
>
> ***MIBG scan** (best test for localizing tumor)*
> > 131-meta-iodobenzylguanidine (MIBG; NE analogue)
> > Can help locate if not on CT scan
>
> *No* **venography** → will cause hypertensive crisis

Pre-op blood pressure control

> ***Alpha-blocker first*
> > **Phenoxybenzamine** (long acting) or **prazosin** (ramp up)
> > > *Avoid* hypertensive crisis by starting the alpha-blocker 1st
> > **Oral hydration** - should **gain weight**
> > **Beta-blocker** if tachycardia or arrhythmias while on alpha blocker
> > > ***Careful* w/ beta-blocker and give after alpha blocker → avoids
> > > > ***hypertensive crisis** (unopposed alpha stimulation→CHF, MI, stroke)

Tx:

> **Resection** (trans-abdominal, open approach if malignant)
>
> **Ligate adrenal vein 1st** to avoid spilling catecholamines w/ surgery
>
> **Debulking** helps sx's w/ unresectable DZ
>
> **Non-adrenal sites** for pheochromocytomas:
> > Proximal to *aortic bifurcation (MC ectopic location)* – organ of Zuckerkandl
> > Others - sympathetic chain ganglia (para-vertebral), bladder
>
> **Persistent hypertension** after removal → check other sites above
>
> **Metyrosine** – inhibits **tyrosine hydroxylase**, resulting in decreased synthesis of catecholamines (used for mets or pre-op prep)
>
> **False positive VMA** – caffeine, fruits, vanilla, iodine, alpha-, beta-blockers

**Hyper-aldosteronism

Primary Disease (↓ renin and ↑ aldosterone; **Conn's Syndrome**)

> **Adenoma** (80%, MCC primary hyperaldosteronism)
> **Adrenal hyperplasia** (20%)
> **Adrenocortical CA** (<1%); **Ovarian Tumors** (< 1%)

Secondary Disease (↑ renin and ↑ aldosterone)

> More common than primary DZ
> 1) **Primary reninism** – renin secreting tumor (Bartter's Syndrome)
> 2) **Secondary reninism** – many causes; CHF, renal artery stenosis

Sx's (primary hyperaldosteronism):

> HTN from sodium retention ___without___ edema
> Hypokalemia, polydipsia, weakness
> Check for hyperaldosteronism in pts w/ HTN _and_ either **low K$^+$**, an **adrenal mass,** or refractory to medical Tx

***Dx of primary hyperaldosteronism:*

> **Serum** (usual findings, but not diagnostic; need both 1 _and_ 2 below)
> > ↓ **renin** and ↑ **aldosterone**
> > **↓ K$^+$** (usually < 3) and ↑ **Na$^+$**; metabolic alkalosis
> 1) ***Plasma aldosterone to renin ratio > 20*
> 2) ***Salt suppression test** (salt loading w/ 24 hr urine aldosterone > 14 mcg)

Localizing studies (DDx - adenoma vs. hyperplasia):
  Abd CT or MRI
  Selective **adrenal venous sampling** for aldosterone - if not
      localized w/ CT/MRI; figures out unilateral vs. bilateral issue
  NP-59 scintigraphy (iodo-cholesterol) is taken up by **adrenal
      adenomas** (DDx adenoma vs. hyperplasia; *not* taken up by
      adrenal CA)
Tx: 1) **Adenoma** (or <u>rare</u> unilateral hyperplasia) - adrenalectomy
      2) **Diffuse hyperplasia**
          a) ***Medical Tx** (*treats <u>majority</u>) - *Spironolactone and
              potassium
          b) **Bilateral adrenalectomy** if above fails:
              MC indication – ***refractory hypokalemia*
              Will need **fludrocortisone** and **hydrocortisone** post-op

**Hypercortisolism (Cushing's Syndrome)
  **MCC – exogenous steroids
  Sx's: abdominal striae, moon face, obesity, buffalo hump, depression,
      insomnia, acne, weakness, hyperglycemia, diastolic HTN
  ****Dx:*
      1st: **24-hour urine free-cortisol** (*most sensitive test*) + **serum ACTH**
          If **ACTH is low** (and cortisol high) → have a cortisol secreting
              lesion (**adrenal hyperplasia** or **adrenal adenoma** → get
              abd CT)
          If **ACTH is high** (and cortisol high) → have either a **pituitary
              adenoma** or **ectopic source** (need to go to 2nd below)
      2nd: **If ACTH is high**→ give high dose **dexamethasone suppression
          test** (suppresses pituitary adenoma) and measure **urine free-
          cortisol:**
          If **urine cortisol suppressed** → **pituitary adenoma**
          If **urine cortisol not suppressed** → **ectopic** producer (eg lung
              CA, etc)
      Abd CT and **MRI** useful for localizing adrenal tumors and
          differentiating adenoma vs. hyperplasia
      NP-59 scintigraphy (iodo-cholesterol) is taken up by **adrenal
          adenomas** (DDx adenoma vs. hyperplasia; *not* taken up by
          adrenal CA)
      If **ectopic** source suspected → chest/abd/pelvic CT scan
      If **pituitary** source suspected → brain MRI
  **Pituitary adenoma (Cushing's Disease)
      **MCC non-iatrogenic Cushing's Syndrome (70% of cases)
      High ACTH and **cortisol suppressed** with high-dose dexamethasone
          suppression test
      MRI and **petrosal sampling** to localize → mostly **micro-adenomas**
      Tx: Most tumors removed w/ **trans-sphenoid** approach
  Ectopic ACTH
      #2 non-iatrogenic cause of Cushing's syndrome (15%)
      *MC source of extra-pituitary ACTH – *small cell lung CA*
      High ACTH and **cortisol <u>not</u> suppressed** with high-dose
          dexamethasone suppression test
      Chest/Abd/Pelvic CT or **MRI** can help localize
      Tx: resection of primary if possible
  Adrenal adenoma
      #3 non-iatrogenic cause of Cushing's syndrome (10%)
      Low ACTH
      Abd CT or MRI to localize (**NP-59 scintigraphy** if that fails)
      Tx: adrenalectomy
  Diffuse adrenal hyperplasia
      Low ACTH
      Tx: ***metyrapone** (inhibits steroid formation); **aminoglutethimide*
          (inhibits cholesterol synthesis); bilateral adrenalectomy

Adrenocortical Carcinoma
Rare; usually large (> 6 cm), usually advanced at dx (ie mets)
Bimodal distribution (before age 5 and in 5th decade)
50% functional (cortisol MC, aldosterone, sex steroids)
Sx's: HTN, abd pain, wt loss, weakness, feminization, masculinization
Tx: **Radical adrenalectomy** (*take __kidney__*; open anterior
approach, not laparoscopic)
Debulking can help pts and prolong survival
Mitotane post-op (adreno-lytic, improves disease free survival)
5-YS – 20%

Give **glucocorticoids** (+ **mineralocorticoid** if bilateral) after
adrenalectomy

Thyroid

266. *All of the following are true except
    a.   T3 is the most active form of thyroid hormone
    b.   Thyroid hormone is <u>not</u> involved in the fight or flight response
    c.   Albumin carries the majority of thyroid hormone in circulation
    d.   TSH is the most sensitive indicator of thyroid function

    Answer c.   Thyroxin-binding globulin (TBG) carries majority of T3/T4.

267. **A 50 yo woman presents to your clinic with a thyroid nodule. After H and P, most appropriate next step in management is:
    a.   Thyroid lobectomy
    b.   Total thyroidectomy
    c.   FNA
    d.   Neck MRI

    **Answer c.   **FNA* *(w/ U/S) is the best initial Dx test for a thyroid nodule.*

268. **Ultrasound on the above pt reveals a 1.2 cm mass. Pathology from the FNA shows follicular cells. The most appropriate next step in management is:
    a.   Thyroid lobectomy
    b.   Nothing
    c.   Neck CT
    d.   Neck MRI

    **Answer a.   **Follicular cells* *on FNA has been shown to result in follicular cell CA in 5-10% of pts. Thyroid lobectomy is required for definitive Dx.*

269. **You take the above patient to the operating room and perform a thyroid lobectomy. Pathology shows this is a 1.9 cm follicular cell carcinoma. The most appropriate next step is:
    a.   Completion total thyroidectomy
    b.   Close
    c.   Post op chemotherapy
    d.   Post-op XRT

    **Answer a.   ***Thyroid CA with a size > 1 cm requires total thyroidectomy.*

270. **The above patient also had palpable lymph nodes in her neck on physical exam prior to surgery. The most appropriate management is:
    a.   Cherry pick the lymph nodes out of the neck
    b.   Radical neck dissection
    c.   Modified radical neck dissection (MRND)
    d.   Post op XRT

    **Answer c.   ***Patients with thyroid CA and clinically positive lymph nodes should undergo total thyroidectomy and MRND.*

271. **After total thyroidectomy and MRND above, post-op this pt should also undergo:
    a.   I-131 therapy
    b.   XRT
    c.   Chemotherapy (5-FU)
    d.   Tamoxifen therapy

    **Answer a.   ***I-131 is a very effective Tx for disseminated thyroid CA.*
    Do <u>not</u> give thyroid replacement until <u>after</u> Tx w/ ^{131}I to avoid suppressing ^{131}I uptake (want TSH level high before Tx w/ ^{131}I)

272. **Post-operatively the above opera singer has a loss of voice pitch. This is most likely due to injury of the:
   a.   Superior laryngeal nerve
   b.   Recurrent laryngeal nerve
   c.   Vagus nerve
   d.   Glossopharyngeal nerve

   Answer a. **Loss of pitch is most consistent with superior laryngeal nerve injury. Careful ligation of the superior thyroid artery branches at the level of the thyroid capsule can help avoid this complication.*

273. **Instead of the above, post-operatively this patient has a hoarse voice. This is most likely due to injury of the:
   a.   Superior laryngeal nerve
   b.   Recurrent laryngeal nerve
   c.   Vagus nerve
   d.   Glossopharyngeal nerve

   Answer b. **Hoarseness is most consistent with recurrent laryngeal nerve injury. This nerve often tracks with the inferior thyroid artery inferiorly. **Hoarseness** may get better (wait 6 mos.), if that fails **medialize vocal cord w/ silicone wedge** or injection (**not re-op repair of nerve**).*

274. **Post-operatively, a patient undergoing a difficult total thyroidectomy has severe respiratory stridor and impending respiratory arrest immediately after extubation in the post-anesthesia care unit. She does not have any signs of hematoma. The most effective way of airway access is:
   a.   Re-intubation
   b.   Open the wound and place emergent tracheostomy
   c.   Take her back to the OR for re-exploration
   d.   Racemic epinephrine

   Answer b. **Given the clinical scenario, this pt likely suffered bilateral RLN injury. Trying to intubate a pt w/ bilateral RLN injury and medialization of both cords is very difficult. The best option is emergent tracheostomy through the collar incision (which you performed for the thyroidectomy).*

275. **Following I-131, the most effective way of suppressing the growth of any residual follicular or papillary thyroid CA is:
   a.   Thyroid hormone replacement
   b.   Daily calcium
   c.   Daily phosphate replacement
   d.   Daily potassium

   Answer a. ***Thyroid hormone** replacement following resection for thyroid CA is a very effective tumor suppressor adjunct. By giving thyroid hormone, you effectively suppress TSH production and inhibit tumor growth*

276. **All of the following are risk factors for metastatic spread and recurrence of papillary and follicular thyroid CA except:
   a.   Males
   b.   Previous XRT
   c.   Age 20-50
   d.   Extra-capsular invasion

   Answer c. ***RFs for thyroid CA mets or recurrence:* Grade (poorly differentiated), **Age** (< 20 or > 50), Male gender, Extra-thyroidal DZ, Size > 1 cm, Previous XRT*

277. **All of the following are true of medullary CA of the thyroid except:

a. Amyloid is found in the tissue
b. Flushing and diarrhea occur
c. Family members of pts w/ MEN IIb should be screened for the RET proto-oncogene
d. MEN IIa pts have the worst prognosis

Answer d. MEN IIb and sporadic forms have the worst prognosis.
Family members of pts w/ MEN IIb should be screened for the **RET proto-oncogene.

278. **All of the following are true of Hurthle cell thyroid tumors except:
a. 80% are malignant
b. MC occurs in elderly
c. Pathology shows Ashkenazi cells
d. Diagnosis is usually made with lobectomy

Answer a. ***80% of **Hurthle cell thyroid tumors** are benign.*

279. *All of the following are true of anaplastic thyroid CA except:
a. Is usually resectable
b. Usually presents in elderly patients with long-standing goiters
c. Has a propensity to invade other structures
d. Is the most aggressive thyroid CA

Answer a. Anaplastic thyroid CA is the most aggressive thyroid CA and is usually beyond surgical management at the time of Dx (5-YS 5%).

280. **A 31 yo woman is 21 1/2 weeks pregnant with her 1st pregnancy and has severe tremors, tachycardia, and sweating. Her endocrinologist makes the diagnosis of hyperthyroidism and starts her on propylthiouracil, however she continues to have symptoms. You advise the physician that the most appropriate next step is:
a. Propranolol
b. I-131
c. Thyroidectomy
d. Methimazole

Answer c. ***The problem in this patient is that you <u>cannot</u> use either I-131 or methimazole because of their teratogenic effects. I-131 will ablate the fetal thyroid. Methimazole causes cretinism (stunted physical and mental growth due to hypothyroidism). Propylthiouracil (PTU) is safe because it does not cross the placenta.*

You could use a beta-blocker, but you would still have hyperthyroidism (albeit with a lower heart rate) and an increased risk of stillbirth. Also, beta-blockers are contra-indicated in the 3rd trimester of pregnancy as they have been associated with fetal growth retardation.

281. **All of the following are true except:
a. The Wolff Chaikoff effect is iodide inhibition of T3 and T4 release
b. The mechanism of propylthiouracil is inhibition of peroxidases and iodide binding
c. The most appropriate initial Tx for thyroid storm is I-131
d. Serum thyroglobulin levels after total thyroidectomy is a very effective for detecting thyroid papillary or follicular cell CA recurrence

Answer c. ***The most appropriate initial Tx for thyroid storm is a **beta-blocker** (eg propranolol). **High doses of **iodine** (Lugol's solution, potassium iodide) inhibit TSH action on thyroid and inhibits organic coupling of iodide to tyrosine, resulting in less T3 and T4 release (**Wolff-Chaikhoff effect**)*

Thyroid Anatomy and Function

Derived from the 1st and 2nd pharyngeal pouches

Post-thyroidectomy stridor due to hematoma – open neck and remove hematoma *emergently* → can cause <u>airway compromise</u>

Vascular supply

- **Superior thyroid artery** – 1st branch off *external carotid artery*
  - At superior pole of thyroid
- **Inferior thyroid artery** – off *thyrocervical trunk* (inferior)
  - Supplies **both inferior** and **superior parathyroids**
  - W/ thyroidectomy, need ligation of inferior thyroid arteries close to thyroid gland to avoid injury to parathyroid glands
- **Superior and middle thyroid veins** – *internal jugular vein* drainage
- **Inferior thyroid vein** – *innominate vein* drainage

**Recurrent laryngeal nerves (RLNs)

- **Motor to entire larynx** <u>except</u> cricothyroid muscle (superior laryngeal nerve)
- In **tracheo-esophageal groove** (posterior to thyroid)
- Can track w/ **inferior thyroid artery**
- **Left RLN** – loops around aorta
- **Right RLN** – loops around right subclavian (or innominate) artery
  1) ****Unilateral injury – hoarseness** (if vocal cord abducts, ie para-median location) or **nothing** (if vocal cord adducts, ie median location);
     - ****Hoarse** – *may get better (wait 6 mos.)*, ****medialize vocal cord** *w/ silicone wedge or injection if persistent sx's* **(**<u>not</u> re-op repair of nerve)**
     - **Asymptomatic** – leave alone
     - **Intra-op RLN injury** – repair at that time
  2) **Bilateral injury**
     - Can **obstruct airway acutely** (vocal cords adducted, Sx's-severe stridor) → need **emergency** **tracheostomy**
       - Can't intubate due to cords blocking airway
     - Can cause **profound aspiration** (vocal cords abducted) → will need **tracheostomy**

**Non-recurrent laryngeal nerve (1%)

- **MC side** – *<u>right</u>*; risk of injury during thyroid surgery

**Superior laryngeal nerve (external branch)

- **External branch** – motor to **cricothyroid** muscle
- Runs superior and lateral to thyroid lobes
- Can track w/ **superior thyroid artery** at upper pole of thyroid
- ***Injury causes in **loss of projection** (or pitch) and **easy voice fatigability** (eg opera singers)*
- Ligating superior thyroid artery branches close to the thyroid capsule helps avoid injury

Function

- **Hypothalamus** – releases **thyrotropin-releasing factor** (TRF) → goes to anterior pituitary gland
- **Anterior pituitary gland** – releases **thyroid-stimulating hormone** (TSH) → goes to thyroid gland
- **Thyroid Gland** – releases T4 and T3
- **T4 and T3** then bind the **thyroid hormone receptor** in the <u>nucleus</u>
- **Thyroid Hormone Function** - ↑ cardiac output, HR, RR, basal metabolic rate and potentates effects of catecholamines
  - ***Although <u>not</u> involved in flight or fight response*
- **TRF** and **TSH** release controlled by T4 + T3 negative feedback loop
- Only **free T4** and **T3** are <u>active</u> (protein bound <u>not</u> active) –
  - Free hormone represents < 1% of total serum T4 and T3
- **T4:T3** serum ratio is **20:1**
- Most T3 from T4 to T3 conversion in periphery (**deiodinases**)
- **T3 is the **more active form** (4x more potent than T4)*

Thyroglobulin – stores T4 and T3 in **colloid**
Peroxidases links tyrosine and iodine
Deiodinases – separate iodine ions (eg T4 to T3 conversion)
Serum thyroid hormone binding proteins (all bind T4 and T3):
> 1) *__Thyroxin-binding globulin__* (TBG)-*_carries majority T4+T3_*
> 2) **Transthyretin** (pre-albumin)
> 3) **Albumin**

Tests of thyroid function
> TSH – <u>most sensitive</u> indicator of gland function
> **T4 and T3 levels**

Thyroxine treatment – TSH levels should fall to 50%
> **S/Es** – osteoporosis long-term

Abnormalities in thyroid descent
> **Pyramidal lobe** (10%) – extends from isthmus toward the thymus
> **Lingual thyroid** and **Thyroglossal duct cyst** (see Head and Neck Chp)

**Thyroid Nodule w/u
> Check for **attachment** to trachea and cervical **adenopathy**
> 1) Get **FNA** *(best initial Dx test)* and U/S
> 2) TFTs (T3, T4, TSH), PTH , Ca
> 3) If **T3/T4 elevated** and FNA shows **thyroid tissue** - likely a **toxic nodule**
> 4) If T3/T4 are <u>not</u> elevated and **FNA + U/S are** →
>> a. **Determinant** (85%) → follow appropriate Tx
>> b. **Indeterminate** (15%) - get radionuclide study (technetium 99)
>>> *Hot nodule* → thyroxin for 6 weeks
>>>> This will decrease TSH and nodule should go away
>>>> If size does not decrease → **lobectomy,**
>>> *Cold nodule* → lobectomy, follow appropriate Tx if CA

> **Thyroid adenomas** - need to differentiate from CA → *requires lobectomy*
> Thyroid CA is the MC **endocrine malignancy** in the US

**Papillary thyroid CA
> <u>MC type</u> - **85%**, psammoma bodies, orphan annie nuclei
> MC Thyroid CA w/ **previous XRT**
> **Long standing goiter** (> 5 years) is a RF for thyroid CA
> **Path**
>> Least aggressive, slow growing, best prognosis; often multi-centric
>> Usually in young women, children
>> **Lymphatic spread 1st** although this is *__not__* **prognostic**
>>> **Positive nodes – children** (75%) > adults (15%); large + firm
>> ***Prognosis based on local invasion (MCC death)*
>> *Can present as a **complex cyst** or **bloody cyst** fluid*
>> Met's go to *__Lung__* (<u>rarely</u> occur)
>> **Overall 5-YS** – 95% (MCC death – local invasion)
>> **__Enlarged lateral neck lymph node__ w/ normal thyroid tissue _(lateral
>> aberrant thyroid tissue)_ = **papillary thyroid CA* w/ lymphatic
>> spread, Tx: **total thyroidectomy**, **ipsilateral MRND**, and [131]I

**Follicular thyroid CA
> More aggressive than papillary
> Older women (> 50); some association w/ **iodine deficiency**
> ***Follicular cells on FNA* – 10% chance of malignancy; need lobectomy
>> → perform **lobectomy**, send for frozen section (FS) and permanent,
>>> if path shows **adenoma or follicular cell hyperplasia**, nothing
>>> else needed; if papillary CA, follow Tx below
> Met's go to *__Bone__* (hematogenous) → 50% have mets at time of Dx
> **Overall 5-YS** – 70% (prognosis based on hematogenous + LN spread)

**The following apply for both *Papillary* and *Follicular Thyroid CA*
Indications for <u>total</u> **thyroidectomy:**
Tumor > 1 cm
Extra-thyroidal Disease (capsular invasion, clinical or positive nodal
disease, or mets)
Multi-centric or bilateral lesions
Previous XRT
Indications for **MRND:**
Extra-thyroidal Disease (capsule invasion, clinical or positive nodal
disease or mets)
Indications for [131]I (6 weeks after surgery, want TSH high for max. uptake):
Tumor > 1cm
Extra-thyroidal Disease (capsule invasion, positive nodes or mets)
Need <u>total thyroidectomy</u> for ^{131}I to be effective
****Do <u>not</u> give thyroid replacement until <u>after</u> Tx w/ [131]I to avoid
suppressing ^{131}I uptake** (want TSH level 3 x normal before [131]I Tx)
XRT only for unresectable disease not responsive to [131]I
Follow **thyroglobulin level** post-op for tumor recurrence (if total
thyroidectomy was performed)
[123]I can be used to look for recurrence late after total thyroidectomy
**After Tx w/ [131]I, give thyroxin to keep TSH levels low
Want TSH ≤ 0.03 and pt mildly thyrotoxic
This is <u>very effective</u> for metastatic DZ

<u>XRT and hormonal therapy for various thyroid CA</u>
XRT – effective for papillary, follicular, medullary and Hurthle cell CA
[131]I – effective for papillary and follicular thyroid CA *only* (<u>not</u> Hurthle, MTC,
or anaplastic); Can cure bone and lung mets
S/Es: sialoadenitis, GI symptoms, infertility, parathyroid dysfunction,
bone marrow suppression (rare), leukemia (rare)
<u>Not</u> used in **children** (CA risk), **during pregnancy** (cretinism, can
traverse placenta) or **lactating mothers** (in milk)

**RFs for thyroid CA mets or recurrence (GAMES-X) - <u>G</u>rade (poorly
differentiated), <u>A</u>ge (< 20 or > 50), <u>M</u>ale gender, <u>E</u>xtra-thyroidal DZ,
<u>S</u>ize > 1 cm, previous <u>X</u>RT

****<u>Medullary thyroid carcinoma</u> (MTC)**
Associated with: **MEN IIa, MEN IIb, Familial MTC** only and **Sporadic MTC**
(ie non-syndrome associated; represents 80% of MTC)
**Associated w/ RET proto-oncogene
Worse prognosis – MEN IIb and sporadic forms
Usually is **1st manifestation** of MEN IIa and MEN IIb (sx's - ****diarrhea,
flushing**)
Path - **parafollicular C cells** which secrete **calcitonin* (diarrhea, flushing)
**Amyloid in gland; more aggressive than follicular, papillary CA
Tx:
Pts w/ MTC as a **palpable thyroid mass:**
Total thyroidectomy
Central neck node dissection
MRND on side of tumor (bilateral if both lobes have tumor)
Pts w/ **Fam Hx** and **RET proto-oncogene** <u>w/o</u> a mass:
MEN IIa → prophylactic total thyroidectomy and central LN
dissection at age **6 years**
MEN IIb → prophylactic total thyroidectomy and central LN
dissection at age **2 years**
Not done earlier due to difficulty in finding recurrent laryngeal
nerves in children (too small); high risk of injury (including
bilateral injury - need for **permanent tracheostomy**)
Monitor post-op **calcitonin levels* for disease recurrence

5-YS for pts who present w/ **palpable MTC**
>> **MEN IIa** – 50% (prognosis based on **distant mets**)
>> **MEN-IIb** – 10%
>> Pts with family Hx of MEN IIa, MEN IIb or Familial MTC should undergo **genetic testing** for *RET proto-oncogene*. Calcitonin is NOT a good screening tool as most pts have already developed MTC if calcitonin is elevated.

Hurthle cell carcinoma
>> **MC benign (80%, adenoma); older patients
>> **Path** – **Ashkenazi cells**; cannot DDx benign vs. malignant based on FNA
>> **Need **lobectomy** to make Dx →
>>> **If benign** – Tx: lobectomy
>>> **If CA** - Tx: total thyroidectomy; MRND for clinically positive nodes

Anaplastic thyroid cancer
>> Elderly pts, long-standing goiters
>> *Most aggressive thyroid CA* – propensity to invade other structures (eg trachea) – rapidly lethal; **Path** – vesicular appearance of nuclei
>> Tx: Total thyroidectomy for rare resectable lesion (possible tracheal rsxn)
>>> Palliative thyroidectomy for compressive symptoms or chemo-XRT
>>> Rapidly lethal (5-YS - 5%); usually beyond surgical Tx at time of Dx

Hashimoto's disease
>> MCC of **hypothyroidism** in adults; MCC **thyroiditis**
>> Sx's: enlarged gland (goiter), painless, chronic thyroiditis
>> Dx: high thyroid *anti-peroxidase* and *anti-thyroglobulin* Ab's
>> Path Autoimmune destruction - **lymphocytic infiltrate**
>>> Goiter from lack of organification of **trapped iodide** in gland
>>> Unusual to have to operate unless there is a suspicious nodule
>>> *Erythrocyte sedimentation rate (ESR) is normal*
>> Tx: **Thyroxine** 1st line (treats vast majority)
>>> **Partial thyroidectomy** (unusual) - for continued growth despite thyroxine, suspicious nodules, or compression sx's

Hyperthyroidism
>> MCC hyperthyroidism – Grave's Disease (80%)
>> DDx Hyperthyroidism:
>>> **Grave's DZ** (autoimmune, **IgG to TSH receptor**); older women
>>>> IgG Ab's – *long acting thyroid stimulator* (LATS) and *thyroid stimulating immunoglobulin* (TSI)
>>> **Toxic adenoma** (single; usually > 2 cm to cause sx's); young women
>>> **Toxic multinodular goiter**
>> Sx's: goiter (Grave's and multi-nodular toxic goiter), heat intolerance, thirst, ↑ed appetite, weight loss, sweating, palpitations, atrial fibrillation
>>> *Sx's only w/ Grave's disease* – exophthalmos, pre-tibial edema
>>> Sx's can worsen w/ **contrast dyes**
>> Dx:
>>> **TFTs** (thyroid function tests - high T3 and T4; low **TSH)**
>>> **Thyroid scan** (RAIU, radio-active iodide uptake)
>>>> High ^{123}I uptake **homogenously** and **diffusely** – Grave's
>>>> High ^{123}I uptake **heterogeneously** and **diffusely** – toxic multinodular goiter
>>>> High ^{123}I uptake **localized** – hot nodule
>>> **U/S** – look for solitary adenoma (hot nodule)
>> Tx-hyperthyroidism (Grave's, toxic adenoma, or toxic multinodular goiter):
>>> **Medical Tx** effective in **95%** (unusual to have to operate)
>>>> **PTU** or **methimazole** (50% recurrence)
>>>> ^{131}I: 5% recurrence (Grave's and toxic adenoma); less effective for toxic multinodular goiter (non-homogenous uptake)
>>>> **Beta-blocker** helps w/ sx's

Indications for surgery: suspicious <u>nodule</u> *(MC indication for operation), <u>failed medical</u> Tx, <u>non-compliance</u>, <u>obstructive</u> goiter, <u>children and pregnant women</u> w/ refractory hyperthyroidism (if PTU fails, <u>cannot use</u> [131]I),*

Make sure **euthyroid** before operating (PTU, Lugol's, beta-blocker)

Surgical options

Subtotal thyroidectomy (5% recurrence; good for multinodular goiters)

Total thyroidectomy with thyroxin replacement

Children – there is general concern for the development of malignancy in young children treated w/ [131]I so it is <u>not used</u>

[131]I should <u>not</u> be used in **children** *(malignancy risk)*, **during pregnancy** *(cretinism, can traverse placenta)* or **lactating mothers** *(in milk)*

Methimazole should <u>not</u> be used **during pregnancy** *(cretinism)*

**<u>Pregnancy and Hyperthyroidism</u>

Tx hyperthyroidism w/ **PTU** until 2nd trimester

If pt still having sx's despite PTU, can add **beta-blocker**

*Cannot use [131]I (will destroy fetal thyroid tissue → cretinism)

If PTU has effectively treated the problem → no surgery

**If PTU has <u>not</u> effectively treated the problem *(ie **still requiring beta-blocker to control sx's)* →

**Thyroidectomy in 2nd trimester (best time, ↓ risk of teratogenic events and premature labor)

Total thyroidectomy or sub-total thyroidectomy

Risk of **still birth** if you let hyperthyroidism go into 3rd trimester

Avoid beta-blockers in 3rd trimester (fetal growth retardation)

PTU - Inhibits peroxidases

S/E's – **aplastic anemia** or **agranulocytosis** (rare)

Safe in **pregnancy** (does not cross the placenta)

Methimazole - Inhibits peroxidases

S/E's – **aplastic anemia** or **agranulocytosis** (rare)

Cretinism in newborns (crosses placenta)

*Do <u>NOT</u> use in pregnancy

*<u>Thyroid storm</u>

Sx's: ↑ HR, fever, irritability, N/V, HTN, diaphoresis

High output cardiac failure (MCC of death)

*MC occurrence – after surgery in pt w/ *undiagnosed Grave's Disease

Other precipitants – anxiety, hard gland palpation, adrenergic drugs

Tx: **Beta-blockers (<u>1st</u> drug to give, esmolol drip)*

*Lugol's Solution (best Tx but takes awhile to have effect;, <u>potassium iodide</u>, give 1 hr after PTU) - **Wolff-Chaikoff effect**

PTU, cooling blankets, oxygen, glucose, steroids

Emergent thyroidectomy <u>rarely</u> indicated

<u>Multi-nodular goiter</u> (can be toxic or non-toxic)

Unusual to have to operate unless **suspicious nodule, cosmesis** issues or **compression** sx's (eg airway compression w/ stridor)

Causes: iodine deficiency (MC world), low-grade TSH stimulation (MC US)

Path – shows colloid

Substernal goiter – when > 50% of gland is below the thoracic inlet

Tx (either for <u>hyperthyroidism</u> or <u>large size</u>) - **PTU,** [131]I**, beta-blocker**

Subtotal (or total) thyroidectomy if **refractory, compressive sx's**, or **suspicious nodule**

95% of **substernal goiters can be removed w/ **neck collar incision** (no sternotomy needed)*

Tracheomalacia is a cx from compressive sx's

Parathyroid

282. *All of the following are true except:
    a. Superior parathyroid glands are derived from the 3rd pharyngeal pouch
    b. Parathyroid hormone (PTH) increases renal absorption of Ca and increases osteoclastic release of Ca from bone
    c. PTH level should drop to 50% or less of the pre-op level within 10 minutes after successfully removing an adenoma
    d. Active Vit D increases gut Ca absorption by increasing calcium binding protein

    Answer a. The **superior parathyroid glands** are from the 4th **pouch**.

    ***PTH level** should drop to 50% or less of pre-op level within 10 minutes after successfully removing an adenoma (drawn from **peripheral vein**).*

283. **All of the following are true except:
    a. The MC location for a missed parathyroid gland at re-exploration is normal anatomic position
    b. The MC location for an ectopic parathyroid gland is thymus
    c. The superior thyroid artery goes to the superior glands and the inferior thyroid artery for the inferior glands
    d. The MCC of hypo-parathyroidism is previous thyroid surgery

    Answer c. **The blood supply to both the superior and inferior parathyroid glands is the **inferior thyroid arteries**.*

    ***MC location of a missing parathyroid gland at re-op is **normal anatomic position**.*
    ***MC location for an ectopic parathyroid gland is **thymus**.*
    The MCC of hypoparathyroidism is **previous thyroid surgery
    *** The MCC of persistent hyperparathyroidism after parathyroid surgery is **missed adenoma**.*

284. *All of the following are true except:
    a. The MCC of hypercalcemia is hyper-parathyroidism
    b. Malignant hypercalcemia is most commonly from osteolysis
    c. Lung CA is the CA with the highest risk of hypercalcemia
    d. PTH related peptide (PTH-rp) causes an increase in urine cAMP

    Answer b. Malignant hypercalcemia is MC from PTH-rp release.
    Squamous cell **lung CA is the CA with the highest risk of hypercalcemia*
    ***PTH related peptide** (PTH-rp) causes an increase in urine cAMP*

285. *Which of the following is most consistent with primary hyperparathyroidism?
    a. Ca 11, PTH 200, elevated urine Ca
    b. Ca 8, PTH 200, elevated urine Ca, serum creatnine 7
    c. Ca 11, PTH 40, low urine calcium
    d. Ca 8, PTH 35, normal urine calcium

    Answer a. Ca 11, PTH 200, elevated urine Ca

286. *Which of the following lab values are most consistent with primary hyperparathyroidism?
    a. Cl 105, phosphate 3 and elevated renal cAMP
    b. Cl 105, phosphate 4 and elevated renal cAMP
    c. Cl 107, phosphate 3 and decreased renal cAMP
    d. Cl 106, phosphate 4 and decreased renal cAMP

Answer a. Primary hyperparathyroidism is associated with an elevated PTH, elevated Ca, elevated renal cAMP (effect of PTH on the PTH receptor in the kidney), and a Cl:PO4 ratio > 33.

287. *Which of the following is most consistent with secondary hyperparathyroidism:
     a.   Ca 11, PTH 200, elevated urine Ca
     b.   Ca 8, PTH 200, elevated urine Ca, serum creatnine 7
     c.   Ca 11, PTH 40, low urine calcium
     d.   Ca 8, PTH 45, normal urine calcium

     Answer b. Secondary hyperparathyroidism occurs primarily in dialysis patients who have chronic loss of Ca.

288. **Which of the following is most consistent with familial hypercalcemic, hypocalciuria (FHH)?
     a.   Ca 11, PTH 200, elevated urine Ca
     b.   Ca 8, PTH 200, elevated urine Ca, serum creatnine 7
     c.   Ca 11, PTH 40, low urine calcium
     d.   Ca 8, PTH 35, normal urine calcium

     Answer c. **Ca 11, PTH 40, low urine Ca. FHH is due to a defect in kidney PTH receptor that results in increased Ca resorption. Urine Ca will be low. **Tx for FHH – nothing (leave alone, Ca level never gets that high)*

289. **You are performing a parathyroidectomy for primary hyperparathyroidism and find 3 normal sized glands. All of the following are true except:
     a.   MC location of a missing gland is normal anatomic position in neck
     b.   The most common location for an ectopic gland is the thymus
     c.   You should resect 2 and 1/2 glands
     d.   If you can't find an adenoma - close and get a sestamibi scan

     Answer d. **You should not resect normal glands. If you cannot find the missing gland, you should close and get a post-op sestamibi scan*

290. **You are performing a parathyroidectomy for primary hyperparathyroidism and find 3 abnormally large glands. All of the following are true except:
     a.   MC location of a missing gland is normal anatomic position in neck
     b.   The most common location for an ectopic gland is the thymus
     c.   You should resect 2 and 1/2 glands
     d.   You should close and get a sestamibi scan

     Answer c. **If the glands are abnormally large, resect 2 and ½ glands.*

291. **All of the following are true of parathyroid CA except:
     a.   The MCC of mortality is airway invasion
     b.   The MC site of mets is lung
     c.   PTH is elevated
     d.   Surgery should include en bloc parathyroidectomy and ipsilateral thyroidectomy

     Answer a. **The MCC mortality w/ parathyroid CA is hypercalcemia – can have extremely high Ca levels (> 15). **Surgery should include en bloc parathyroidectomy and ipsilateral thyroidectomy*

292. **A 30 yo woman recently diagnosed with MEN I syndrome develops confusion, somnolence, and a shortened QT on EKG. The next appropriate step is:
     a.   Alpha-blockade
     b.   Beta-blockade
     c.   Calcium
     d.   Intravenous fluids and lasix

Answer d. **MEN I includes parathyroid hyperplasia, pancreatic tumors, and pituitary tumors. Of these, only **hypercalcemia** from hyper-parathyroidism is associated with confusion, somnolence, and short QT. **Tx - **rapid normal saline bolus** (200-300 cc/hr) and **Lasix**

293. **Which of the following is characteristic of MEN I:
    a.   Parathyroid hyperplasia, pancreatic tumors (MC –gastrinoma), pituitary tumors
    b.   Parathyroid hyperplasia, medullary carcinoma of the thyroid, and pheochromocytoma
    c.   Medullary carcinoma of the thyroid, pheochromocytoma, marfanoid habitus, mucosal neuroma
    d.   Von Recklinghausen's Disease

Answer a. MEN I consists of parathyroid hyperplasia, pancreatic tumors (gastrinoma is MC for this syndrome), and pituitary tumors (prolactinoma MC). ****Gastrinoma** is the MC MEN I tumor overall. (Note insulinoma is the MC endocrine pancreatic tumor in general population but not in the MEN I).

294. **All of the following are true except:
    a.   MENIN inactivation is associated w/ MEN IIa
    b.   Urine catecholamines should be checked in MEN IIa and IIb pts before elective surgery
    c.   Ca levels should be checked in MEN I and MEN IIa pts before elective surgery
    d.   Ret proto-oncogene is associated w/ MEN IIa and IIb

Answer a. ****MENIN** inactivation is associated w/ MEN I
****Ret proto-oncogene** is associated w/ MEN IIa and IIb
****Urine catecholamines** should be checked in MEN IIa and IIb pts before elective surgery (R/O pheochromocytoma)
****Ca levels** should be checked in MEN I and MEN IIa pts before elective surgery (R/O parathyroid hyperplasia)

295. **All of the following are true except:
    a.   MEN I pts w/ simultaneous tumors should have the hyperparathyroidism corrected 1st
    b.   MEN IIa pts w/ simultaneous tumors should have the pheochromocytoma corrected 1st
    c.   MEN IIb pts w/ simultaneous tumors should have the medullary thyroid CA corrected 1st
    d.   Gastrinoma is the MC pancreatic tumor in MEN I pts

Answer c. **MEN IIb pts w/ simultaneous tumors should have the **pheochromocytoma** corrected 1st ****Gastrinoma** is the MC pancreatic tumor in MEN I pts

Anatomy
Superior parathyroids
> Near posterior and superior portion of thyroid, often lateral to RLNs
> Above inferior thyroid artery
> *Derived from 4th pouch* (associated w/ **thyroid complex**)
> Can migrate to **posterior** mediastinum

Inferior parathyroids
> More anterior, often medal to RLNs
> Below inferior thyroid artery
> *Derived from 3rd pouch* (associated w/ **thymus**)
> *Inferior parathyroids have more **variable location** and are more likely to be **ectopic** (aberrant) compared to superior parathyroids*
> Occasionally in **tail of thymus** (MC ectopic site)
> Can migrate to **anterior** mediastinum

PTH – *increases* serum Ca by 3 mechanisms:
1) **Kidney Ca reabsorption** in distal tubules, also ↓s kidney PO_4 absorption (all mediated by **cAMP**)
2) **Osteoclast release of Ca in bone** (also releases PO_4)
3) **Vitamin D production in kidney** (↑s Vit D 1-alpha hydroxylation)
Net serum PO_4 *decreases* due to PTH

Vit D (1,25-dihydroxy-cholecalciferol)
Synthesis: 7-dehydrocholesterol → *UV light* → Vit D3 → *liver (25-hydroxylation)*→Vit D3-25OH→ *kidney (1-hydroxylation)*→Vit D
Active Vit D *increases* intestinal Ca and PO_4 absorption by increasing *calcium binding protein*

Calcitonin - *decreases* serum Ca by 2 mechanisms:
1) **Bone Ca resorption** (osteoclast inhibition)
2) **Kidney Ca and PO_4 excretion**

Normal Values

Normal Ca:	2.2 - 2.6 mmol/L (8.5-10.5 mg/dL)
Normal Ionized Ca (1/2 above)	1.1 - 1.5 mmol/L (4.5 - 5.5 mg/dL)
Normal PTH:	10 - 60 (pg/ml)
Normal PO_4:	2.5 - 5.0
Normal Cl⁻:	98 - 107
Parathyroid weight	60 - 80 gm

Hypercalcemia (90% from **hyperparathyroidism or **CA**):
1) **Hyperparathyroidism** (MCC overall)
2) **CA** (*MC due to PTH-rp*)
   a) **PTH-related peptide** (lung CA #1) – not picked up on PTH assay
      high **urine cAMP** w/ PTH-rp (acts on kidney PTH receptor)
   b) **Cytokines + excess Vit D precursors** (hematologic CA)
   c) **Osteolysis**
   **CA w/ *highest risk* of hypercalcemia overall – small cell lung CA

<u>Primary Hyperparathyroidism</u>
PRAD-1 oncogene increases risk for parathyroid adenomas
Genetic Syndromes - MEN I and IIA, familial hyperparathyroidism
Sx's:
   Muscle weakness, nephrolithiasis, pancreatitis, GI ulcers, depression, bone pain, pathologic Fx, bone loss on densitometry scan
   *Most patients are **asymptomatic*** – high Ca found on routine lab work
   Osteitis fibrosa cystica (brown tumor, bone lesion from Ca resorption)
   Hypertension can result from renal impairment
Dx: ↑ **PTH** and ↑ **Ca** (*ionized* best test)
   Other:↓ phos, ↑ urine Ca, ↑ renal cAMP (action on PTH receptor);
      **Cl⁻ to phos ratio >33 (hyperchloremic <u>metabolic acidosis</u>)
Path - <u>Single adenoma</u> (80%); diffuse <u>hyperplasia</u> (15%); <u>multiple adenomas</u> (4%); parathyroid <u>adenocarcinoma</u> (< 1%, very rare),
Indications for surgery:
1) **Symptomatic** - pancreatitis, ulcers, joint or bone pain, Fx, weakness, kidney stones
2) **Asymptomatic** w/: **Ca > 13,** low **Cr** clearance (> 30%; from chronic Ca overload), decreased **bone mass** (densitometry t-**score < −2.5**, any site)**, Age < 50** (lowers lifetime risk of cx's)
Tx:
   Adenoma – resection
   Parathyroid hyperplasia - resect 3 1/2 glands (<u>form the 1/2 gland 1ˢᵗ</u>) or total para-thyroidectomy and auto-implantation (in strap muscles or forearm); ****Do *not* biopsy all glands** → risks hemorrhage and hypoparathyroidism
   Parathyroid CA – radical parathyroidectomy (take ipsilateral **thyroid**)
   Pregnancy – surgery in 2ⁿᵈ trimester; ↑ **stillbirth** if not resected

Intra-op PTH level: see if you got correct gland (peripheral blood draw) ***PTH should go to **50% of pre-op value in **10 minutes***
If you find 3 fairly big glands (ie have **hyperplasia and missing a gland or you have hyperplasia and pt was born w/ 3 glands)
Check missing gland locations
Take **2 ½ glands** (or 3 glands w/ auto-implantation)
Check **intra-op PTH**, if still high PTH → check missing gland locations + thymectomy; if still high PTH → close, post-op sestamibi scan
If you find 3 totally normal sized glands (ie can't find the adenoma); check missing gland locations + **thymectomy
*Still not found, close, post-op **sestamibi scan** to find gland*
Missing Gland locations:
    **Thymus tissue (MC ectopic location for parathyroid gland)
    Near **carotid bifurcation** (open carotid sheath)
    Anterior to **vertebral bodies**
    Superior and **posterior to pharynx**
    Tracheo-esophageal groove
    Intra-thyroid (use U/S to find it)
    Anterior and **posterior mediastinum** *(can't reach from neck)*
Follow Ca post-op (remember to give Ca post-op)
    Post-op hypocalcemia etiologies:
        Bone hunger (early) – normal PTH, decreased HCO3-
        Graft/Remnant failure (late) – low PTH, normal HCO3-
Persistent hyperparathyroidism post-op (1%)
    MCC – missed adenoma in neck
    Sestamibi scan to localize missing gland, re-operate

Secondary hyperparathyroidism
MCC – **chronic renal failure**
Dx: ↑ **PTH** and ↓ **Ca** (may be near normal), ↑ **urine Ca**, ↑ **serum PO₄**
Most do not need surgery (95%)
Indications for Surgery: refractory **Bone Pain** (MC indication) or **pruritis** also for **fractures** (85% get relief)
    Tx: subtotal (3 1/2 glands) or total parathyroidectomy w/ auto-implant
*Cinacalcet (mimics action of Ca) - activates calcium-sensing receptor in parathyroid and **decreases PTH secretion**
*Calciphylaxis (calcific uremic arteriopathy)
    Associated w/ **chronic renal failure**; very poor prognosis
    Calcification and **thrombosis** of small to medium sized blood vessels; can occur in any tissue
    1st manifestation usually is **skin ischemia** and **necrosis;** painful
    Dx: **skin biopsy (calcification and thrombosis of blood vessels)*
    Tx: Dialysis, aggressive wound care

Tertiary hyperparathyroidism
*Renal failure now corrected w/ **kidney TXP** but still have high PTH*
Lab values same as primary hyperparathyroidism (ie ↑ **PTH** and ↑ **Ca)**
Surgical indications same as primary hyperparathyroidism
Tx: subtotal (3 1/2 glands) or total parathyroidectomy w/ auto-implantation

**Familial hypercalcemic hypocalciuria (FHH)
Defect in **PTH receptor** in distal convoluted tubule of **kidney** that increases resorption of Ca (increased binding of PTH to the receptor)
Dx: ↑ **serum Ca** (only to 11 or so, never symptomatic)
    PTH is normal (5-40)
    **Urine Ca is low (key to Dx, this is opposite of primary hyperparathyroidism)
**Tx: nothing (Ca not that high); ***No parathyroidectomy*

**Hypercalcemic Crisis

Ca usually needs to be **> 13** (ionized > 6) for sx's to occur

MCC hypercalcemic crisis – *previous primary hyperparathyroidism undergoing another procedure*

Sx's: lethargy, oliguria, hypotension, arrhythmias

Tx: ****1st - rapid _normal saline_ Infusion** (200-300 cc/hr)

    **No lactated ringers (contains Ca)

    2nd _lasix_ (**do _not_ use thiazide diuretics which cause Ca resorption)

    Dialysis if refractory to above

    ***Chronic Tx in malignancy → *Bisphosphonates** [eg **alendronate** (Fosamax)]; Inhibits osteoclast bone resorption

Just to re-state: **lactated ringers** and **thiazide diuretics** are _contraindicated_ in pts w/ hypercalcemia

**_Parathyroid cancer_ *(Rare)*

Mortality from **hypercalcemia** – can have extremely high Ca levels (> 15)

↑ **PTH** and ↑ **Ca**; ↑ **alkaline phosphatase**

MC site for mets – lung

Tx wide en bloc excision (parathyroidectomy and **ipsilateral *thyroidectomy); recurrence – 50%; 5-YS – 50%*

**_MEN Syndromes_

MEN I (MENIN inactivation)

    Parathyroid hyperplasia

        Usually 1st part to be **symptomatic**; (kidney stones)

        Tx: four-gland resection w/ auto-transplantation in forearm

            Don't leave gland in neck – hard re-op if recurrence

    Pancreatic islet cell tumors

        **Gastrinoma MC for MEN I (50% multiple, 50% malignant)

        MCC death in these pts (also MCC morbidity)

    Pituitary adenoma - Prolactinoma MC

    Simultaneous tumors - need to correct **hyperparathyroidism 1st

MEN IIa (RET proto-oncogene)

    Parathyroid hyperplasia

        Tx: four-gland resection w/ auto-transplantation in forearm

            Don't leave gland in neck – hard re-op if recurrence

    Medullary CA of thyroid

        Usually 1st part to be **symptomatic** (MC Sx - diarrhea)

        Nearly all pts w/ MEN IIa get this (> 95%); often bilateral

        MCC death in these pts

    Pheochromocytoma - often bilateral, nearly always benign

    Simultaneous tumors - need to correct **pheochromocytoma 1st

MEN IIb (RET proto-oncogene)

    -

    Medullary CA of thyroid

        Usually 1st part to be **symptomatic (**MC Sx - diarrhea**)**

        Nearly all patients w/ MEN IIb get this (95%); often bilateral

        MCC of death in these pts

        More aggressive than MEN IIa

    Pheochromocytoma - often bilateral, nearly always benign

    Mucosal ganglioneuromas (anywhere in GI tract)

    Marfan's habitus, musculoskeletal abnormalities

    Simultaneous tumors - need to correct **pheochromocytoma 1st

** Need to check **Ca level** before operating on pts w/ MEN I or IIa

** Need to check for **urine catecholamines** (pheochromocytoma) before operating on pts w/ MEN-IIa or IIb

Pituitary Gland

296. **All of the following are true except
   a. A calcified cyst near the sella turcica in a 5 yo boy is most consistent w/ meningioma
   b. Trouble lactating following peri-partum hypotension is consistent w/ Sheehan's syndrome
   c. Most prolactinomas can be treated w/ bromocriptine
   d. ADH is released primarily in response to high plasma osmolarity

   Answer a. A calcified cyst near the sella turcica is most consistent w/ **craniopharyngioma**. Tx – resection if symptomatic (benign cyst)

Hypothalamus
Releases **TRH, CRH, GnRH, GHRH,** and **dopamine** into median eminence
Hormones then pass through the posterior pituitary (neurohypophysis) on their way to the anterior pituitary (adenohypophysis)
Dopamine – inhibits prolactin secretion (constitutive inhibitor)

Posterior pituitary (neurohypophysis)
Consists of axons extending from **supraoptic** and **paraventricular nuclei** of **hypothalamus** into the posterior pituitary gland
Secrete 2 hormones into capillaries of the hypophyseal circulation:
   1) **ADH** (ie vasopressin)
      Release controlled by **supraoptic nuclei** mostly
      Primarily regulated by **osmolar receptors** in hypothalamus;
         Released in response to **high plasma osmolarity**
      Causes increased **water absorption** in **kidney collecting ducts**
   2) **Oxytocin** – release controlled by **paraventricular nuclei** mostly
Posterior pituitary does <u>NOT</u> contain cell bodies

Anterior pituitary (80% of gland, adenohypophysis)
ACTH, TSH, GH, LH, FSH, and **prolactin** released
NO direct blood supply; has **portal system** w/ blood passing through neurohypophysis 1st

Pituitary gland found in **sella turcica**

Bi-temporal hemianopia (visual problems w/ pituitary mass) – from a pituitary mass compressing optic nerve (CN II) at the chiasm
Contraindications to trans-sphenoid resection of tumors – supra-cellar (dumbbell-shaped tumor) extension, massive lateral extension
Bromocriptine – can be used reduce all endocrine secreting pituitary tumors *except* ACTH secreting

Pituitary tumors
Prolactinoma
MC pituitary tumor; MC are ***micro*-adenomas**
Sx's: amenorrhea, galactorrhea, infertility, poor libido, visual problems
Dx: ↑ **prolactin** (> 150 usual); MRI + visual field testing
Tx: ***Most prolactinomas do not need surgery***
   1) **Asymptomatic** and **micro-adenoma** (≤ 10 mm) – follow w/ MRI
   2) **Symptomatic** or **macro-adenoma** (> 10 mm):
      Bromocriptine (dopa agonist) - 85% success (safe w/ pregnancy)
      Trans-sphenoid surgery (for failed medical Tx, hemorrhage, visual loss, wants pregnancy, CSF leak) – 85% successful (15% recurrence)

Acromegaly (excessive growth hormone, GH)

> GH stimulates secretion of **insulin-like growth factor-1**
>
> MC are *macro*-adenomas
>
> Sx's: jaw enlargement (macroglossia), HA, ↑ soft tissue, HTN,
>> amenorrhea, DM, gigantism; visual problems related to size
>>
>> Can have **life-threatening cardiac issues** (valves, cardiomyopathy)
>
> Dx: *↑ IGF-1 level* (*best test*, random GH level <u>not</u> useful)
>> **MRI** to look for tumor
>
> Tx:
>> **Surgery 1ˢᵗ** choice if not invading surrounding tissues (→ trans-
>>> sphenoid resection)
>>
>> **Octreotide** and **bromocriptine** can shrink tumor and relieve sx's
>>> **Pegvisomant** (GH receptor antagonist)

Other conditions

Sheehan's syndrome

> Pituitary insufficiency in mother after childbirth
>
> From hypovolemia or shock following childbirth causing pituitary ischemia
>
> **1ˢᵗ sign** – *postpartum **trouble lactating***; can also have amenorrhea,
>> adrenal insufficiency, hypothyroidism
>
> Affects **anterior pituitary** (portal venous blood supply), posterior pituitary
>> usually not affected (direct arterial blood supply)
>
> Tx: replace deficiencies

Craniopharyngioma

> **Benign**
>
> MC children aged 5-10 years
>
> ***Calcified cyst*** near anterior pituitary, remnants of **Rathke's pouch**
>
> Sx's: headaches, growth failure, bi-temporal hemianopia, endocrine
>> abnormalities, hydrocephalus
>
> Tx: surgery if symptomatic; **Diabetes insipidus** – frequent Cx post-op

Bilateral pituitary masses – if non-endocrine producing → probably metastases

Breast

297. *All of the following are true except:
    a. Laceration of the long thoracic nerve will result in a winged scapula
    b. Laceration of the thoracodorsal nerve will result in weak adduction
    c. The MC injured nerve w/ MRM or ALND is intercostobrachial nerve
    d. The MCC of malignant axillary adenopathy is metastatic breast CA

    Answer d. *The MCC of malignant axillary adenopathy is **lymphoma**.*

298. *A 46 yo woman undergoes breast biopsy and the pathology comes back as phyllodes tumor. You find no evidence of metastatic disease. The most appropriate management is:
    a. Modified radical mastectomy
    b. Lumpectomy and axillary lymph node dissection
    c. Radical mastectomy
    d. Wide local excision and no axillary node dissection

    Answer d. *Phyllodes tumors* consist of stromal cells and can be hard to differentiate from fibroadenomas. These behave like sarcomas and nodal mets are extremely rare. **Tx - wide local excision** w/ 1 cm margin, **No ALND**

299. **A 54 yo woman presents to your office w/ bloody nipple discharge. All of the following are true except:
    a. This patient needs bilateral mammograms
    b. This most commonly occurs with invasive ductal CA
    c. This patient likely requires a ductogram and directed excision
    d. This patient should have a breast U/S

    Answer b. **The MCC of bloody nipple discharge is **intra-ductal papilloma**. **Tx is **ductogram** to locate the papilloma and **wire localized excision**.*

300. **A 40 yo woman presents to you with breast pain and lumpy breast tissue that seems to vary with her hormonal cycle. She thinks she feels a dominant area that she hadn't felt before. All of the following are true except:
    a. She needs bilateral mammograms
    b. She needs an U/S
    c. She needs a core needle biopsy of the dominant area
    d. In patient's with fibrocystic disease, atypical hyperplasia does not increase cancer risk

    Answer d. **Atypical ductal hyperplasia** and **atypical lobular hyperplasia** increase the risk for breast CA. These lesions do not require negative margins.

301. **A 55 yo woman presents w/ a BiRAD 4 lesion on mammogram has suspicious linear calcifications. You perform a needle localization excisional biopsy which comes back ductal carcinoma in situ (DCIS). All of the following are true except:
    a. Comedo type DCIS is an indication for subcutaneous mastectomy
    b. Males w/ DCIS should undergo simple mastectomy
    c. This patient should receive an axillary lymph node dissection (ALND)
    d. Negative margins should be obtained for DCIS

    Answer c. **ALND is NOT indicated for DCIS.**
    **Lumpectomy with XRT is an option for most DCIS lesions*
    Comedo type DCIS is an indication for **simple mastectomy***
    Males w/ DCIS should undergo **simple mastectomy***
    Negative margins are required for DCIS (avoids sampling error)*

302. **A 40 yo woman undergoes a stereotactic excisional biopsy for a suspicious lesion on mammogram. The suspicious area is completely resected however the pathology comes back <u>LCIS</u> with positive margins. Her mother had breast CA at age 60. All of the following are true except:
   a. Re-excision for negative margins is required
   b. Observation with repeat mammography and examination in 6 months can be performed
   c. Tamoxifen can be used to Tx this pt
   d. Ductal CA is the most likely CA to occur w/ pre-existent LCIS

   Answer a. **LCIS does <u>not</u> require negative margins.*
   **LCIS does <u>not</u> form calcifications*
   Ductal CA* is the most likely CA to occur iin pts w/ **pre-existent LCIS
   **Tx options for LCIS:*
      1) **Nothing** and **careful F/U**
      2) **Hormonal Therapy** - 50% reduction in risk of breast CA
         Pre-menopausal – Tamoxifen, careful F/U (5 years maximum)
         Post-menopausal – Raloxifene, careful F/U
            Decreased DVT/PE and cataracts compared to Tamoxifen
      3) **Bilateral simple mastectomy** (<u>No</u> ALND or SLNB)

303. **All of the following are true of the BRCA gene except:
   a. Total abdominal hysterectomy and bilateral salpingo-oophrectomy decreases breast CA risk by 70%
   b. BRCA I gene equates with an ovarian cancer risk of 40% (lifetime)
   c. BRCA gene confers a worse prognosis in comparable staged non-BRCA breast CA
   d. BRCA II gene equates w/ a male breast cancer risk of 10% (lifetime)

   Answer c. **Women w/ BRCA* and breast CA have the **same prognosis** as comparable-stage breast CA in pts not having BRCA. **HER receptor* confers a **worse prognosis** for comparable-stage breast CA.

   **BRCA Tx options:*
      1) **Careful F/U** (± **Tamoxifen**) or;
      2) **Prophylactic mastectomy** (± TAH and BSO)
   **TAH and BSO* w/ BRCA gene → decreases breast CA risk by 70%
   **Bilateral prophylactic mastectomy* w/ BRCA gene → decreases breast CA risk by 90%
   **Bilateral prophylactic mastectomy and TAH and BSO w/ BRCA gene* → decreases breast CA risk by 95%

304. **A 60 yo woman presents with a 6 cm infiltrating ductal CA along with palpable but moveable axillary adenopathy. She has no signs of metastatic disease. All of the following are true in this patient except:
   a. This patient is a candidate for primary (neoadjuvant) chemotherapy
   b. She will ultimately require a modified radical mastectomy regardless of her response to chemotherapy
   c. She needs a chest/abdomen/pelvic CT scan for systemic work-up
   d. She is a candidate for lumpectomy and axillary lymph node dissection if the tumor shrinks with chemotherapy

   Answer b. **This pt has Stage IIIa* disease (T3, N1, M0). For Stage IIIa w/ T3N1M0, the initial therapy can be surgery or chemo. If the pt wishes to have BCT, primary chemo can be given in an attempt to shrink the tumor, followed by lumpectomy and ALND. The other option is MRM w/ post-op chemo-XRT (tumor is > 6 cm so you need XRT after MRM). For **Stage IIIb**, neoadjuvant chemo, followed by surgery (uaully MRM), then post-op chemo-XRT is standard Tx.

305. **All of the following are true of adjuvant Tx for breast CA except:

a. TAC (taxanes, Adriamycin and cyclophosphamide) is indicated for either 1) tumors > 1 cm, 2) positive nodes or 3) ER/PR negative tumors
b. Trastuzumab is indicated for breast CA that is 1) HER2 positive and 2) is either > 1 cm or has positive nodes
c. Post-menopausal breast CA < 1 cm with negative nodes and having positive ER/PR receptors should receive aromatase inhibitor Tx only as post-op therapy (no chemotherapy)
d. BCT is always contra-indicated after neoadjuvant therapy for T3 and T4 tumors

Answer d. MRM is not always required after neoadjuvant chemo for T3 or T4 tumor. If the tumor shrinks can go w/ BCT including ALND (no SLNB due to neoadjuvant Tx). *An exception to this is inflammatory breast CA which always requires MRM after neoadjuvant Tx*

TAC (taxanes, Adriamycin and cyclophosphamide) is indicated for either 1) tumors > 1 cm, 2) positive nodes or 3) ER/PR negative tumors
Trastuzumab is indicated for breast CA that is 1) HER2 positive and 2) is either > 1 cm or has positive nodes
Post-menopausal breast CA < 1 cm with negative nodes and having positive ER/PR receptors should receive aromatase inhibitor Tx only as post-op therapy (no chemotherapy)

306. *A 50 yo woman comes to clinic and has a 4 cm ductal carcinoma on mammography. You perform a physical exam on the patient and you notice the lymph nodes in her axilla are fixed and matted. Work up for metastatic disease is negative. This patients clinical stage is:
    a. Stage IB
    b. Stage IIA
    c. Stage IIB
    d. Stage IIIA

Answer d. A 4 cm CA is T2 and fixed nodes is N2a, T2N2M0, stage IIIa.

307. All of the following are surgical options in the above pt except:
    a. Lumpectomy and axillary lymph node dissection
    b. Modified radical mastectomy
    c. Lumpectomy and sentinel lymph node biopsy
    d. Quadrectomy and axillary lymph node dissection

Answer c. **Pts w/ clinically positive nodes** are not candidates for SLNB.

308. **The following are contraindications to breast conserving therapy (BCT) except:
    a. Pregnancy
    b. Lobular CA
    c. Previous XRT that would result in excessive XRT dose
    d. Multi-focal disease

Answer b. *Lobular CA is not a contra-indication to BCT*

309. *A 56 yo woman has a 2 cm ductal carcinoma on CNBx and negative nodes on exam. You decide to perform SLNB using lymphazurin blue dye and technetium labeled sulfur colloid . All of the following are true except:
    a. If you do not find blue or radio-labeled nodes, ALND is indicated
    b. If 3 blue nodes are found, they should all be taken
    c. If one node has a gamma count of 1500, another node has 200, and 4 other nodes have 10-20, then resection of the highest count node and any nodes 10% or greater than that node is indicated
    d. A supraclavicular node w/ a high gamma count should be left alone

Answer d. ***This node should be sampled. Unusually, you find a node that is hot which is outside the area you were expecting. You need to go after that node for staging purposes.*

> ***If you cannot find any blue nodes, you cannot accurately stage the patient. You need to perform an **ALND**.*
> ***You should **take all of the blue nodes**. Typically, w/ sentinel lymph node biopsy you find 1-3 nodes.*
> ***Resect the **highest count node** and any nodes 10% or greater than that Node.*

310. **All of the following are true of sentinel lymph node biopsy (SLNB) except:
     a. The major concern is the false negative rate
     b. Inflammatory breast CA is a contra-indication to SLNB
     c. The risk of lymphedema is lower w/ SLNB
     d. Lymphazurin blue dye has been associated with type II hypersensitivity reaction

     Answer d. ***Type I hypersensitivity reaction occurs in 1% of pts receiving lymphazurin blue dye. **T3 and T4 lesions (eg inflammatory breast CA) are <u>contraindications</u> to SLNB.*

311. **All the following are true of axillary lymph node dissection for beast CA except:
     a. Nodes beneath and lateral to pectoralis minor should be taken (level I and II nodes)
     b. The superior border for dissection is the axillary vein
     c. The posterior border is the scapula
     d. The anterior border is the pectoralis muscle

     Answer c. ***The posterior border is the **latissimus dorsi muscle**.*

     **Node levels
     > I – lateral to pectoralis minor muscle
     > II – beneath pectoralis minor muscle
     > III – medial to pectoralis minor muscle, extends to thoracic inlet (Halsted's ligament)
     > Remove **Level I and II nodes** en bloc w/ ALND for breast CA

312. *A 63 yo woman undergoes lumpectomy + SLNB for a T3N0M0 ductal CA. Six months later, she feels a nodule underneath the lumpectomy suture line. FNA comes back ductal carcinoma. The most appropriate next step is:
     a. Repeat lumpectomy including the lump
     b. Sentinel lymph node biopsy
     c. XRT
     d. Modified radical mastectomy (MRM)

     Answer d. **Tx for breast CA recurrence after lumpectomy is **MRM**. There is a 2-3% chance of recurrence after appropriate lumpectomy.*

313. **All of the following are true of Trastuzumab (Herceptin) except:
     a. The major S/E is neurotoxicity
     b. HER receptor is associated with a worse prognosis for breast CA
     c. Has a 50% reduction in breast CA recurrence when combined w/ chemo
     d. It is given after chemotherapy if both are indicated

     Answer a. **Trastuzumab major S/E - cardio-toxicity*
     *Taxol major S/E - neurotoxicity

314. *After a MRM, pathology shows a tumor that is 4 cm and 6 lymph nodes are positive. Estrogen receptors are positive but progesterone receptors are negative. The most appropriate post-op management is:
    a. Chemo, XRT and hormonal therapy
    b. Tamoxifen only
    c. XRT only
    d. Chemotherapy followed by Tamoxifen

    Answer a. ** ≥ 4 positive nodes is an indication for **XRT after MRM**

315. *A 60 yo woman has a palpable node in her axilla. You get a bilateral mammogram and CXR which are both negative. You decide to excise the node and you find adenocarcinoma that is positive for estrogen receptors. The most appropriate next step is:
    a. Chemotherapy (Adriamycin and cyclophosphamide)
    b. XRT
    c. Modified radical mastectomy
    d. Sentinel lymph node biopsy

    Answer c. *Occult breast CA* can present as an enlarged lymph node in the axilla. With the finding of breast CA in the axillary node, you should perform MRM on the same side. In 70%, you will find breast CA in the breast. Instead of excisional Bx above, core needle could be performed.

316. **A 56 yo woman with no PMHx presents to your office with a <u>weepy, scaly lesion</u> on her right nipple. Mammogram and U/S do not show any mass. You get a wedge biopsy of the <u>skin and breast tissue</u> which shows Paget cells and DCIS. The appropriate next step is:
    a. Modified radical mastectomy
    b. Simple mastectomy (including the nipple areolar complex)
    c. Lumpectomy and axillary lymph node biopsy
    d. XRT

    Answer b. **DCIS w/ Paget's → **simple mastectomy including <u>nipple areolar complex</u>** (classic answer). ALND is <u>not</u> indicated for Paget's w/ DCIS.

    Breast CA w/ Paget's → simple mastectomy <u>and</u> ALND or SLNB (including nipple areolar complex resection) or **MRM**

317. **All of the following are true except:
    a. The majority of male breast CA is lobular CA
    b. The mechanism is inflammatory breast CA is dermal lymphatic invasion by tumor
    c. The usual Tx sequence for inflammatory breast CA is neoadjuvant chemo → then surgery (usually MRM) → then adjuvant chemo-XRT
    d. XRT is good for metastatic flare-ups

    Answer a. The majority of male breast CA is ductal CA
    The usual Tx sequence for **inflammatory breast CA is neoadjuvant chemo → then surgery (usually MRM) → then adjuvant chemo-XRT*

318. *All the following are true of transverse rectus abdominal (TRAM) flaps except:
    a. The timing of TRAM flap should be months after XRT
    b. Peri-umbilical muscle perforators are the most important blood supply to the skin overlying the flap
    c. CABG w/ left IMA is a contraindication to left sided pedicle TRAM flap
    d. Laparoscopic cholecystectomy is a contra-indication to TRAM flap

    Answer d. *Lap cholecystectomy is <u>not</u> a contraindication to TRAM flap.

319. **A 55 yo woman undergoes MRM for breast CA and develops chronic lymphedema. Five years later she comes to your office with a dark purple raised lesion underneath her arm. Which of the following is true of this likely condition:
   a. This represents a breast cancer recurrence
   b. This is a sarcoma
   c. This is melanoma
   d. The patient has contra-lateral breast CA

   Answer b. **This is classic for *lymphangiosarcoma* following axillary dissection and **chronic lymphedema** (Stewart Treves Syndrome).

Nerves
   Long thoracic nerve – innervates **serratus anterior**
      Injury results in winged scapula; trouble lifting arm above head
      Lateral thoracic artery goes to serratus anterior
   Thoracodorsal nerve – innervates **latissimus dorsi**
      Injury results in weak pull-ups and weak arm adduction
      Thoracodorsal artery goes to latissimus dorsi
   ***Intercostal brachiocutaneous nerve**
      Lateral cutaneous branch of 2nd intercostal nerve
      Provides sensation to medial arm and axilla
      Found just below axillary vein w/ axillary lymph node dissection
      Can transect without serious consequences (can get numbness)
      **MC injured nerve w/ MRM or axillary node dissection

*MCC of malignant axillary adenopathy – lymphoma

*Mastodynia (pain in breast) - *rarely breast CA* (< 1%)
      Tx: Danazol, OCP's, NSAID's, *evening primrose oil*, bromocriptine, thyroxine, Vit E, low fat diet
   Avoid nicotine and methylxanthines (caffeine)
Accessory breast tissue – MC in axilla
*Accessory nipples (polythelia) – anywhere from axilla to groin (MC breast anomaly)
Breast asymmetry – common finding in women
Breast reduction – ability to lactate usually not compromised

*Mondor's disease - sclerosing superficial vein thrombophlebitis of breast
      from trauma or strenuous exercise; cordlike, can be painful
   MC location – lower outer quadrant
   Tx: NSAIDs

*Fibroadenoma
   MC breast lesion in adolescent and young women
   Can change in size w/ menstrual cycle and enlarge w/ pregnancy
   Can have large, coarse calcifications
   Sx's: usually painless, slow-growing, well circumscribed, firm, rubbery
   Path – prominent fibrous tissue compressing epithelial cells
   Pts aged < 30 → if feels benign (firm, rubbery, not fixed) and; U/S is c/w fibroadenoma (distinct borders, homogenous, hyper-echoic) and FNA or core needle biopsy shows fibroadenoma → can follow the mass
      If above 3 criteria not full-filled → excisional Bx
      If the mass continues to grow → excisional Bx
      *Avoid resection in teenagers and younger → can affect breast development and very rare breast CA in this group
   Pts aged ≥ 30 → bilateral mammogram and U/S
      Tx: excisional biopsy of fibroadenoma to ensure diagnosis

**_Phyllodes Tumor_ (1% of breast CA)
>> Can be very fast growing, and can increase in size in just a few weeks
>> 10% malignant (**cystosarcoma phyllodes**) – based on mitoses per high-power field (> 5-10)
>> ****_No nodal spread;_** hematogenous spread in any (although rare)
>> Resembles giant fibroadenoma
>> **Path** – has stromal and epithelial elements (mesenchymal tissue)
>> Considered a low grade sarcoma if malignant
>> ****_Tx: WLE w/ 1 cm margins;_** ****_No ALND_**

**_Nipple discharge_
>> Majority of nipple discharge is **benign**
>> Need bilateral mammogram and U/S; on breast exam look for trigger point
>> **Non-spontaneous** and **Yellow-Green Discharge**
>>> MCC – fibrocystic disease
>>> Should have lumpy tissue c/w **fibrocystic DZ**
>>> *Should be cyclical and non-spontaneous*
>>> Tx: reassure patient
>>> **If there is any doubt** → excisional Bx
>>> **Any other type of discharge** (spontaneous or another color) → needs some sort of **resection**
>> ****_Bloody_** nipple discharge
>>> MCC – intra-ductal papilloma; occasionally ductal CA
>>> Dx: ductogram to find papilloma, place wire in duct and resect area
>> **Serous, spontaneous** or **bloody** (w/ no associated papilloma) discharge – each **worrisome for CA**
>>> Tx: Wire guided excisional Bx of ductal area + any associated mass

**_Intra-ductal papilloma_
>> ****_MCC bloody discharge from nipple_**
>> Papilloma usually small, non-palpable, and close to nipple
>> *Benign lesion* – <u>NOT</u> pre-malignant
>> Dx and Tx: ****contrast *ductogram* to localize** – leave wire in responsible duct and resect ductal area

**Fibrocystic Disease
>> **Lots of types** – fibromatosis, sclerosing adenosis (cluster calcifications resembling breast CA), apocrine metaplasia, duct adenosis, epithelial hyperplasia, ductal hyperplasia, lobular hyperplasia
>> ****_Only significant breast CA risk is in atypical ductal hyperplasia or atypical lobular hyperplasia_** *(unusual findings, **relative risk 4-5**)*
>> Sx's: breast pain, nipple discharge (yellow to brown), masses, lumpy tissue
>>> Often varies w/ hormonal cycle
>> Tx: **Reassurance** (unless suspicious breast exam, mammogram, or U/S)
>>> Repeat in studies in 3 months
>> ****_Do not need negative margins w/ atypical ductal hyperplasia or atypical lobular hyperplasia_**

**_Lobular Carcinoma In Situ_ (LCIS)
>> **30% lifetime risk** for breast CA (***both breasts at risk**; **1%/year**)
>> Considered **marker** for breast CA → **_NOT_ pre-malignant itself**
>> ****_Does not form calcifications_**, <u>No</u> invasion of basement membrane, <u>Not</u> usually palpable, <u>Not</u> usually seen on mammography
>> Usually an **incidental finding**; multifocal DZ is common
>> MC in **pre-menopausal** women
>> ****_Pts that subsequently develop breast CA are most likely to develop a ductal CA (70%)_**
>> 5% risk of **synchronous breast CA** at time of Dx of LCIS (MC **ductal CA**)
>> ****_Do not need negative margins with LCIS_**

**Tx options for LCIS:
    1) **Nothing** and **careful F/U**
    2) **Hormonal Therapy** - 50% reduction in risk of breast CA
        Pre-menopausal – Tamoxifen, careful F/U (5 years maximum)
        Post-menopausal – Raloxifene, careful F/U
            Decreased DVT/PE and cataracts compared to Tamoxifen
    3) **Bilateral simple mastectomy** *(No ALND or SLNB)*

**Ductal Carcinoma In Situ (DCIS)
    Usually <u>not</u> palpable, presents as a **cluster of calcifications** on
        mammography; calcifications can be **linear** or **branching**
    Path
        In situ - no invasion of basement membrane
        Malignant cells of ductal epithelium
        50% get CA if not resected *(*ipsilateral breast at risk)*
        Considered pre-malignant
        Comedo subtype – most aggressive
            High risk of multi-centricity, micro-invasion, and recurrence
            Tx: total mastectomy (see below)
    Recurrence risk – increased w/ comedo type and lesions > 2.5 cm
    **DCIS Tx options (2):
        1) **Lumpectomy + XRT** (usually needle localization, get all the
            calcifications, need 1 cm margin; **XRT** decreases **local**
            recurrence for DCIS but <u>no</u> change in survival)
        2) **Simple mastectomy** (indications below)
            **Males
            **Comedo necrosis
            Diffuse malignant appearing calcifications (hard to follow)
            Multi-centric or multi-focal DCIS
            Inability to get **margins** despite re-resection
            Inability to get **good cosmetic result**
            Pt preference
            Previous XRT that would result in excessive total XRT dose
            High grade
            DCIS recurrence
    **Need negative margins for DCIS
    **NO ALND or SLNB w/ lumpectomy or mastectomy for DCIS
        (classic answer), *controversial whether pts undergoing*
        mastectomy should have SLNB (last chance to sample nodes)
    Subcutaneous mastectomy (ie simple or total mastectomy)
        Leaves 1% of breast tissue; **preserves nipple-areolar complex*
        <u>Not</u> indicated for breast CA Tx → used only for DCIS and LCIS
    Tamoxifen for 5 years after resected DCIS (optional)
        Decreases risk of breast CA in DCIS pts by 45%
        Only for ER or PR positive lesions

Breast CA
    BRCA I and II (+ family history of breast CA) and **CA risk:
    BRCA I

Female breast CA	**60%** lifetime risk
Ovarian CA	**40%** lifetime risk
Male Breast CA	**1%** lifetime risk

    BRCA II

Female breast CA	**60%** lifetime risk
Ovarian CA	**10%** lifetime risk
Male Breast CA	**10%** lifetime risk

    50% of females will get CA in the other breast w/ CA in the 1st breast
    BRCA I and II found in < 5% of all breast CA (is autosomal dominant)
    **BRCA is the largest RF for breast CA

Women with BRCA and breast CA have the **same prognosis as
comparable-stage breast CA in pts not having BRCA

Screening in pts w/ BRCA
Yearly mammograms + MRI starting age 25
Yearly pelvic exam, pelvic U/S, and CA-125 starting age 25

**_Prophylaxis for BRCA_ – reduction in breast CA risk
****TAH and BSO** w/ BRCA gene → decreases breast CA risk by **70%**
****Bilateral prophylactic mastectomy** w/ BRCA gene → decreases
breast CA risk by **90%**
****Bilateral prophylactic mastectomy and TAH and BSO** w/ BRCA
gene → decreases breast CA risk by 95%

**_BRCA Tx options:_
1) **Careful F/U** (± ****Tamoxifen**) _or;_
2) **Prophylactic mastectomy** (± TAH and BSO)

Consideration for prophylactic mastectomy:
1) Family history + BRCA gene _or:_
2) LCIS
Also need either: 1) high pt anxiety, 2) poor access for F/U, 3)
difficult lesion to follow on exam, mammography, or U/S, _or_ 4)
pt preference

**_TNM_
Tis – LCIS, DCIS, Paget's DZ of nipple w/o tumor
T1: < 2 cm, **T2**: 2–5 cm, **T3**: > 5 cm
T4: **T4a** – chest wall involvement (does <u>not</u> include pectoral muscles)
T4b – skin (edema, ulceration, or satellite nodules), peau d'orange
T4c – both above
T4d – inflammatory breast CA (erythema)
N1: ipsilateral movable axillary nodes
N2: **N2a** – fixed ipsilateral axillary nodes
N2b – clinically positive internal mammary nodes in absence of axillary
nodes
N3: **N3a** – ipsilateral infraclavicular nodes
N3b – ipsilateral axillary and internal mammary nodes
N3c – ipsilateral supraclavicular nodes
M1: distant metastasis

Stages

Stage	
Stage I	T1, N0, M0
Stage IIa	T0-1, N1, M0 or T2, N0, M0
Stage IIb	T2, N1, M0 or T3, N0, M0
Stage IIIa	T0-3, N2, M0 or T3, N1, M0
Stage IIIb	T4, N0-2, M0
Stage IIIc	N3
Stage IV	M1

5-YS: Stage I - 90%, Stage II - 75%, Stage III - 50%, Stage IV - 15%

**_Node status_– _single most impt prognostic factor in pts w/o systemic mets_
Survival directly related to number of positive nodes

Receptors
Positive PR and **ER receptors** – better overall prognosis
Better response to hormones, chemo, surgery, and overall prognosis
PR–positive tumors better prognosis than ER–positive
Tumor that is both PR and ER–positive has best prognosis
10% of breast CA is _negative_ for both receptors
**_HER2/neu receptor_ – _associated w/ worst prognosis for breast CA_
Trastuzumab (Herceptin) blocks this receptor

MC site breast CA mets – bone (axial skeleton)
MC type of breast CA – ductal CA (85%)

*_Adenocarcinoma in axillary node in woman w/ no identifiable source_
Check for **ER** and **PR** receptors → if positive → ipsilateral MRM (70% will
have ipsilateral breast CA)

Treatment by Stage

Stage I, II, IIIa, and IIIc (only N3a or N3b)
- **1st Surgery** (usually)
  - **Stage I and II** – BCT or MRM; **exception** is T3N0M0 and pt wants BCT, can undergo primary (neoadjuvant) chemo 1st to shrink tumor, then BCT
  - **Stage IIIa** – MRM usual, **exception** is T3N1M0 and pt wants BCT, then give *primary chemo 1st* to shrink tumor, then BCT w/ ALND
  - **Stage IIIc** (only N3a or N3b) – MRM
- **2nd Adjuvant chemo** (TAC, see below) – indicated for tumors > 1 cm, positive nodes, or ER/PR negative tumors
- **Trastuzumab** – if HER2 positive and tumor > 1 cm or positive nodes
- **Hormonal Tx** – for ER or PR positive tumor (or unknown status)
  - **Pre-menopausal** – *Tamoxifen* (2-3 yrs)
  - **Post-menopausal** – *Aromatase inhibitor* (anastrozole, 5 yrs)
- **XRT** follows chemo (eg w/ lumpectomy *or* if indicated after MRM)

Stage IIIb (T4 tumor)
- **1st Neoadjuvant chemo** → then **surgery** (usually MRM)** → then **adjuvant chemo-XRT** (MC scenario)
- **Trastuzumab** – if HER2 positive
- **Hormonal therapy** - for ER or PR positive tumor (or unknown status)
  - **Pre-menopausal** – *Tamoxifen* (2-3 years)
  - **Post-menopausal** – *Aromatase inhibitor* (5 years)
  - **MRM not always required after neoadjuvant chemo for T4 tumor** – if tumor shrinks can go w/ BCT (*except* for inflammatory CA which always requires MRM)

Stage IIIc (only N3c) and **Stage IV** (mets)
- Both non-operable disease; Tx - chemo **+** hormonal therapy
- **Bony mets** – bisphosphonates (eg alendronate) → ↓ skeletal cx's
- Can consider MRM for **palliation** (eg ulcerative, fungating lesion)

Chemo
TAC
- **Taxanes** (Docetaxel or Paclitaxel, S/E – neuropathy)
- **Adriamycin** (S/Es - cardiomyopathy)
  - Max dose – 500 mg/cm^2 body surface area
- **Cyclophosphamide** (S/Es - hemorrhagic cystitis)
- Chemo given before XRT
- Tumors < 1 cm, negative nodes and positive ER/PR receptors – no chemo (*hormonal therapy only*)

BCT (includes SLNB or ALND) and **XRT** – need **1 cm margin**
- **Breast conserving therapy** (BCT) – lumpectomy, quadrectomy, ect
- *Need to have **negative margins** before starting XRT*
- No real difference in **survival** compared to MRM
- **2% risk of local recurrence** →**Need salvage MRM** for local recurrence
- **Absolute contraindications** to BCT
  1) **2 or more primaries** in separate quadrants
  2) **Positive margins despite re-resection** (can re-resect x 1 for negative margins) – need negative margins
  3) **Pregnancy** (1st trimester + early 2nd trimester)
  4) **Previous XRT** that would result in excessive total XRT dose
  5) **Multi-focal** or **multi-centric DZ**
  6) **Diffuse malignant appearing calcifications**
- **Relative contraindications** to BCT
  1) **Unacceptable cosmetic result** from large tumor (eg T3/T4)
     - **If neoadjuvant Tx shrinks T3/T4 down → can go w/ BCT*
  2) **Scleroderma** or **SLE**
  3) **Inflammatory breast CA**

**_SLNB_ *(sentinel lymph node biopsy)*
    Fewer cx's than ALND
    ***Indicated only for malignant tumors **> 1 cm** (generally T1 and T2)*
    **<u>Not</u> indicated in pts w/ clinically positive nodes → need ALND
    Accuracy best when **primary tumor present** (gets correct lymphatic
        channels)
    Lymphazurin blue dye and **technetium labeled sulfur colloid**
        radiotracer used (injected around tumor area):
        Need 1-4 hours for technetium uptake
        Type I hypersensitivity reactions w/ lymphazurin blue dye (1%)
    Usually find **1-3 nodes** (in 95% sentinel node found) - get <u>permanent stains</u>
    Can't find dye or tracer in OR → **formal ALND**
    Tumor found in LN's on path → **formal ALND**
    If SLNB is **positive** for tumor → **formal ALND**
        Exception is small <u>isolated</u> foci of tumor (< 0.2 mm)
    **Contraindications to SLNBx:
        1) **Pregnancy**
        2) **Neoadjuvant therapy**
        3) **T4 - Advanced Disease** (eg inflammatory breast CA)
        4) **T3 - Large tumor** (> 5 cm, T3) – blocks lymphatics
        5) **Palpable nodes** (clinically positive)
        6) **Previous axillary dissection**
        7) **Tumor already taken out** (relative)
        8) **Multi-centric DZ** (relative)
    **Can perform SLNBx even if planning on mastectomy

**_ALND_ (axillary lymph node dissection)
    For **clinically positive nodes, positive SLNBx** or **contraindication to
        SLNBx**
    Superior border – axillary vein
    Medial border – chest wall (watch for the long thoracic nerve)
    Lateral border – skin flap
    Anterior border – pectoralis minor muscle
    Posterior border – latissimus dorsi (find thoracodorsal nerve)
    **Node levels
        I – lateral to pectoralis minor muscle
        II – beneath pectoralis minor muscle
        III – medial to pectoralis minor muscle, extends to thoracic inlet
            (Halsted's ligament)
        Rotter's nodes – between the pectoralis major and minor muscles
        Remove **Level I and II nodes** en bloc w/ ALND for breast CA
        Level III nodes are removed only if grossly involved
        Lymphedema and other cx's are increased w/ level III dissection
        Node dissection does <u>not</u> improve survival

*Modified radical mastectomy
    Removes all breast tissue, muscle fascia, nipple-areolar complex, and level
        I and II nodes (ALND) en bloc; remove drains when < 30-40 cc/day
    Radical mastectomy – <u>rarely</u> performed anymore; includes MRM and
        overlying skin, pectoralis major and minor muscles, level I/II/III nodes
    Complications (Cx's)
        Cx's of mastectomy – infection, flap necrosis, seromas
        Cx's of ALND – infection, lymphedema, lymphangiosarcoma
        Cx's of XRT – edema, erythema, ulceration, rib Fx's, pneumonitis,
            bone or soft tissue sarcoma, contra-lateral breast CA
        Axillary vein thrombosis – early, sudden, post-op arm swelling
        Lymphatic fibrosis – slow arm swelling over 1-2 years
        **Intercostal brachiocutaneous nerve
            MC injured nerve after mastectomy; no significant sequelae
            Hyperesthesia / numbness of inner arm and lateral chest wall
        Long thoracic nerve or **thoracodorsal nerve injury**

**Hormonal Therapy
Tamoxifen
For **pre-menopausal** breast CA
50% decrease in **recurrence** and 35% decrease in **mortality**
Need positive ER or PR receptors for benefit
Mechanism - blocks ER and PR receptors
Decreases **osteoporosis**
S/Es: **thromboembolism (1%; DVT. PE, stroke)*, **endometrial CA**
Duration of Tx – 20 mg/d for 2-3 years
Raloxifene not approved for adjuvant breast CA Tx
Contraindications – previous thromboembolism, Coumadin Tx, pregnancy
*Aromatase inhibitors (anastrozole, letrozole)
For **post-menopausal** breast CA
50% decrease in **recurrence**
Need positive ER or PR receptors for benefit
Mechanism - blocks conversion of testosterone to estrogen in peripheral tissues
Lower **DVT, stroke** and **endometrial CA** compared to Tamoxifen
S/Es – **fractures*
Duration of Tx – 5 years
Oophrectomy also an option instead of oral agents

**Trastuzumab (Herceptin, anti-HER2/neu receptor monoclonal Ab)
50% decrease in **recurrence** for HER positive tumors
Blocks HER2/neu receptor – human epidermal growth factor receptor 2 (receptor tyrosine kinase)
S/Es – cardiac disease (heart failure)
Duration of Tx – 1 year;
Contraindications – previous cardiac disease

XRT (5000 rads total) - decreases **local recurrence
**Indications for XRT after MRM:
Skin or **chest wall involvement** (not pectoral muscle)
Positive margins
Tumor > 5 cm (T3)
Inflammatory CA
Advanced Nodal Disease (XRT to nodal area) - $\geq$ 4 nodes positive extra-capsular invasion, N2 or N3
Contraindications to **XRT:**
Scleroderma or **collagen vascular DZ** (get severe fibrosis, necrosis)
Previous XRT (and would exceed total max dose)
Pregnancy
SLE (Lupus, relative), Active **rheumatoid arthritis** (relative)

**Paget's Disease of Breast
Sx's: scaly, weepy skin lesion on nipple (areolar)
Look for underlying mass or suspicious calcifications on mammograpy
almost *all pts* have either underlying DCIS or ductal CA
Dx: **full thickness incisional breast Bx** (including skin) – shows **Paget's cells in skin**, may show DCIS or CA cells
Tx: ***DCIS w/ Paget's → **simple mastectomy including nipple areolar complex (classic answer). ALND not indicated for Paget's w/ DCIS*
Breast CA w/ Paget's → simple mastectomy and ALND or SLNB (including nipple areolar complex resection) or MRM
Some are using central lumpectomy (include nipple-areolar complex) + post-op XRT instead of simple mastectomy

**Lobular CA (10% of all breast CA)
  Does not form calcifications
  Extensively **infiltrative** (often **bilateral, multi-focal,** and **multi-centric**)
  Signet ring cells – worse prognosis
Ductal CA (85% of all breast CA) – scirrhotic CA worse prognosis of all subtypes

**Inflammatory breast CA *(T4d)*
  Very aggressive - median survival is 36 mos (worse than other breast CA)
  **Dermal lymphatic invasion causes peau d'orange lymphedema w/
    erythema (T4d)
  Sx's: pain, erythema, warmth
  Dx ****Need Full thickness incisional biopsy** including skin
  Tx: ***follow* **stage IIIb protocol *(neoadjuvant chemo → then surgery
    (usually MRM)*** → then **adjuvant chemo-XRT** *(MC scenario)*
  BCT not really an option here because you should take the skin w/
    resection *(inflammatory breast CA considered relative
    contraindication to BCT)*

*Male breast CA (<1% of all breast CA) - almost always **ductal CA**
  Worse prognosis due to **late presentation**
  Increased **pectoral muscle** involvement

*Metastatic flare – pain, swelling, erythema in mets areas; spinal compression
  Tx: ***XRT** (eg bone mets) ± steroids
Recurrence along mastectomy scar - resection if no mets (1 cm margin)

TRAM pedicle flap - MC flap used for breast reconstruction
  Based off the **superior epigastric artery**
  Avoid left sided TRAM if previous CABG with left IMA use
  Avoid with previous incisions that have transected the upper abdominal
    wall (laparoscopic cholecystectomy not a contra-indication)
  Use contra-lateral rectus muscle if chest XRT for breast CA (IMA is
    compromised by XRT)

**Stewart-Treves syndrome
  Lymphangiosarcoma from chronic lymphedema following ALND
  Dark purple nodule or lesion on arm 5 - 10 years after surgery
  Tx: sarcoma w/u and resection

Thoracic

320. **All of the following are true except:
    a. Right angled rigid bronchoscopy is useful for looking into the right upper lobe
    b. The thoracic duct crosses the mediastinum right to left at T4-5
    c. The greatest change in dimension w/ inspiration is anterior and posterior
    d. Type II pneumocytes produce surfactant

    Answer c. The greatest change in dimension w/ inspiration is superior and inferior (diaphragm movement)

    Right angled rigid bronchoscopy* is useful for looking into the **right upper lobe
    The thoracic duct **crosses the mediastinum right to left at **T4-5**
    Type II pneumocytes* produce **surfactant (reduces alveolar surface tension)

321. **All of the following are true except:
    a. The main function of surfactant is to reduce alveolar surface tension
    b. A decrease in cardiac output is likely to increase the carbon monoxide diffusion capacity (DLCO) of the lung
    c. Pre-op FEV_1 is the single best predictor of being able to wean off the ventilator after pulmonary resection
    d. The MCC of hypoxia following lung resection is alveolar hypoventilation (atelectasis)

    Answer b. A decrease in C.O. is likely to decrease DLCO.

    The MCC of **hypoxia following lung resection is **alveolar hypoventilation (atelectasis)**
    **Pre-op FEV_1* is the single best predictor of being able to wean off the ventilator after pulmonary resection
    The MCC of **hypercarbia following surgery is **poor minute ventilation**
    The MC complication following lobectomy is **atelectasis

322. *All of the following are true of thoracic outlet syndrome (TOS) except:
    a. The subclavian vein is the MC involved structure
    b. Resection of the first and any cervical ribs is the key part of surgery
    c. The phrenic nerve is located anterior to the anterior scalene muscle.
    d. The long thoracic nerve is located posterior to the middle scalene

    Answer a. The **brachial plexus** is the MC structure involved in thoracic outlet syndrome (usually involving the ulnar distribution, C8-T1). This results in weakness and paraesthesias in the 4th and 5th digits of the hand along w/ pain and paraesthesias along the medial part of the forearm.

323. **A 24 yo college pitcher is in the ED w/ acute pain and swelling in his right arm. U/S shows clot in the subclavian vein. The next appropriate step is:
    a. Catheter directed thrombolytic therapy
    b. Thrombectomy
    c. Resection of the 1st rib
    d. Resection of the subclavian vein and reconstruction w/ 10 mm graft

    Answer a. **Paget von Schrotter's disease is acute thrombosis of the subclavian vein. Classically, it presents in pitchers, or pts who have a lot of strenuous repetitive motion in the arm. **The initial Tx is **thrombolytic therapy** to open up the vein followed by 1st **rib resection** during the **same hospital admission** and not wait for a repeat episode.

324. *Which lung CA is most likely to be associated with a paraneoplastic syndrome?
   a.   Small cell lung CA
   b.   Adenocarcinoma
   c.   Squamous cell CA
   d.   Large cell CA

   Answer a. *Small cell lung CA* is MC involved in **paraneoplastic syndromes** (MC - **ACTH**, also **ADH**). Squamous cell CA can have **PTH-rp** release.

325. **A 65 yo cachectic man with an apical lung cancer presents with acutely swollen face, arms and hands. The best treatment for this patient's condition is:
   a.   Chemotherapy
   b.   Emergent XRT
   c.   Resection
   d.   Antibiotics

   Answer b. **This pt most likely has **Superior Vena Cava (SVC) syndrome** due to CA in-growth into the SVC. **Tx requires **emergent XRT** which will rapidly shrink the tumor and open up the SVC

326. *A 65 yo cachectic man with an apical lung cancer presents with ptosis, miosis, and anhydrosis. These symptoms are most likely from:
   a.   A paraneoplastic syndrome
   b.   Invasion of the brachial plexus
   c.   Invasion of the SVC
   d.   Invasion of the sympathetic chain at T1

   Answer d. Pancoast Tumors (superior sulcus) can present w/ either:
       1) Invasion of the **sympathetic chain** at T1, which results in ptosis, miosis, and anhydrosis (Horner's syndrome)
       2) Invasion of the **brachial plexus** (MC - **ulnar nerve** sx's)

327. **A 65 yo man w/ COPD has right lung CA that you are contemplating resecting. You get PFTs which show an FEV-1 of 1400 cc. This pt likely:
   a.   Could tolerate either a pneumonectomy or lobectomy
   b.   Could tolerate a lobectomy but not pneumonectomy
   c.   Could tolerate wedge resection but not lobectomy
   d.   Could not tolerate any surgery

   Answer b. A pneumonectomy would leave this patient with an **FEV-1** of about 700 (roughly 50% of the initial 1400). The predicted post-op FEV-1 needs to be ≥ 800 to give a reasonable chance of not being ventilator dependent.

   Due to differences in individual patient's height, weight, and lung size, a more accurate guide is to use percent predicted FEV-1. That is, the post-operative FEV-1 should be at least 40% of the normal FEV-1 for that patient's size and age.

328. *A 57 yo man has a 3 cm mass in the RLL on chest CT. Bx of the mass shows adenocarcinoma. You perform a mediastinoscopy and a right paratracheal lymph node is positive for CA. The most appropriate next step is:
   a.   Perform right lower lobe resection only
   b.   Perform RLL resection and mediastinal lymph node dissection
   c.   Perform pneumonectomy and mediastinal lymph node dissection
   d.   Chemo-XRT

   Answer d. Positive paratracheal nodes identified on mediastinoscopy are considered N2 disease and the pt is unresectable. Chemo-XRT only is indicated.

329. **All of the following are true of mediastinal tumors except:
   a. The best method for Dx of an anterior mediastinal tumor that is non-diagnostic on needle Bx is anterior thoracotomy (parasternal mediastinotomy, Chamberlain procedure)
   b. Thymomas are the MC mediastinal tumor overall
   c. Median sternotomy is generally the best operative approach for anterior mediastinal tumors
   d. The MC anterior mediastinal tumor in children is germ cell tumor

Answer b. Neurogenic tumors are the MC mediastinal tumor overall

The best method for Dx of an anterior mediastinal tumor that is non-diagnostic on needle Bx is **anterior thoracotomy (also called parasternal mediastinotomy or Chamberlain procedure, usually at 2nd **costal cartilage**)*

****Median sternotomy** is he best approach for anterior mediastinal tumors*

Lung Anatomy and Physiology
Airways (trachea to level of terminal bronchiole)
   Conducting airways – 150 cc of anatomic dead space
Blood supply
   Upper 2/3 trachea – inferior thyroid arteries
   Lower 1/3 trachea and **lung parenchyma** – bronchial arteries
Mediastinal Structures
   Azygos vein is along right side, dumps into **superior vena cava**
   Thoracic duct runs along right side, **crosses midline at T4-T5**, goes into **left neck*, turns around and dumps into **left subclavian vein* at junction w/ internal jugular vein
   Phrenic nerve – runs anterior to hilum
   Vagus nerve – runs posterior to hilum
Lung
   Right lung volume   55% (3 lobes: RUL, RML, and RLL)
   Left lung volume   45% (2 lobes: LUL and LLL; lingula)
   Quiet inspiration – diaphragm 80%, intercostals 20%
   Greatest change in dimension – superior and inferior (diaphragm)
   Accessory muscles – sternocleidomastoid muscle (SCM), levators, serratus posterior, scalenes
   *Type I pneumocytes – gas exchange (diffusion in **alveoli**)
   *Type II pneumocytes – surfactant production
   Surfactant – **phosphatidylcholine** main agent; decreases **alveolar surface tension** and keeps **alveoli open**

**Pulmonary function tests before pulmonary resection
   **Need predicted <u>post-op</u> FEV_1 > 0.8 L (> 40% of predicted value)
      If close → get qualitative V/Q scan (*use <u>perfusion</u> measurement*)
         Find the contribution of that portion of lung to overall FEV_1 and the predicted FEV_1 after resection
      FEV_1 single best predictor of being able to **wean off ventilator after pulmonary resection*
      FEV_1 best predictor for post-op **pulmonary complications*
   Need following <u>pre-op</u> values before resection
      **DLCO > 11-12 ml/min/mmHg CO (> 50% of predicted value)
         DLCO – carbon monoxide diffusion capacity
         Measures lung's ability to **transfer gases** (**especially oxygen*)
         Causes of **decreased DLCO** - lowered capillary surface area, low Hgb, poor alveolar architecture, increased dead space, low C.O., pulmonary hypertension
      pCO_2 < 45 (at rest)
      pO_2 > 60 (at rest, not on oxygen)
      VO_2 max > 10-12 ml/kg/min (maximum oxygen consumption (10-15 intermediate risk, need pt discussion)

Pulmonary Resection Complications
Pulmonary cx's cause **most deaths** after lung surgery (eg resp. failure)
**MCC post-op hypoxemia – *alveolar hypoventilation (causes atelectasis) get shunt*
**MCC post-op hypercarbia – *poor minute ventilation*
MC resection resulting in:
    Persistent air leak – segmentectomy/wedge
    Atelectasis – lobectomy **(MC Cx following lobectomy)**
    Arrhythmias – pneumonectomy
    Broncho-pleural fistula – pneumonectomy
Mortality - wedge 1%, lobectomy 3%, pneumonectomy 6%

Persistent air leak
1) Make sure **chest tube on suction** and **check system** → repeat CXR
2) **Place 2nd chest tube anteriorly**
3) **Bronch** if still having a problem w/ re-expansion [look for foreign body or bronchus problem (eg BPF, mucus plug)]
Consider chest CT
Wait it out if lung re-expanded and just simple air-leak (7 days)
Not resolved →
    If after spontaneous PTX - staple bleb, mechanical pleurodesis
    If after pulmonary resection - mechanical pleurodesis

Atelectasis (lung collapse from ****alveolar hypoventilation)
**MC Cx following lung resection
**MCC hypoxemia following lung resection
Results in **hypoxemia** and **pulmonary shunting**
Tx: incentive spirometer, cough, pain control, walk pt, epidural
    If refractory consider bronch to look for **mucus plugging**
    If already on the ventilator, may need to ↑ TV's

Empyema
MCC empyema – pneumonia w/ subsequent infection of parapneumonic effusion; also occurs after thoracic surgery (pulmonary, esophageal)
Sx's: pleuritic chest pain, fever, cough, SOB
Pleural fluid - WBCs >500 cells/cc, bacteria on GS, pH < 7.4, glucose < 60
Most do not require decortication
Has **3 stages:**
1) **Exudative** - swelling of pleura (low protein and cell count)
    Tx: **chest tube** (bedside thoracostomy) **+ Abx's**
2) **Fibrinopurulent** - fibrin deposits, purulent fluid; ↑PMNs (pus)
    Tx: **chest tube + Abx's**
    Failure to re-expand the lung → VATS deloculation
3) **Organized** (chronic phase) - occurs after 3-4 weeks
    In-growth of fibroblasts and capillaries w/ **lung trapping** by collagen; *lung can't expand* → pus and thick fibrous peel
    Tx: **Decortication** (removes fibrous peel) *If can't tolerate decortication* → place **Eloesser flap** (open thoracic window - direct external opening, allows drainage)

Hamartomas
*MC benign adult lung tumor (represent 75% of all benign adult tumors)
Contain **fat, cartilage, and **connective tissue*** (eg muscle)
Dx: **chest CT** (can be diagnostic w/o need for Bx)
Calcifications can appear as a ***popcorn lesion** on chest CT
Do not require resection
Repeat chest CT in 3 months to confirm diagnosis

Upper airway tumors (trachea and main bronchi)
> **Children** – 90% benign
>> **MC benign** – hemangioma (usually resolves on its own)
>> **MC malignant** – carcinoid
>
> **Adults** – 90% malignant
>> **MC benign** – papilloma (usually resolves on its own)
>> **MC malignant** – SCCA (others-bronchial gland tumors)
>
> **Bronchial gland tumors** – carcinoid, mucoepidermoid and adenoid cystic
>> CA; MC slow growing and unusual to rare mets
>
> **Carcinoid**
>> Represent 90% of all bronchial gland tumors in adults
>> **Typical** carcinoids (90%) – 5% mets; homogenous, 5-YS – 95%
>> **Atypical** carcinoid (10%) – 50% mets; necrosis, disorganized, $\geq$ 1
>>> mitosis/2HPF, heterogeneous, 5-YS – 50%
>>
>> **Strongest RF for survival** – atypical vs. typical
>
> **Adenoid cystic CA** (cylindroma)
>> Mucosa frequently intact, predilection to **peri-neural** invasion
>> CA spread often **well beyond endoluminal component**
>> ***Very responsive to XRT***
>> **Slow growing** – can survive decades even w/ mets
>> ***If you can't get complete rsxn* – give XRT *(very sensitive to XRT)***
>
> **Mucoepidermoid CA** – can be low or high grade
> Tx: resection (1 cm margin) for all if resectable primary and no distant mets

Want tracheostomy between the 2nd and 3rd tracheal rings
> Too high – vocal cord problems
> Too low – tracheo-innominate fistula

<u>**Lung Abscess**</u>
> **MCC** – aspiration PNA; **MC location** – *superior segment of RLL*
> **MC organism** – staph aureus (usually polymicrobial)
> RFs – ETOH
> Dx: chest CT (*best test*)
> *Tx: **Abx's only** (first line Tx, cures 95%)* ; **CT guided drainage** if that fails

<u>**Exudative Effusion**</u>: Protein > 3, Specific gravity > 1.016, LDH ratio > 0.6
> (fluid:serum)

<u>**Spontaneous Pneumothorax**</u>
> **Typical pt** – tall, healthy, thin, young, males, smoking Hx
> **Recurrence:**
>> After 1st PTX   **20%**
>> After 2nd PTX   **60%**
>> After 3rd PTX   **80%**
>
> **Etiology** – rupture of a **lung bleb**; MC in **upper lobe apex**; MC **right side**
> Tx - **chest tube**
> **Surgery for:** recurrence, large blebs on CT scan, persistent air-leak > 7
>> days despite 2 good chest tubes, non-reexpansion of lung despite 2
>> good chest tubes, tension PTX, bilateral PTX, hemothorax, previous
>> pneumonectomy, high risk profession (pilot, diver, mountain climber,
>> or lives in remote area)
>
> **Surgery** – thoracoscopy, blebectomy and mechanical pleurodesis

<u>**Pulmonary AVMs**</u> – between pulmonary arteries and pulmonary veins
> **MC site** – lower lobes
> Sx's: hemoptysis and SOB; can occur w/ **Osler-Weber-Rendu Syndrome**
> Tx: *embolization*

Thoracic outlet syndrome (TOS)
> Scalene triangle – anterior scalene, middle scalene, 1st rib
>> Subclavian vein is anterior to the anterior scalene
>> Subclavian artery + brachial plexus are between anterior and middle
>>> scalenes
>
> **MC anatomic abnormality for TOS – <u>cervical rib</u>*
> Neurogenic *(*MC type of TOS)*
>> **Pain + paresthesias** (present in 95%) in medial forearm and fingers
>> Usually **normal** neuro exam; sx's **worse w/ manipulation**
>> **Tinsel's test** – tapping reproduces symptoms (neurogenic TOS)
>> **MC nerve distribution** – <u>ulnar nerve</u> (C8-T1)
>> Dx: nerve conduction velocity < 60 m/S
>> Tx Physiotherapy for 3 mos. <u>(all pts);</u> – *don't rush to operate*
>>> **If above fails** and **nerve conduction velocity < 60 m/S** → <u>**1**st</u>
>>>> **rib resection**, cervical rib resection if present, anterior
>>>> and middle scalenes divided
>
> **Arterial** (Subclavian Artery)
>> Compression usually secondary to **anterior scalene hypertrophy**
>> Can get **aneurysms** or **acute occlusion** (No pulse, arm **white + cold**)
>> **Adson's, hyper-abduction, costoclavicular tests** – all result in loss
>>> of radial pulse; hand cold and pale
>> Dx: **angiogram** (gold standard), **duplex U/S**
>> Tx:1st rib and cervical rib resection; possible bypass graft if artery
>>> too damaged or aneurysm present
>>> **Acute thrombosis** - balloon thrombectomy via brachial artery if
>>>> threatened limb; catheter directed intra-arterial thrombolytics if
>>>> non-threatened; 1st rib resection on same admission
>
> ***Venous (Subclavian Vein; Paget Von Schrotter's)*
>> Sx's: usually presents as ***effort-induced thrombosis of
>>> subclavian vein (eg baseball pitchers, excessive use of arm)*
>>> Arm **acutely swollen** and **blue**
>> **Venous thrombosis** much more common than arterial
>> Dx: **Duplex U/S (venogram is Gold Standard but takes too long)*
>> Tx: ***Acute occlusion – TPA 1st (intra-vein directed lysis of clot),
>>> heparin*, then ***1st rib resection* on <u>*same hospital admission*</u>

*Chylothorax
> **Milky white fluid** – sudan red stains the TAG's
> Has ↑ lymphocytes + TAGs (>110 ml/µl) - *fluid is <u>resistant</u> to infection*
> **MCC** – lymphoma
> Can also occur after injury to thoracic duct w/ surgery or trauma
> **Injury above T5–6** – left-sided chylothorax.
> **Injury below T5–6** – in right-sided chylothorax
> **Thoracic duct crosses mediastinum right to left at T5-6*
> **Tx:**
>> **1-3 weeks of conservative Tx → chest tube, NPO TPN, octreotide*
>> 1) If above fails, surgery w/ **ligation of thoracic duct** on **right side
>>> low in mediastinum* if due to **trauma or iatrogenic** injury
>> 2) If **CA** (lymphoma MC), chemo and/or XRT or **talc pleurodesis**

Solitary Pulmonary Nodule (coin lesion)
> **Overall 5-10% are malignant**
>> Age < 50   < 5% malignant
>> Age > 50   > 50% malignant
> **MC lesion overall** – <u>granuloma</u> (histoplasmosis MC,)
> **MC tumor overall** – <u>hamartoma</u> (benign, 10% of all cases)
> **MC malignant tumor** – <u>bronchogenic CA</u> (MC adenocarcinoma)
>> **#2 mets** (breast CA MC)

Lung cancer
MC CA related death in US for men and women (30% of all CA deaths)
Risk proportional to smoking pack-years (biggest RF)
Risk ↓s after quitting smoking but not back to baseline
Path: ****MC type** – adenocarcinoma (not squamous)
*Strongest prognostic indicator – lymph node involvement
MC site of mets – brain
Overall 5-YS rate – 10% (35% w/ resection for cure)
Small cell lung CA – vast majority not resectable due to early spread
Mediastinal adenopathy (> 1.0 cm) or **central mass** – need
mediastinoscopy
Assesses **mediastinal nodes** – If positive, tumor unresectable
Looking into **middle mediastinum** w/ mediastinoscopy
Para-aortic or **AP** (aorto-pulmonary) **window adenopathy**
→ **Chamberlain** (go through left 2nd rib cartilage)
Mediastinoscopy does not assess AP window nodes
Supra-clavicular or scalene adenopathy → **FNA** of node
Tx: **Formal lung resection** (lobectomy or pneumonectomy) if resectable
(no distant mets or mediastinal nodes) and pt can tolerate resection
XRT – ↓s local recurrence; painful mets; no change in survival
Chemo-XRT (carboplatin + paclitaxel) does not change 5-YS

Special Issues
**Superior vena cava syndrome
MCC - lung CA (others – lymphoma)
Sx's: head, neck fullness, dyspnea, dizziness
**Tx: emergent XRT if CA source (best Tx: dramatic effect within
hours; raise head, O2, lasix, steroids)
**Pancoast tumors (superior sulcus: tumor invades chest wall apex, T4)
Can get **Horner's syndrome** (invasion of **T1 sympathetic chain* →
ptosis, miosis, anhidrosis) and/or **ulnar** nerve sx's (brachial
plexus invasion)
*Paraneoplastic syndromes
*Squamous cell CA – PTH-related peptide
*Small cell CA – ACTH and ADH
MC paraneoplastic syndrome – small cell ACTH
Mesothelioma
Asbestos exposure (↑s risk 90x)
Poor prognosis from aggressive nodal invasion and distant mets
Cell types
Non-small cell CA (NSCC) – 80%
Adenocarcinoma (MC overall)- usually peripheral, forms gland
Squamous cell CA - usually central, obstructive, keratin pearls
Bronchoalveolar - can look like pneumonia
Small Cell (neuroendocrine, Kulchitsky cells) – 20%
Usually **unresectable** at Dx (<5 % resectable)
Often **mets** to mediastinum, median survival 1-2 years
Chemo main Tx: Cisplatin + etoposide; add XRT if low stage
Mets to lung → if isolated may be resected for colon, renal cell CA,
sarcoma, melanoma, ovarian, or endometrial CA
**Right angle rigid bronch – good for looking into the right upper lobe

**Mediastinum
Normal Structures
Anterior – thymus
Middle – heart, great vessels, phrenic, vagus, trachea, main bronchi
Posterior – esophagus, descending aorta, vertebral bodies, thoracic
duct, azygos vein, hemi-azygos
Mediastinal mass sx's (any location can cause sx's)
Often **asymptomatic**
Respiratory insufficiency (MC Sx), chest pain, and dysphagia

Tumors (majority benign)

      *MC mediastinal tumor in adults and **children** – <u>neurogenic</u> (MC posterior)

      *MC location for mediastinal tumor in adults and **children** – <u>anterior</u>

      Adult solitary mediastinal mass

MC mediastinal overall	**neurogenic**
MC anterior	thymoma*
MC middle	cyst
MC posterior	neurogenic

      Children solitary mediastinal mass

MC mediastinal overall	**neurogenic**
MC anterior	germ cell*
MC middle	cyst
MC posterior	neurogenic

      Anterior (T's) – Thyroid, parathyroid, T-cell lymphoma, Thymoma, Teratoma (and other germ cell), cystic hygroma

      Middle – cysts (bronchogenic and pericardial), lymphoma, teratoma

      Posterior – neurogenic, lymphoma, enteric duplication cysts

      **Procedure for Dx on anterior mediastinal mass – <u>*Chamberlain procedure*</u> (anterior thoracotomy also called parasternal mediastinotomy, go through 2nd rib cartilage)

      **Incision for removal of anterior mediastinal mass – <u>*median sternotomy*</u>

Thymoma

      All thymomas need resection

      Thymus too big or associated w/ myasthenia gravis→ resection

      50% are **malignant**

      50% are **symptomatic**

      50% of pts w/ thymomas have **myasthenia gravis**.

      10% of pts w/ myasthenia gravis have **thymomas**.

      Children *almost never* get thymomas

      Tx: **resection** *(**<u>median sternotomy)</u>*

      Myasthenia Gravis pt w/ **severe refractory sx's** and a normal size thymus should undergo thymectomy (80% get improvement)

Lymphoma (MCC mediastinal **adenopathy**) - **NHL** (MC) and **Hodgkin's**

Germ cell tumors

      Teratoma - MC germ cell tumor in mediastinum (hair, cartilage, fat)

            <u>Benign</u> - marker negative; <u>malignant</u> - elevated AFP, beta-HCG

            Tx: resection; chemotherapy if malignant

      Others – Seminoma, Non-seminoma (see Urology Chp for Tx)

Cysts

      Bronchogenic + Enteric Cysts – posterior to carina, not connected to airway; can get infected and small CA risk; Tx - resection

      Pericardial Cyst- MC right costophrenic angle; Tx: leave (no CA risk)

Neurogenic tumors

      MC in **paravertebral sulcus** (sympathetic chain or intercostal nerve) 10% have intra-spinal involvement (**MRI** if suspected)

      Tx: <u>resection</u> (may need spinal surgery for removal if intra-spinal)

      Neurolemma (MC; schwannoma, benign nerve sheath tumor)

      Neurofibroma (nerve sheath) – assoc. w/ von Recklinghausen's (café-au-lait macules, freckles, optic gliomas); 5% malignant

      Others - ganglioneuroma (benign), ganglioneuroblastoma (malignant), neuroblastoma (very malignant, children)

Cardiac

330. **Three days after a large anterior myocardial infarction, a pt develops a new holo-systolic murmur and cardiogenic shock. He is intubated due to respiratory distress and is started on multiple inotropes and pressors. CVP is 20 and PA pressures are 60/30. Despite support, his pressure continues to be 80/50 with a HR of 130. The most important next step in this pts Tx is:
    a. Obtain an ECHO
    b. Fluid resuscitation
    c. Place an IABP
    d. tPA

    Answer c. A pt in persistent cardiogenic shock despite maximal support should have an IABP placed. The pt does not need fluid resuscitation as his CVP is 20. An ECHO would make the Dx (likely a **ventricular septal rupture** or possible blown papillary muscle w/ acute mitral regurgitation) but the pt should be stabilized first. Use of IABPs have improved survival for cardiogenic shock following MI.

    ***ventricular septal rupture** will show a **set-up in oxygenation saturation** from the right atrium to pulmonary artery as a result of the hole in the ventricular septum.*

331. **The MCC of death following heart transplant is:
    a. Reperfusion injury
    b. Chronic allograft vasculopathy (accelerated arteriosclerosis)
    c. Infection
    d. Acute rejection

    Answer b. ***Chronic allograft vasculopathy** (accelerated arteriosclerosis) is the MCC of death following **heart TXP**.

332. **All of the following are true of congenital heart disease except:
    a. Tetralogy of Fallot results in decreased pulmonary perfusion and is the MC cyanotic congenital heart disease
    b. Ventricular septal defect is the MC congenital heart defect
    c. Tet spells are often self treated by squatting
    d. Trans-esophageal echo is better than a swan ganz catheter at assessing pulmonary vascular resistance (PVR)

    Answer d. **ECHO cannot assess PVR** *(cannot figure out pulmonary artery and wedge pressure which is required for calculation.*
    $PVR = [(PA\ pressure - wedge)\ /cardiac\ output] \times 80$
    ***Tetralogy of Fallot** results in decreased pulmonary perfusion and is the MC cyanotic congenital heart disease*

333. **The most important determinant of oxygen consumption is:
    a. Heart rate
    b. Wall tension
    c. Stroke volume
    d. Preload

    Answer b. **Although both HR and wall tension are the factors involved in myocardial oxygen consumption, **wall tension** is the primary determinant.*

334. *Which of the following risk factors is highest for mortality after CABG surgery?
    a. Older age
    b. History of congestive heart failure
    c. Prior myocardial infarction
    d. Pre-operative cardiogenic shock

Answer d. *The biggest risk factor for mortality after CABG is pre-operative **cardiogenic shock**.*

335. **The patency rate of an internal mammary artery to the left anterior descending artery and saphenous vein graft to any other coronary artery are:
    a.   IMA – 90% 20 year patency, SVG – 80% 5 year patency
    b.   SVG – 90% 20 year patency, IMA – 80% 5 year patency
    c.   IMA – 50% 20 year patency, SVG – 40% 5 year patency
    d.   SVG – 50% 20 year patency, IMA – 40% 5 year patency

    Answer a. ***A left internal mammary artery graft to the left anterior descending artery** has a patency of about 90% at 20 years. This has the best patency of any coronary graft.* Saphenous vein grafts have patency rates of 80% at 5 years.

336. **A 62 yo woman presents with tearing like chest pain radiating to her back. Her blood pressure is 190/100 in her right arm and 90/50 in her left arm. Her HR is 95. EKG shows some non-specific T wave changes and CXR looks normal. CK-MB and troponins are not back yet. All of the following are appropriate at this stage in the patient's management except:
    a.   tPA
    b.   Chest CT
    c.   BP control
    d.   Radial a-line

    Answer a. You need to R/O dissection is this pt before assuming it is an MI. The tearing like chest pain radiating to the back is highly suggestive of aortic dissection. ***Control of HTN** is the best initial Tx for aortic dissections (IV beta-blocker best, eg esmolol)*

337. **You obtain an emergent chest CT which shows a dissection involving only her ascending aorta. You place a radial a-line and start an esmolol drip The most appropriate next step in this patients care is:
    a.   Dissection repair
    b.   observation
    c.   heparin drip
    d.   place a stent graft

    Answer a.
    Ascending aortic dissections** (Type A) all need repair through a **median sternotomy.

    ***Descending aortic dissections** (Type B) require open repair only 10% of the time (repair through a **left posterolateral thoracotomy**).*

338. **All of the following are true except
    a.   Chronic left main disease is an indication for PTCA and stent
    b.   3 vessel disease is generally an indication for CABG
    c.   Acute ST elevation MI is an indication for PTCA w/ stent
    d.   Door to balloon time should be under 90 minutes for ST elevation MI

    Answer a. Significant left main disease should be treated w/ CABG.
    ***Acute ST elevation MI** is an indication for PTCA w/ stent.*

339. **Which of the following predicts the worst survival in a pt w/ aortic stenosis not undergoing valve replacement:
    a.   Dyspnea on exertion
    b.   Syncope
    c.   Angina
    d.   Loud murmur

Answer b. ***Of the items listed, **syncope** has the worst natural history for aortic stenosis is terms of survival (mean survival 3 years).*

Congenital heart disease
  In utero circulation
  Ductus arteriosus – connection between descending aorta and left pulmonary artery (PA); blood shunted away from lungs
  Ductus venosum – connection between portal vein and IVC
    Blood shunted away from liver
  Fetal circulation to placenta – 2 umbilical arteries
  Fetal circulation from placenta – 1 umbilical vein
  Ventricular septal defect (VSD)
    *MC congenital heart defect
    L→R shunt (CHF is severe); 80% **close spontaneously** by age 1 yr
    Timing of repair:
      Large VSDs (shunt > 2.5) – **at 1 year*
      Medium VSDs (shunt 2-2.5) – **at 5 years*
      Small VSDs usually *left alone*
    FTT – MC reason for early repair
  Atrial septal defect (ASD) – repair at 1-2 yrs of age
  **Tetralogy of Fallot
    **MC cyanotic congenital heart defect
    R→L shunt; ***4 anomalies* – VSD, pulmonary stenosis, overriding aorta, right ventricular (RV) hypertrophy
    ***Causes **decreased pulmonary perfusion** + shunting across VSD*
    Sx's: Tet spells (cyanosis – child then squats to ↑ SVR and ↑ blood flow to lung – essentially ↓s blood flow through VSD)
    Timing of operation: 3-6 months (earlier if ↑ cyanosis)

Coronary artery disease - MCC of death in US
  RFs – smoking, HTN, males, family history, hyperlipidemia, diabetes
  Medical Tx – nitrates, smoking cessation, weight loss, statin drugs, ASA
  Anatomy; 1) **Left main coronary artery** (branches into left anterior descending and circumflex arteries); 2) **right coronary artery**
  Most atherosclerotic lesions are **proximal**
  **Revascularization
    PTCA and stent – 90% patency at 1 year
    Saphenous vein graft – 80% 5-year patency
    **Internal mammary arteries (IMA) – off subclavian arteries
      **Best conduit for CABG – 90% 20-year patency rate
      *Usually placed on the **left anterior descending** artery*
    **Acute ST elevation MI is an indication for PTCA w/ stent.
  CABG procedure
    Cold potassium solution (cardioplegia) **arrests heart in diastole**
      Keeps heart **protected** and **still** while grafts are placed
    General indications (stenosis needs to be ≥ 70%)
      1) **Left main** disease
      2) **3-vessel** disease
      3) **2-vessel** disease w/ **proximal LAD stenosis**
  **High mortality RFs: ***pre-op cardiogenic shock* (#1), emergency surgery, age, reoperation, and low EF

Mechanical complications of myocardial infarction
  MC occur **3-7 days** after myocardial infarction
  Sx's: hypotension; if VSR or acute MR have new systolic murmur
  DDx:
    1. ***Ventricular septal rupture* (VSR, holo-systolic murmur heard best at right sternal border; *post-infarct heart defect*)
    2. **Papillary muscle rupture** [causes acute mitral regurgitation (MR), holo-systolic murmur heard best in axilla]
    3. **Free wall rupture** (usually quickly fatal)

185

Dx: **ECHO** - *best test* to figure out which of the above
      PA catheter – ***step-up in oxygen content*** between right atrium
            and pulmonary artery secondary to L→R shunt will occur w/
            **VSR (not w/ papillary muscle rupture and acute MR)
Tx: **Intra-aortic balloon pumps** (IABP) have ↑ed survival for VSR and
            acute MR due to acute papillary muscle rupture following MI
      VSR Tx – patch
      Papillary muscle rupture Tx – replace valve
      Free wall rupture Tx – patch

****Aortic stenosis**
   MC valve lesion
   MCC – calcification of aortic valve (RFs – age, bicuspid aortic valve)
   **Cardinal sx's (overall mean survival after onset of sx's 2-3 years)

Dyspnea on exertion	5 year mean survival
Angina	4 year mean survival
**Syncope	3 year mean survival
Dyspnea at rest (from heart failure)	2 year mean survival

   Valve area < 1.0 cm^2 – considered severe
   Indications for surgery (only for severe AS, valve is replaced):
      1) **Symptomatic AS** or:
      2) **Asymptomatic w/ valve area < 0.6 cm2** (critical AS)

****Aortic Dissection**
   MC location for intimal tear – ascending aorta
   Dissection occurs in **media layer* of blood vessel wall
   Cx's of ascending aortic dissection: aortic valve insufficiency,
         coronary or aortic branch occlusion, tamponade, aortic rupture
   Sx's *tearing chest pain* radiating to back (knife-like); 95% have severe HTN
   RFs – **HTN**, connective tissue D/Os, family Hx, aneurysms, atherosclerosis
   Dx: **Chest CT** *(best test)* – see flap
   **Initial medical Tx (*control HTN*, stabilize dissection) – IV beta-blocker
         (best Tx, eg esmolol)
   Tx:
         Ascending Aortic Dissections – **all need repair (*median
               sternotomy*)**; graft attempts to obliterate the false lumen
         Descending Aortic Dissection – surgery **only if complication
               (eg limb or organ ischemia, rupture, uncontrollable HTN or pain,
               extensive hemothorax) – *****left posterior-lateral thoracotomy*
               if undergoing open repair

Cardiac Tamponade Post-op from cardiac surgery
   Sx's *(classic)* high chest tube drainage that suddenly stops, followed by
         increasing filling pressures (PA, CVP), low BP and low UOP
   Dx: often clinical Dx, **CXR** - widened mediastinum; **ECHO** - tamponade
   Tx: **If pt has pulse** - emergent re-exploration in OR
         No pulse - open pts chest at bedside
   1st ECHO sign of cardiac tamponade – right atrial diastolic compression
   Mechanism of tamponade – ****decreased ventricular filling due
         pericardial fluid (blood)

Cardiac Tumors
   MC tumor (and MC benign tumor) – **myxoma**; 80% in left atrium
         Can present w/ distal emboli (eg stroke, leg ischemia)
   MC primary malignant tumor – angiosarcoma
   MC metastatic tumor to heart – lung CA
   MC primary pediatric cardiac tumor – rhabdomyoma

Vascular

340. *All of the following are true of thromboangitis obliterans (Buerger's) except:
    a. MC in young men
    b. Characterized by thrombotic occlusions of small and medium sized vessels, resulting in severe rest pain + ulceration/gangrene of digits
    c. Is curable with nicotine cessation
    d. Involves major occlusions proximal to brachial and popliteal arteries

    Answer d. The major vessels proximal to the brachial and popliteal arteries are normal. Small to medium sized arteries are affected.

341. **All of the following are true except::
    a. A normal carotid artery has continuous forward flow
    b. The MC site of carotid stenosis is the bifurcation of internal and external carotid arteries
    c. A healthy 60 yo man with TIA's and a carotid stenosis of 80% should receive medical therapy ASA
    d. PTA is generally the best Tx for symptomatic carotid stenosis from fibromuscular dysplasia

    Answer c. **Pts w/ symptoms from carotid disease and a stenosis $\geq$ 60-70% should have CEA. **Asymptomatic pts and stenosis $\geq$ 70-80% should have CEA.

    **PTA (not CEA) is the best Tx for carotid stenosis from fibromuscular dysplasia (angiogram shows 'sting of beads' appearance)

342. **All of the following are true except:
    a. The vagus is the MC injured nerve w/ CEA and results in hoarseness
    b. The MCC of death after CEA is myocardial infarction
    c. The facial vein can be routinely ligated
    d. CEA involves removing the intima only

    Answer d. CEA involves removing the intima and part of medial layers.

    **The vagus is the MC injured nerve w/ CEA and results in hoarseness.

343. *A 56 yo woman is suffering from vertigo, syncope and frequent falls. You get a duplex U/S which shows minimal carotid stenosis bilaterally (0-49%) and reversal of flow in the left vertebral artery and antegrade flow in the right vertebral artery. Which of the following is most appropriate in this patient:
    a. Left carotid endarterectomy
    b. Left vertebral artery stent
    c. Left subclavian stent
    d. Basilar artery stent

    Answer c. The pt has **subclavian steal syndrome** from subclavian artery stenosis as evidenced by the retrograde flow through the left vertebral artery. Tx – left subclavian stent or carotid to subclavian artery bypass.

344. **All of the following are true except:
    a. ASA is the Tx of choice for improving long term vascular graft patency
    b. Best predictor of long term patency in extremity vein grafts is surgical technique
    c. Duplex U/S is the best technique for surveillance of bypass grafts
    d. Rest pain typically begins w/ an ABI < 0.5

    Answer b. **The best predictor of long term patency in extremity vein bypass grafts is **vein quality.

***ASA is the Tx of choice for improving vascular **graft patency**.*
***Duplex U/S is the best technique for **surveillance** of bypass grafts.*

345. *A 55 yo golfer presents w/ a 40-pack year smoking history and pain is his calfs after walking 150 feet. The most appropriate next step in management is:
    a. Angiogram and PTA
    b. Coumadin
    c. Smoking cessation and exercise therapy
    d. Angiogram and bypass

    Answer c. Medical Tx is the initial Tx for **intermittent claudication**.

346. **All of the following are true except:
    a. The right renal artery MC goes posterior to the IVC
    b. The left renal vein MC goes anterior to the aorta
    c. Renal fibromuscular dysplasia (FMD) is best treated w/ open bypass
    d. Isolated iliac artery stenosis is best treated w/ PTA and stent

    Answer c. Renal FMD is best treated w/ PTA and stent.

    ***The **right renal artery** MC goes posterior to the IVC.*
    **The left renal vein MC goes anterior to the aorta.
    ***Symptomatic isolated iliac artery stenosis is best treated w/ **PTA and iliac stent** (80% 5-year patency).*

347. **All of the following are true except
    a. Maintenance of flow to at least one hypogastric artery is indicated for both open and endovascular aorto-bifemoral repairs
    b. AAA's measuring 4.9 cm should be repaired
    c. Hematemesis 6 months after open AAA repair is worrisome for aorto-enteric fistula (MC aorto-duodenal)
    d. Chylous ascites following open AAA repair is best treated initially w/ a drainage catheter and if that fails ligation of the cisterna chyli

    Answer c. ***AAA measuring 4.9 cm should be observed (> 5.5 cm indication for repair)*
    Maintenance of flow to at least **one hypogastric artery** (internal iliac artery) is indicated for both open and endovascular aorto-bifemoral repairs to **prevent pelvic ischemic cx's
    *****Hematemesis** 6 months after open AAA repair is worrisome for **aorto-enteric fistula** (MC aorto-duodenal); Dx – CT scan, Tx - graft resection and extra-anatomic bypass*
    *****Chylous ascites** following open AAA repair is best treated initially w/ a **drainage catheter** and of that fails **ligation of the cisterna chili***
    *****Bloody diarrhea** following AAA repair is worrisome for **ischemic colitis** (Dx – colonoscopy)*

348. **Two years after an aorto-bifemoral graft (ABF) for AAA, your pt presents w/ an acutely painful right groin. U/S which shows a pseudoaneurysm and a large fluid collection. What is the most likely cause of this pts problem:
    a. Trauma
    b. Infection
    c. Poor surgical technique
    d. Graft thrombosis

    Answer b. **Late pseudoaneurysm after vascular bypass graft is most consistent w/ **graft infection**. **The **MC organism** overall in graft infections is __staph epidermidis__.*

349. **All of the following are true of pseudoaneurysms except:
   a.   Initial Tx for a femoral artery pseudoaneurysm following angiography is U/S guided thrombin injection
   b.   Tx for a femoral artery pseudoaneurysm following an aortic bifemoral graft is open repair
   c.   There are no collateral vessels around the knee
   d.   Tx for a distal femoral artery pseudoaneurysm in an IVDA pt is ligation _without_ bypass

   Answer c. **Geniculate collaterals** *exist around the knee.*

   ****IVDA pts** w/ **distal femoral pseudoaneurysms** *can undergo* **simple ligation** *of superficial femoral artery as the* **profunda artery** *has collateral circulation to lower leg through* **geniculate collaterals**

350. **Six weeks after an ABF for an AAA, your pt returns to clinic w/ mild pain in his left groin. His femoral artery tissue was poor on that side and you are worried about a pseudoaneurysm. The study of choice for this is:
   a.   MRI
   b.   Abdominal CT
   c.   Duplex ultrasound (U/S)
   d.   Angiogram

   Answer c. ***Color flow duplex U/S** is the most cost effective option to study post-op AAA repairs (estimates blood flow + delineates anatomy).*

   ****Duplex U/S** is also the best method for peripheral bypass graft surveillance.*

351. **All of the following are true of popliteal artery aneurysms except:
   a.   The MC complication is rupture
   b.   Thrombosis can occur
   c.   They are often bilateral
   d.   Pts w/ compressive sx's should undergo aneurysmorrhaphy w/ interposition graft, as opposed to exclusion w/ bypass

   Answer a. Aneurysms below the inguinal ligament _rarely_ rupture. Popliteal artery aneurysms are more likely to have thrombosis or form emboli.

   ****Pts** w/ **compressive sx's** *(venous congestion edema, paresthesias, numbness) should undergo* **aneurysmorrhaphy w/ interposition graft** *(open aneurysm, place bypass graft in aneurysm sac), as opposed to just exclusion of the aneurysm w/ bypass, to alleviate sx's.* **Geniculate collaterals** *can continue to fill the aneurysm sac if it is just ligated, causing recurrent sx's*

352. *A 22 yo woman is evaluated in the ED for vague sx's of abd pain and is found to have a 2.5 cm splenic artery aneurysm. The most appropriate next step is:
   a.   Coumadin
   b.   Careful follow-up
   c.   Exclusion with covered stent placement or open procedure
   d.   Splenectomy

   Answer c. All **visceral artery aneurysms (> 2 cm**, > 1.5 cm for renal artery aneurysms) need repair except for splenic artery aneurysms. The rupture rate for visceral artery aneurysms is 50% for those other than splenic. The majority of these are repaired using **covered stents**.

   ***Women in child bearing age** should have splenic artery aneurysms repaired due to a specific risk of **rupture w/ pregnancy**.

353. *You perform a lower arm brachial artery to cephalic vein PTFE loop fistula in a 65 yo man with established chronic kidney disease (end stage renal disease). There is a palpable thrill and doppler signal at the end of the case. On POD#1, you inspect the graft and there is a poor thrill and poor doppler signal. The most appropriate next step in this patients management is:
   a. Heparin
   b. Fistulogram
   c. Graft ligation
   d. Graft excision

   Answer b. Take the pt back to the OR, de-clot the graft, and perform a **fistulogram** to figure out the issue.   .

354. **In the above pt, you place a PTFE hood patch at the site of the PTFE-venous anastomosis and the flow through the graft improves. Two days later your pt starts to develop arm swelling. Initially you try conservative Tx (eg elevating the arm). The arm continues to swell. The most appropriate next step is:
   a. Heparin
   b. Compressive wraps
   c. Re-do the venous anastomosis
   d. Angiogram and shoot run-off

   Answer d. Arm swelling after AV fistula (or AV graft) placement is due to **venous HTN**. The initial Tx is arm elevation and as collaterals develop, the swelling goes down. If major arm swelling persists, it suggests major outflow obstruction (eg axillary, subclavian, or innominate vein stenosis). Get an angiogram and look at the shunt run-off. Tx for the stenotic area is ****PTA and stent placement**.

355. **All of the following suggest venous outflow obstruction for an AV fistula except:
   a. Increase in returning line pressure
   b. Acute hand ischemia early following AV fistula placement
   c. High outflow pressure > 200
   d. Increase in re-circulation

   Answer b. Acute hand ischemia following AV fistula placement suggests **inflow** obstruction.

   **Pts w/ late venous outflow obstruction can present w/ an **increase in pressure in returning line, high outflow pressure (> 200) or increase in recirculation. Tx is placement of a venous stent at the obstruction or redo the venous anastomosis depending on level of obstruction (venogram to figure it out)

356. *A 21 yo man is shot in the leg. Five years later he presents to your clinic with right groin discomfort and a "vibration feeling" in his groin. All of the following are true of this patient's most likely condition except:
   a. Mild left ventricle hypertrophy
   b. A thrill over the groin is likely present
   c. This is best diagnosed w/ ultrasound
   d. He will likely need a femoral to popliteal bypass

   Answer d. Open repair is indicated for acquired AV fistulas. (primary closure of vein w/ **lateral venous suture**, patch for artery; interpose some sartorius muscle between vein and artery so fistula does not recur)

357. *A 62 yo man w/ severe type II DM presents with a heal ulcer. There is skin breakdown but it does not seem to be involving the bone. X-ray shows no signs of osteomyelitis. All of the following are appropriate for this patient except:
   a. Aggressive wound care
   b. Debride
   c. Keep wound moist
   d. Patient will likely need a below the knee amputation

   Answer d. Because the bone is not involved, the heel can be potentially salvaged. **Heel ulceration w/ *exposed calcaneus* would be an indication for *amputation*.*

358. **A 56 yo obese man with significant smoking history has multiple large ulcerations on the antero-medial aspect of his left lower leg just above the medial malleolus. The surrounding skin has a **brawny appearance** due to hemosiderin deposition. The most effective initial therapy for healing these ulcers is:
   a. Unna Boot (Zinc oxide paste gauze)
   b. Duoderm (hydrocolloid)
   c. Wound VAC
   d. Vein stripping

   Answer a. The most effective Tx for venous insufficiency w/ severe venous ulcers is Unna Boot. **Brawny edema *occurs from high capillary venous pressure and leakage of RBCs that are eventually get destroyed w/ hemosiderin deposition (*brown appearance*)*

359. **All of the following are contraindications to vein stripping except:
   a. DVT
   b. Sapheno-femoral and sapheno-popliteal valve incompetence
   c. Venous outflow obstruction
   d. Varicosities with pregnancy

   Answer b. Sapheno-femoral and sapheno-popliteal valve incompetence are the indications for vein stripping.

360. *Which organ does not contain lymphatics:
   a. Lung
   b. Liver
   c. Spleen
   d. Muscle

   Answer d. Muscle does not contain lymphatics.

361. **All of the following are true of thrombophlebitis except:
   a. A palpable cord is consistent w/ superficial thrombophlebitis
   b. Staph aureus is the MCC of bacterial thrombophlebitis
   c. Removal of any intravenous catheter is the 1st step in Tx of thrombophlebitis
   d. Continued bacteremia or purulence at the site indicates need for vein resection

   Answer a. A palpable cord is consistent w/ **suppurative** thrombophlebitis (ie pus in the vein). **Continued *bacteremia or purulence* at the site of thrombophlebitis indicates need for **vein resection *(excise entire vein)*.

362. **Following a prolonged ischemia period (6 hours), you successfully perform a femoral to posterior tibial artery bypass for an acutely threatened leg. Several hours post-op, your pt develops an acute swollen painful right leg that feels tight to exam. He has pain w/ passive motion of the leg. The most appropriate next step in management is:

a. Fasciotomy
b. Arterial bypass
c. Lasix
d. Heparin

Answer a. ***Reperfusion injury resulting in* **compartment syndrome** *can occur after restoration of blood flow if occlusion time is > 4-6 hours. Tx is* **fasciotomy** *of the muscle compartment.*

363. **The MC injured nerve w/ lower extremity (calf) fasciotomy for compartment syndrome is
     a. Superficial peroneal
     b. Common peroneal
     c. Tibial
     d. Peroneal

Answer a. ***The* **superficial peroneal nerve** *is very superficial at the area between the anterior and lateral compartments near the proximal fibula. When performing the 2 incision technique for 4 compartment fasciotomy, the lateral incision comes very close to the superficial peroneal nerve.*

364. **A 54 yo woman presents with an acutely cold and painful right foot. Posterior tibial and dorsalis pedis pulses are gone on the right and intact on the left. You cannot feel a right femoral pulse. She has never had pain like this before and has lost sensation and motor function in her right foot. Which of the following is the most appropriate next step
     a. Catheter directed TPA
     b. Heparin only
     c. Cut-down and embolectomy
     d. Careful observation

Answer c. This pt has a threatened lower extremity (loss of motor function and sensation) and should be taken to the OR for emergent embolectomy. This scenario is most consistent with **embolus**.

> ***MC source of emboli to extremities or viscera* – <u>heart</u> *(usually due to* **atrial fibrillation**).
> ***MC source of emboli to head (ie stroke, TIAs) –* <u>carotid bifurcation</u> *(from atherosclerosis)*

Atherosclerosis stages
Normal arterial wall – intima, media, and adventitia
LDL cholesterol becomes **oxidized** in blood and **damages** arterial wall
Macrophages come to repair damage, causing an **inflammatory reaction**
Macrophages cannot process cholesterol, so **cholesterol builds up** in wall, attracting more macrophages (macrophages become **foam cells** w/ absorption of LDL)
Initially starts as a **fatty streak** and then cholesterol builds up
Smooth muscle proliferation in media occurs, further narrowing the arterial wall *(causes HTN)*
Thrombus can form on the damaged arterial wall, which if already narrowed, will completely **occlude the vessel** *(etiology of myocardial infarction)*
RFs: smoking, HTN, ↑ LDL or VLDL, DM, age, males, family Hx
Prevention and **Tx of atherosclerosis:**
    Statin drugs (eg simvastatin, *best preventive Tx for atherosclerosis*)
    Dietary change – less fat and cholesterol; ↑omega 3 fatty acids
    D/C smoking, control HTN, DM control, ASA
Homocysteinemia can ↑ risk of atherosclerosis. Tx: **folate, B-6, B-12**

*Buerger's disease (from tobacco; *thromboangiitis obliterans*)
Young men, **smokers**, can also occur w/ smokeless tobacco
Severe **rest pain** w/ bilateral **ulceration** + **gangrene of digits** (esp fingers)
Criteria:
Age < 45 years
Current (or recent) history of **tobacco** use
Distal extremity **ischemia** (claudication, rest pain, ulcers, gangrene)
Consistent **angio findings** (see below)
Dx: **angiogram**
1) **Corkscrew collaterals** w/ severe distal disease
2) **Normal arterial tree proximal** to popliteal / brachial arteries (ie small vessel disease)
Tx: stop smoking or will require continued amputations

*Fibromuscular dysplasia (FMD)
Young females; HTN occurs if renal involved
Medial fibrodysplasia most common variant (85%)
MC involved vessels – <u>renal arteries</u> (right side), then carotid and iliac
Usually causes **stenosis**; 50% **bilateral**; stenosis more **distal** then atherosclerosis; can also cause aneurysms
Dx: **angiogram** *(best for Dx)* – 'string of beads' appearance
Tx: **PTA** ± stent (*best Tx*, <u>not</u> endarterectomy) or **bypass**

**Carotid Anatomy
Normal internal carotid artery has **continuous forward flow**
Normal external carotid artery has **tri-phasic flow** (late-phase reverse flow)
1st branch of external carotid artery (ECA) – superior thyroid artery
1st branch of the internal carotid artery (ICA) – ophthalmic artery
Communication between internal and external carotid arteries is through **ophthalmic artery** (off ICA) and **internal maxillary artery** (off ECA)

MC diseased intracranial artery – middle cerebral artery
MC site of stenosis – carotid bifurcation
Stroke usually from arterial **embolization** (not thrombosis) from **ICA**
Heart 2nd MC source of emboli
Most important RF for cerebrovascular disease – HTN

Amaurosis fugax
Occlusion of ophthalmic branch of ICA (sign of carotid disease)
Get *transient* **visual changes** → shade coming down over pts eyes
Hollenhorst plaques on ophthalmologic exam
Transient ischemia attacks (TIA's) → sx's for < 24 hours

Dx: **Carotid Duplex U/S** every 6 months (measures carotid flow velocities; ICA/CCA ratio, want a certified lab)
Angiography *(best test; although many operate just on U/S findings)*

**Recommendations for Surgery
Asymptomatic ≥ 70-80%
Symptomatic ≥ 60-70%

Carotid endarterectomy - *removing **intima** and part of **media** from internal carotid*
Most impt technical concern** – getting a **good distal end-point (want to avoid an intimal flap)
Facial vein – can be routinely divided
***Occluded internal carotid artery** – do <u>NOT</u> repair (no benefit)*
Completed stroke → CEA 6 weeks later if stenosis meets criteria
Crescendo TIA's (or fluctuating neuro sx's) → emergent CEA
Vertebral artery disease Tx – PTA w/ stent best option

Criteria for Shunting during CEA (some always shunt)
  Pressure < 40
  You are operating on pt awake and they have neuro changes
  EEG changes (slowing)
  Contralateral tight stenosis or occlusion
**Nerve injuries
  Vagus
    **MC injured nerve w/ CEA
    Between IJ and carotid
    Injury causes **hoarseness** (recurrent laryngeal nerve off vagus)
    MC from **vascular clamping** during endarterectomy
  Marginal mandibular branch of facial nerve
    Injury causes droop in corner of mouth
    Catch this w/ **retractor** at angle of jaw
    Often recovers in 3 weeks
  Hypoglossal
    Near digastrics (2 cm above carotid bifurcation)
    Injury w/ high dissection
    *Tongues deviation to side of injury
    Difficulty w/ speech and mastication
  Ansa cervicalis – strap muscles; no serious deficits
  HTN post-op – from injury to carotid body
  Neuro event early post-op – go back to OR and re-explore
  Pseudoaneurysm post-op (pulsatile, bleeding mass after CEA) –
      emergent re-op (drape and prep before intubation)
  **MCC death after CEA – *myocardial infarction*

*Subclavian steal syndrome
  Subclavian artery is the MC site of upper extremity stenosis
  Proximal subclavian artery stenosis resulting in ***reversal of flow** through
      ipsilateral vertebral artery into subclavian artery
  Sx's – syncope, vertigo, falls, ocular problems (all vertebrobasilar) arm pain
  Repair with limb or neurologic sx's (MC Sx's – vertebrobasilar)
  Dx: angiogram
  Tx: PTA + stent (*best Tx*); common carotid to subclavian bypass if that fails

Medical Tx for Intermittent Claudication - ***smoking cessation** (best Tx; offer
  nicotine patch); graded exercise program; Tx lipid / cholesterol issues,
  HTN and DM; ASA or plavix (helps prevent cardiovascular events)

  Amputation risk: 10% lifetime
  Need for revascularization (surgical or percutaneous): 20% lifetime
  Increased risk of **cardiovascular events** (stroke, MI sudden death)
      *Need to be on ASA or plavix
  5-year mortality for intermittent claudication – 30%

Peripheral Arterial Disease (PAD)
  MCC – atherosclerosis
  MC atherosclerotic occlusion in lower extremities – Hunter's canal
    Distal superficial femoral artery exits here
    Sartorius muscle covers Hunter's canal
  Sx's: cramping, pain w/ exercise (ie intermittent claudication); pallor, hair
    loss, abnormal nail growth, poor capillary refill
    Severe Disease →
      If leg is **dependent →** rubor + pain relieved
      If leg is **elevated →** pallor + pain worsens (blood flow can't be
        sustained against gravity)
  Leriche syndrome (lesion at aortic bifurcation or above)
    1) **No femoral pulses**
    2) **Buttock or thigh claudication**
    3) **Impotence** (↓ flow in internal iliac arteries)

ABI's (ankle-brachial index; normal 1-1.2)

Claudication	< 0.9 (**same distance** each time)
Rest pain	< 0.5 (usually starts across **distal foot/arch**)
Ulcers	< 0.4 (starts in **toes, non-healing**)
Gangrene	< 0.3 (starts in **toes**)

ABI's can be very **inaccurate w/ DM** secondary to **incompressibility of vessels**; have to go off PVRs and angio

ABI based on return of systolic blood pressure after application of blood pressure cuff

PVRs (pulse volume recording) – finds occlusion and at what level

Arteriogram (*best test* for PVD)

Needed if PVRs and/or ABI's suggest significant disease

Can possibly **intervene** w/ angio as well

Collateral circulation – forms from abnormal pressure gradients

Circumflex iliac arteries to subcostal arteries

Circumflex femoral arteries to gluteal arteries

Geniculate arteries around the knee

Leg compartments

Anterior- Deep peroneal nerve (dorsiflexion, sensation 1st + 2^{nd}toes)

Anterior tibial artery

Lateral- Superficial peroneal nerve (eversion, lateral foot sensation)

Deep posterior- Tibial nerve (plantar-flexion)

Posterior tibial artery and peroneal artery

Superficial posterior – sural nerve

Revascularization procedure indications:

1) Significant **lifestyle limitation** despite maximal medical Tx

2) **Rest pain** (implies threatened limb, ie ABI < 0.5)

3) **Tissue loss, non-healing ulcers**, or **limb salvage**

→ Get angio, correct most proximal problem 1st

Use **saphenous vein graft** below the knee (PTFE has low patency below knee)

Femoral-distal grafts (eg peroneal, anterior tibial or posterior tibial artery) - need to have *run-off below the ankle* (ie a native vessel needs to go past the ankle joint) for this to be effective

Indications – bypasses distal to knee only for **limb** or **tissue salvage** (eg non-healing ulcer)

Best predictor of long term patency in extremity vein graft – vein quality

ASA *is Tx of choice following lower extremity bypass grafting to reduce cardiovascular events and improve graft patency.*

Duplex U/S *is the best technique for graft surveillance after bypass.*

Cx's

Early swelling (hours) following lower extremity bypass – edema from *reperfusion injury* (can get **compartment syndrome**)

Late swelling (days) following lower extremity bypass – likely *DVT*, get U/S

MCC early failure of reversed saphenous vein graft for lower extremity bypass - *technical problem*

MCC late failure of reversed saphenous vein graft for lower extremity bypass - *vein atherosclerosis*

Late hemorrhage or pseudoaneurysm *(weeks to years)* → likely **graft infection**; eroding into suture line

Isolated Iliac stenosis Tx - <u>PTA + stent</u> *(Tx of choice, 80% 5-year patency)*

PTA - intima **ruptured** and media **stretched**; pushes plaque out

Requires passage of wire 1st

PTFE (Gortex) – decreased patency when crosses knee

Have to use <u>saphenous vein graft</u> below knee

Dacron – good for aorta and large vessels

Renal atherosclerosis – left side MC, proximal ⅓ of artery; Tx: PTA w/ stent

Renal fibromuscular dysplasia (FMD) – right side MC, distal ⅓ of artery, women; Tx: PTA w/ stent

**Abdominal aortic aneurysms (AAA)

Normal aorta **2-3 cm**; 90% AAAs are infra-renal
**MCC - *atherosclerosis*
Sx's: **MC** found incidentally; can present w/ rupture, distal embolization
Rupture

Sx's: back or abd pain; hypotension

Dx: ***duplex U/S in ER best*** *(avoid sending hypotensive pt to CT)*
CT - retroperitoneal fluid, extra-luminal contrast
MC site of rupture – left posterolateral wall, 2–4 cm below renals
↑ rupture risk w/ **diastolic HTN** or **COPD** (coughing→expansion)
50% mortality w/ rupture (if pt reaches hospital alive)
**AAA repair criteria:

**Size ≥ 5.5 cm
Infected (mycotic)
Symptomatic
Growth > 0.5 cm/yr
*Open Repair Issues:

1) ***Inferior mesenteric artery** (IMA) **re-implantation** criteria:
Back pressure < 40 mmHg (poor back-bleeding)
Previous **colonic surgery**
SMA stenosis
If **flow to left colon appears inadequate**
2) ***Internal iliac artery** (hypogastric) **re-implantation:**
Need to maintain at least one open internal iliac artery
Absence of retrograde flow in internal iliac arteries (ie absence
of back-bleeding) → re-implant one internal iliac artery
Avoids buttock claudication (MC symptom), vasculogenic
impotence, spinal cord ischemia, recto-sigmoid ischemia

Mortality with elective open repair – 3-4%
MCC post-op death (and MCC of acute death) – myocardial infarction
MCC late post-op death – renal failure
Major vein injury w/ proximal cross-clamp – retro-aortic left renal vein
Impotence – 50% (disruption of autonomic nerves and blood flow to pelvis)
*Diarrhea (esp. bloody) after AAA worrisome for **ischemic colitis**
IMA often sacrificed w/ AAA repair, can cause **left colon ischemia**
Dx: **colonoscopy** (*best test*, need to go to splenic flexure)
*Chylous Ascites following ABF repair
White drainage, high in lipids, high lymphocyte count
Drainage catheter, conservative Tx for 2-3 wks (same Tx as
chylothorax – NPO, TPN, octreotide)
If that fails, re-op to ***ligate cisterna chili** area (located on **right side**
of aorta near right renal artery)
MC late Cx after aortic graft placement – atherosclerotic occlusion

**Infected ABF graft

Sx's – fever, elevated WBCs
Dx: **Abd CT** w/ oral and IV contrast (micro-bubbles sign of infection)
Consider **diagnostic tap** of fluid if unsure
May have positive blood cultures
Tx: Extra-anatomic bypass - **Axillary to femoral bypass**, then **femoral-
femoral cross-over** through non-infected planes, remove graft
Blood flow doubles to donor artery for fem-fem cross-over
Late hemorrhage or **late pseudoaneurysm** (years) after vascular bypass
graft is most consistent w/ ***graft infection*** (breaks down suture line)
**MCC of graft infection overall   *staph epidermidis*
    **MCC early *(< 1 month)*   *staph aureus*
    MCC late   staph epidermidis

Infections are increased in grafts going to **groin**
Most sensitive test for Dx of graft infection – tagged WBC scan

Femoral Pseudoaneurysm

Sx's: **groin or leg pain** and **swelling,** bleeding

Collection of blood in continuity w/ arterial system but not enclosed by all 3 layers of arterial wall

2 MC causes:
1) Percutaneous interventions <u>or</u>:
2) Disruption of a suture line between graft and artery

Dx: **Duplex U/S** *(best test)*

Tx:
1) If from **percutaneous intervention → U/S guided compression w/ thrombin injection**; open repair if acutely expanding, nerve compression, compromising skin or failure of conservative Tx
2) If from **disrupted suture line** (eg technical error, not getting full thickness bites) → ***emergent operative repair** (can have massive blood loss if this bursts)
3) **Late pseudoaneurysm** (years; can have bleeding) → MC related to *infection* and suture line breakdown, *Tx- resection of graft*

***Tx for distal femoral artery pseudoaneurysm in IV drug user** – ligation <u>without</u> reconstruction (**profunda femoris** artery has collaterals to **geniculate arteries** around the knee to support leg)*

Aorto-enteric fistula (eg aorto-duodenal fistula)

Pt's have history of abdominal vascular surgery, now w/ UGI bleeding

Sx's: herald bleed w/ **hematemesis**, then **blood per rectum**, then **exsanguination** *(classic)*

MC site – **duodenum** (3rd or 4th portion) erodes into **proximal suture line** leading to **UGI bleed**

Dx: **CT scan** *(best test)* – fluid around graft, thickened bowel wall, graft possibly in bowel lumen

Tx: same as aortic graft infections above (ie extra-anatomic bypass) + duodenum closure

Ischemic colitis

Sx's: **LLQ pain** and **bloody diarrhea** (can be non-bloody)

RFs:
Ligation of IMA at surgery (eg AAA repair)
Recent **low flow state** (eg CHF, MI, sepsis, cardiac surgery)

Results in **left colon ischemia**

Dx: **Colonoscopy** *(best test)* - **cyanotic edematous mucosa** w/ exudates
Splenic flexure and **lower sigmoid / upper rectum** most vulnerable with low flow states (watershed areas)
Griffith's Point (splenic flexure) – SMA (middle colic) and IMA (left colic) junction
Sudeck's Point – superior rectal (off IMA) and middle rectal (off internal iliac's) artery junction
Middle and Lower Rectum are <u>spared</u>
Supplied by middle (off internal iliac) and inferior (off internal pudendal, which is branch of internal iliac) rectal arteries

Indications for colectomy - full thickness ischemia (black bowel), pneumotosis intestinalis, clinical deterioration (eg sepsis, uncontrolled hemorrhage), perforation, diffuse peritoneal signs

Late strictures can occur from ischemia - Tx dilatation 1st, resection if refractory

**Popliteal Artery Aneurysms
  MC peripheral aneurysm
  MCC – atherosclerosis
  Leg exam has prominent popliteal pulses
  50% bilateral
  50% have another aneurysm elsewhere (MC - AAA)
  Sx's: Most likely to get emboli (MC) or thrombosis w/ limb ischemia
     Can present w/ an acutely threatened leg
        **rare rupture
  Intervention indications: symptomatic, > 2 cm, mycotic
  Tx: **Bypass w/ exclusion
  Acute thrombosis – tPA or open thrombectomy to restore blood flow;
     repair later
  **Pts w/ compressive sx's (venous congestion edema, paresthesias,
     numbness) should have **aneurysmorrhaphy w/ interposition graft
     (open aneurysm, place bypass graft in aneurysm sac), as opposed to
     exclusion w/ bypass, to alleviate compressive sx's. Geniculate
     arteries can continue to fill the aneurysm and cause compressive
     sx's if just ligation w/ bypass is performed.

     Iliac / femoral artery aneurysm repair indications - > 3.0 cm and > 2.5
        cm respectively, symptomatic or mycotic. They are usually
        associated with other aneurysms (MC – AAA).

     Rupture – MC Cx of aneurysms above inguinal ligament
     Thrombosis and emboli – MC Cx's of aneurysms below inguinal ligament

*Popliteal entrapment syndrome
  Sx's: *intermittent lower extremity claudication in young pts (< 30)
        *loss of pulse w/ plantar-flexion; can be bilateral
  Dx: angiogram
  Usually have medial deviation of popliteal artery around medial head of
     gastrocnemius muscle
  Tx: *resection of gastrocnemius muscle medial head

*Adventitial cystic disease
  Sx's: intermittent claudication, usually middle aged males, 40-50
  *Loss of pulse w/ knee flexion and extension (sx's also increase)
  MC area – popliteal, often bilateral
  Ganglia from adjacent joint capsule or tendon sheath compress artery
  Dx: angiogram
  Tx: *resection of cyst

Visceral Artery Aneurysms
  *Repair all splanchnic aneurysms when diagnosed (50% rupture) except
     splenic (< 2% rupture, see below)
  Diameters > 2 cm considered aneurysmal (renal > 1.5 cm)
  RFs: medial fibrodysplasia, portal HTN, inflammation (eg pancreatitis)
  Tx: covered stent or exclusion w/ bypass

  Splenic artery aneurysm
     MC visceral artery aneurysm (> 2 cm aneurysmal); MC in women
     1-2% rupture risk (much lower than other visceral aneurysms)
     Splenic artery aneurysms have a specific propensity to rupture w/
        pregnancy (MC in 3rd trimester – 90% rupture in some reports)
     Repair indications – symptomatic, pregnancy, child bearing age,
        > 3-4 cm (higher rupture risk)
     Tx: covered stent or open exclusion (can exclude w/o bypass graft
        or splenectomy - has collaterals)

AV Fistulas and Grafts for Dialysis
MCC AV graft failure – venous obstruction from **intimal hyperplasia**
*Early failure – *technical problem*
*Late failure – *intimal hyperplasia* on venous side
Early thrombosis → suspect technical problem
De-clot and get a **fistulogram** to help figure out problem
Arm swelling after AV fistula
Results from venous HTN
Initial Tx: elevation, as collaterals develop swelling goes down
Persistence of major swelling suggests obstruction of a <u>major</u>
outflow vein (axillary, subclavian, innominate) → **need
angiogram w/ shunt run-off** (venogram)
Tx - PTA w/ stent of stenotic area *(best Tx)*
Arm ischemia after AV fistula:
Mild form - Sx's: cool, numbness, pain in hand w/ HD
Usually reverses in a few weeks after starting HD
Severe form
Sx's: can start immediately after placing graft, gross ischemia
(mottling, cyanotic)
Usually associated w/ upper arm graft
Associated w/ *arterial obstruction* *(inflow obstruction)*
proximal to graft (eg subclavian artery stenosis)
Dx: **angiogram** – check for arterial obstruction proximally
Tx:*Band venous end of graft* (do this acutely if hand
threatened, W/U cause later)
Revascularize inflow problem if present
Graft ligation (last resort)
Late venous outflow obstruction
Can have an **increase in pressure in returning line,** high **outflow
pressure** (> 200) or an increase in **recirculation** (all signs of
venous outflow problem and impending graft failure)
Dx: **fistulogram w/ shunt run-off** (venogram, figure out level of
obstruction)
Tx: **stent** venous outflow obstruction (may need to redo the venous
anastomosis if intimal hyperplasia there is the problem)

Traumatic AV fistula
Sx's **arterial insufficiency** (eg claudication), **CHF** (high output cardiac
failure due to shunt), **aneurysm**
Dx: **Duplex U/S** *(best test)* or angio; May feel **thrill** or hear **bruit**
Tx: **Open Repair** → lateral venous suture; patch arterial side (may
need bypass graft), interpose muscle (eg sartorius muscle)
or tissue between artery and vein so that it does not recur

Diabetic foot ulcer
Diabetics can't feel feet, so **plantar ulcers** form at pressure areas
Usually at **metatarsal heads** and **heel**
Tx: debridement, keep moist, leg elevation, non-weight bearing, abx's
Malperforans ulcer (at **metatarsal heads**, MC 2nd MTP joint)
Often have osteomyelitis; Tx: as above but also need cartilage
debridement of metatarsal head if osteomyelitis present
Heel ulceration to bone (exposed calcaneus) → Tx: amputation
Wound Biopsy (wound curettage base of wound) – send cultures
Best Dx test for organisms
Best Dx test for osteomyelitis
Tx of wet gangrene (erythema, pus, red streaks) - *Early, aggressive,
debridement of ulcerated area → surgical emergency*
Severe cellulitis spreading past ulcerated area (red streaks, erythema
and swollen toe or extremity, pus coming out of ulcer, possibly septic)
→ *early amputation at appropriate level (can be life saving)*

**<u>Compartment</u> syndrome
　　Reperfusion injury *(PMNs) following prolonged (4-6 hrs)* **ischemia and
　　　　the restoration of blood flow *(eg acutely ischemic leg for 6 hours, pt*
　　　　undergoes fem-tibial bypass, now has acute leg swelling)
　　MC affects ***anterior compartment** of leg (get foot-drop)
　　Sx's: **1ˢᵗ - pain w/ passive motion**; early post-op extremity **swelling**,
　　　　paresthesias, paralysis; loss of pulse is a <u>late finding</u>
　　Dx: based on **clinical suspicion**
　　　　Compartment pressure **> 20 mmHg** abnormal → fasciotomy
　　Tx: **Fasciotomies** → leave open 5–10 days (skin graft after that)

　　**Lower Extremity Fasciotomy - **Watch for superficial peroneal nerve
　　　　w/ lateral incision on lower leg (injury would cause decreased eversion
　　　　of foot) – ****MC injured nerve w/ lower extremity fasciotomy**

**<u>Acute lower extremity ischemia</u>
　　**MCC - *embolism from <u>heart</u> (usually from atrial fibrillation)*

　　Emboli (MC) - **No collaterals, No PMHx of claudication, contra-lateral leg*
　　　　pulses are normal, often have arrhythmias
　　　　Sx's: pain, paresthesias, paralysis, poikiothermia, pulseless
　　　　Leg Exam: **pallor** (white)→ **cyanosis** (blue)→ **marbling**
　　　　MCC arterial emboli – <u>heart</u> *due to atrial fibrillation (70%)*
　　　　MC site of obstruction– <u>common femoral artery</u>
　　　　Tx: embolectomy usual

　　Thrombosis – **usually have chronic PAD (no hair on legs, shiny surface),*
　　　　Hx of claudication or previous bypass graft, No arrhythmias, weak
　　　　contra-lateral pulses (from diffuse atherosclerosis)
　　　　Exam: usually have collaterals (so <u>less likely</u> leg will be threatened)
　　　　Tx: **Non-threatened leg** (motor + sensation intact)
　　　　　　Mild sx's (good collateral perfusion) – heparin only
　　　　　　Moderate sx's - catheter directed intra-arterial tPA + heparin
　　　　　Threatened leg (loss of motor or sensation) - OR thrombectomy

**<u>Mesenteric ischemia</u>
　　**MCC – *embolism from <u>heart</u> (usually from atrial fibrillation)*

　　Superior Mesenteric Artery Embolism
　　　　**MC source – <u>heart</u>, *(from atrial fibrillation)*
　　　　Pain out of proportion to exam *(hallmark)*, sudden onset
　　　　Tx: open embolectomy usual

　　Superior Mesenteric Artery Thrombosis
　　　　*MCC – <u>atherosclerosis</u> *(usually chronic sx's of PAD)*
　　　　Tx: catheter-directed tPA or open thrombectomy

　　Non-Occlusive Mesenteric Ischemia (NOMI)
　　　　Etiologies – low flow state, hypovolemia, hemoconcentration, Digoxin,
　　　　　　high dose pressors, cocaine, sepsis → ****final common**
　　　　　　pathway is low cardiac output to visceral vessels
　　　　RFs – prolonged shock, CHF, prolonged cardiopulmonary bypass
　　　　Sx's: abd pain
　　　　Angio – shows constricted vessels
　　　　Tx: ***Optimize C.O.** (<u>best Tx</u> **for NOMI** - fluid, Dopamine,
　　　　　　Dobutamine); **papaverine** or **nitrates** to increase visceral blood
　　　　　　flow (catheter directed into visceral vessels)

**Primary Venous Insufficiency

Sx's: edema, ulceration, aching, heaviness, bleeding, thrombophlebitis

**Brawny edema – *suggests severe disease, hemosiderin deposition causes color change*

Ulceration occurs above and posterior to **medial malleoli**

Edema – secondary to incompetent perforators

Elevation brings relief

RFs: obesity, low activity, smoking

Dx: **Duplex U/S** *(best Dx study)* w/ pt standing, look for:

1) **Incompetent sapheno-femoral** or **sapheno-popliteal valve** - diagnosis of **valve incompetence** made if relief of muscle pressure proximally (eg thigh) causes retrograde flow in vein

2) **Incompetent perforator valves**

3) **DVT** - need to make sure pt does **not** have a DVT

**DVT Is a contraindication to vein stripping and avulsion

U/S gives **location**, **vein size**, and **direction of blood flow**

Normal venous Duplex U/S – augmentation of flow with distal compression (eg calf) or release of proximal compression (eg thigh)

Medical Tx 1ˢᵗ (aimed at **reducing venous hypertension*) - avoid long standing, weight loss, D/C smoking, elevate legs, stockings

Unna Boot *for severe disease* - Zinc oxide triple layer wrap for severe ulcers or significant edema; ****90% of ulcers cured this way

Surgical Tx (for failure of medical Tx)

Fundamentals of surgical Tx of varicose veins is **ablation of reflux source** (escape point)

Varicosities < 1 mm (eg varicose veins) – sclerotherapy

Varicosities > 4 mm

1) If the sapheno-femoral (GSV) + sapheno-popliteal (LSV) valves are <u>competent</u> (just have **incompetent perforators**) → *stab avulsion technique* to remove varicosities (removes perforators)

2) If sapheno-femoral (GSV) and sapheno-popliteal (LSV) valves are <u>not competent</u> (reflux along entire length of vein) → *vein stripping*

**Contraindications to vein stripping – *DVT, venous outflow obstruction, pregnancy (varicosities go away after delivery)*

**Superficial thrombophlebitis (nonbacterial inflammation)

MC in setting of **previous peripheral IV**

Tx: NSAIDs, warm packs, arm elevation

**Suppurative thrombophlebitis – fever and ↑WBCs

Sx's: **erythema, red streaking** up arm, and **fluctuance** at site **palpable cord;** MC w/ previous peripheral IV

MC organism – staph aureus

Dx: U/S will show **cord**; blood cultures may show organism

Tx: 1) **Remove IV** and **abx's;** warm compress, elevation

2) ****Need to resect entire vein** for continued **purulence** or **bacteremia** *despite abx's*

*Lymphatics <u>not</u> found in bone, muscle, tendon, cartilage, brain, or cornea

Gastrointestinal Hormones

365. *Parietal cells of the stomach secrete:
   - a. HCL and intrinsic factor
   - b. Pepsinogen
   - c. Secretin
   - d. Cholecystokinin

   Answer a. The parietal cells secrete HCL and intrinsic factor.

366. *Chief cells of the stomach secrete:
   - a. HCL and intrinsic factor
   - b. Pepsinogen
   - c. Secretin
   - d. Cholecystokinin

   Answer b. Chief cells primarily secrete **pepsinogen**.
   1st enzyme in protein digestion – pepsin
   1st enzyme in carbohydrate digestion - salivary amylase

367. **Intrinsic factor binds:
   - a. Fe
   - b. Cu
   - c. B-12
   - d. B-6

   Answer c. Intrinsic factor binds B-12.
   **Deficiencies in B-12 can occur w/:*
      1) ****gastric bypass** (intrinsic factor needs acid to bind B-12)
      2) ****terminal ileum resection** (B-12 absorbed there)
      3) pernicious anemia and blind loop syndrome

368. *Omeprazole works by:
   - a. Inhibiting the parietal cell H/K ATPase
   - b. Blocking histamine receptor
   - c. Blocking acetylcholine receptors
   - d. Blocking TSH receptors

   Answer a. *Omeprazole* works by inhibiting the parietal cell H/K ATPase
   (proton pump). *Ranitidine* works by inhibiting the parietal cell histamine
   receptor.

369. **Gastrin:
   - a. Is primarily produced in the fundus
   - b. Increases secretion of HCL from parietal cells (via enterochromaffin cells which release histamine)
   - c. Increases secretion of intrinsic factor from parietal cells
   - d. Increases secretion of pepsinogen from chief cells

   Answer a. *Gastrin is primarily produced by G cells in <u>antrum</u> + <u>duodenum</u>*

370. **All of the following are true of motilin except:
   - a. The highest concentration of receptors is in the stomach antrum
   - b. Motilin exerts its effect on the migrating motor complex during phase III (peristalsis)
   - c. The primary response is increasing antrum and duodenal motility
   - d. Secretion is stimulated by somatostatin

   Answer d. Secretion is inhibited by somatostatin
   **The highest concentration of motilin receptors is in the stomach antrum
   **Motilin enhances the migrating motor complex during phase III (peristalsis)
   **The primary response to motilin is increased antrum + duodenal motility

**Gastrin

Produced <u>G cells</u> in stomach **antrum and **duodenum**
Secretion stimulated by – protein, vagal input (acetylcholine), ETOH,
    antral distention, pH > 3.0
Secretion inhibited by – pH < 3.0, somatostatin, secretin, CCK
Target cells – <u>parietal cells</u> (**via *enterochromaffin cells* which release
    histamine) and <u>chief cells</u>
**Response
    Secretion of **HCl, intrinsic factor** and **pepsinogen** (*strongest*
        stimulator for all)
    ↑s **gastric motility**
**Proton pump inhibitors (*eg Omeprazole*) *block H^+/K^+ ATPase of parietal*
    cell (final pathway for H^+ release).
Parietal cells – release HCl and Intrinsic Factor
Chief cells – release pepsinogen
**Intrinsic Factor – *binds B-12 for absorption in the terminal ileum*

**Somatostatin

Produced by <u>D cells</u> in stomach **antrum, small intestine** and **pancreas**
Secretion stimulated by – acid in duodenum
**Target cells – *many "the great inhibitor"*
Response:
    Inhibits gastrin and HCl release
    Inhibits release of insulin, glucagon, secretin, CCK, GIP, VIP, motilin
    ↓s pancreatic and biliary output
    Slows gastric emptying
Octreotide (somatostatin analogue) – can ↓ pancreatic fistula output

**CCK (*cholecystokinin*)

Produced by <u>I cells</u> of **duodenum** (MC site)
Secretion stimulated by – protein and fat in duodenum
Response:
    **Relaxation of sphincter of Oddi
    Gallbladder contraction
    ↑ed **pancreatic **acinar <u>enzyme</u> secretion** (acinar cells, zymogen
        granules)
    ↑ed **intestinal motility**

**Secretin

Produced by <u>S cells</u> of **duodenum** (MC site)
Secretion stimulated by – acid (pH < 4), fat, bile
Secretion inhibited by – pH > 4.0, gastrin
Endocrine (primarily) + **exocrine** effects
Response:
    Inhibits HCl (*primary duty*) and **gastrin release
    ↑s **pancreatic **ductal <u>HCO_3^-</u> secretion**
    ↑s **bile flow**
    <u>High</u> pancreatic duct output has – ↑ HCO_3^-, ↓ Cl^-
    <u>Slow</u> pancreatic duct output has – ↓ HCO_3^-, ↑ Cl^-
    Carbonic anhydrase in duct exchanges HCO_3^- for Cl^-

**Motilin

Release by <u>M cells</u> primarily from ***duodenum**
**Highest concentration of motilin receptors – *stomach* **antrum*, also
    in duodenum, colon
Secretion stimulated by – duodenal acid, vagus input
    Released during **fasting** or **inter-digestive phase** (not while eating)
Secretion inhibited by – somatostatin, secretin, pancreatic polypeptide,
    duodenal fat
Primary Response – *increases* **antrum *and* **duodenal motility** *[initiates*
    phase III (<u>peristalsis</u>) of the migrating motor complex (MMC)]
**Erythromycin *acts on this receptor*

**Glucagon
Released by <u>alpha cells</u> of the **pancreas** (also stomach, intestine)
Secretion stimulated by – ↓ serum glucose, ↑ amino acids (to protect
from hypoglycemia w/ all protein meal), acetylcholine (vagus),
catecholamines (beta adrenergic)
Secretion inhibited by – ↑ serum glucose, ↑ insulin, somatostatin
Response:
**Relaxes sphincter of Oddi
Glycogenolysis and **gluconeogenesis**
Lipolysis and **ketogenesis**
Proteolysis
All decreased → gastric acid secretion, pancreatic secretion, intestinal
motility, stomach motility, myenteric motor complexes
Alpha and **beta cells** = G.I. (glucagon and insulin)

Insulin
Released by <u>beta cells</u> of the **pancreas**
Secretion stimulated by – serum glucose, glucagon, protein ingestion
Secretion inhibited by – somatostatin
Response:
Cellular glucose uptake
Protein, glycogen and fat <u>synthesis</u> (anabolic)
Type I diabetes – pancreatic beta islet cells destroyed
Type II diabetes – insulin resistance

*Pancreatic polypeptide
Secreted by islet cells in **pancreas**
Response – *<u>decreases</u> pancreatic endocrine and exocrine function
Peptide YY - released from terminal ileum after fatty meal
Response - <u>decreases</u> gastric emptying, gastric acid secretion, pancreatic
function, and gallbladder contraction

*Bombesin (gastrin-releasing peptide)
Release from post-ganglionic fibers of vagus nerve
Response – *<u>increases</u> gastric acid secretion, intestinal motility, and
pancreatic enzyme secretion
Vasoactive intestinal peptide (VIP)
Produced by cells in **gut** and **pancreas**
Secretion stimulated by – fat, acetylcholine
Response: <u>increases</u> intestinal secretion (water, electrolytes) and motility

Bowel recovery after surgery
Small bowel recovers in <u>24 hours</u>
stomach recovers in <u>48 hours</u>,
large bowel recovers in <u>3-5 days</u>

Anorexia – mediated by hypothalamous (CCK, peptide YY)

**Deficiencies in B-12 can occur w/:
1) ****gastric bypass** (intrinsic factor needs acid to bind B-12)
2) ****terminal ileum resection** (B-12 absorbed there)
3) pernicious anemia and blind loop syndrome

Esophagus

371. *All of the following are true except:
    a. The upper thoracic esophagus is best approached w/ a right thoracotomy
    b. The MC site of esophageal perforation is near the cricopharyngeus
    c. The lower esophagus is predominantly smooth muscle
    d. The indentation on EGD at 25 mm from the incisors is likely the diaphragmatic hiatus

    Answer d. The indentation on EGD at 25 mm from the incisors is the aortic arch. The indentation for the diaphragmatic hiatus occurs at 45 cm.

372. **All of the following are true except:
    a. The UES pressure at rest and during the early part of the swallow are approximately 70 mmHg and 15 mmHg
    b. LES pressure at rest and during a swallow are approximately 15 mmHg and 0 mmHg
    c. The LES relaxes soon after initiation of a swallow through a vagally mediated process
    d. The lower esophageal sphincter (LES) is normally seen on EGD at about 40 cm from the incisors

    Answer d. The LES is not seen on EGD. It is a physiologic area found with manometry. **The LES relaxes soon after initiation of a swallow through a vagally mediated process.**

373. **All of the following are true except:
    a. Diffuse esophageal spasm is characterized by high amplitude repetitive *non-peristaltic* contractions
    b. Nutcracker esophagus is characterized by high amplitude *peristaltic* contractions
    c. Scleroderma of the esophagus is characterized by aperistalsis and high LES pressure
    d. Achalasia is characterized by high LES pressure and absence of peristalsis

    Answer c. **Scleroderma of the esophagus is characterized by aperistalsis and low LES pressure** w/ concomitant massive reflux and severe esophagitis.

    Achalasia is characterized by high LES pressure and absence of peristalsis.
    Diffuse esophageal spasm is characterized by high amplitude repetitive non-peristaltic contractions.
    Nutcracker esophagus is characterized by very high amplitude peristaltic contractions.
    Manometry is the best test for **primary esophageal dysmotility D/Os** (achalasia, diffuse esophageal spasm, and nutcracker esophagus) and scleroderma of the esophagus.

374. **The most important step in treatment of a pt with a Zenker's diverticulum is:
    a. Resection of the diverticulum
    b. Division of the superior laryngeal constrictor muscles
    c. Esophagectomy
    d. Division of the cricopharyngeus muscle

    Answer d. **The most important step in treatment of a Zenker's diverticulum is performing a **cricopharyngomyotomy**. The anatomic problem with a Zenker's diverticulum is failure of the UES to relax with swallowing.

The diverticulum is usually resected but in some situations when the diverticulum would be too hard to remove, it can be suspended upward such that it drains into the esophagus.

375. **All of the following are true except:
   a. The most sensitive test for GERD is a 24 hour pH study
   b. The MC problem leading to GERD is inadequate LES pressure.
   c. Barrett's with high grade dysplasia should be treated w/ PPI
   d. The relative risk for esophageal CA in pts w/ Barrett's is 50

   Answer c. Barrett's is *squamous to columnar metaplasia* of the esophagus. The specialized, *intestinal-type* columnar epithelium (have intestinal **Goblet cells**) is felt to be the type at risk for **malignant degeneration** to adenocarcinoma.

   High grade Barrett's dysplasia *is an indication for* **esophagectomy**. *Up to 20% of pts w/* **high grade dysplasia** *actually have esophageal CA somewhere in the Barrett's portion.*

   Barrett's increases the relative risk of **esophageal CA** to 50 (50 x more likely to get esophageal CA compared to general population).

376. **All of the following are true to Schatzki's Ring except:
   a. These patients almost universally have hiatal hernias
   b. These patients usually have GERD
   c. Dysphagia is the most common symptom
   d. These lesions should undergo resection

   Answer d. **Schatzki's Ring** *occurs in pts w/ hiatal hernias. Tx for sx's includes* **ring dilatation + PPI**. *Resection of these rings is* never *indicated.*

377. **The all of the following are true of laparoscopic fundoplication except:
   a. The key to hiatal dissection is finding the right crura and the key to the wrap is finding the left crura
   b. The best test for recurrent reflux or dysphagia following Nissen is barium esophagogram
   c. MCC of dysphagia following laparoscopic fundoplication is that the wrap is too tight
   d. Shortened esophagus requires esophagectomy and gastric replacement

   Answer d. *Shortened esophagus requires* **Collis gastroplasty** *to lengthen the esophageal tube (forms neo-esophagus out of stomach).*

   The best test for **dysphagia** *or* **recurrent reflux** *following Nissen is* **barium esophagogram** *(assesses wrap cx's)*
   The MCC of dysphagia *following laparoscopic fundoplication is that the* **wrap is too tight**

378. **A 48 yo male who drinks a case of beer per day devours a large meal, develops nausea, and then vomits. Five hours after this, he develops severe chest pain and is brought to the ED. His BP is 100/50 and has a HR of 110 so you get 2 IVs him and give him a fluid bolus. All of the following are true of the pts likely condition except:
   a. Gastrografin, followed by thin barium swallow is the best study for diagnosis
   b. The MC location for the problem in the left lower esophagus
   c. A left thoracotomy is usually the best incision given the MC location
   d. Simple full thickness esophageal bites are all that is needed for repair

Answer d. ***Be careful here. After washing out the vomited material w/ **Boerhaave's Syndrome**, you need to perform a myotomy to see the extent of the injury in the mucosa. Classically, the mucosal injury will extend farther than the muscle injury. So what you see at first glance is <u>not</u> the full extent of the injury. **Gastrografin swallow, followed by thin barium swallow is the best study for Dx of an esophageal perforation.*

379. **A 65 yo man undergoes routine EGD for GERD. After the procedure, he develops chest pain. CXR is negative. The most appropriate next step is:
    a. Chest CT
    b. Abdominal CT
    c. Gastrografin followed by thin barium swallow
    d. Chest MRI

    Answer c. ***The Dx study of choice for possible esophageal perforation is **gastrografin** followed by thin **barium swallow**.*

380. **Treatment of esophageal leiomyoma involves:
    a. Extra-mucosal enucleation via thoracotomy
    b. Segmental resection
    c. XRT
    d. Chemotherapy

    Answer a. ***Tx of **esophageal leiomyoma** is **extra-mucosal enucleation** through a thoracotomy. Notably, you do <u>not</u> want to try and biopsy leiomyomas on EGD - can create mucosal scar tissue and make enucleation difficult and increase risk of disrupting the mucosa.*

381. **A 55 yo man presents w/ dysphagia and weight loss. Esophagogram shows a lesion at the gastro-esophageal junction and biopsies come back as adenocarcinoma. Given the likely Dx, all of the following are true except:
    a. The right gastroepiploic artery is the main blood supply to the stomach after trans-hiatal esophagectomy
    b. This patient should have endoscopic U/S (best test for T status)
    c. The most important prognostic factor is depth of lesion
    d. In general, lesions > T1 should undergo neoadjuvant chemo-XRT

    Answer c. ***The most important prognostic factor for esophageal CA devoid of systemic mets is **nodal involvement**.*
    ***In general, lesions > T1 should undergo **neoadjuvant chemo-XRT**.*
    *****GE junction tumors** are treated like **esophageal CA** and 10 cm margins are generally indicated.*
    *Adenocarcinoma is the MC type of esophageal CA
    ***The **right gastroepiploic artery** is the main blood supply to the stomach after trans-hiatal esophagectomy*

382. **The best test for suspected caustic esophageal injury due to ingestion is:
    a. CXR
    b. Endoscopy
    c. Chest CT
    d. Barium swallow

    Answer b. ***The best test for suspected **caustic esophageal injury** is **endoscopy**. Do <u>NOT</u> go past the point of severe injuries as you may cause a perforation – just making the diagnosis and assessing injury here.*

Normal Anatomy and Function
Layers: Mucosa (squamous epithelium), **Submucosa**
      Muscularis propria
            Upper 1/3 esophagus – *striated muscle
            Lower 2/3 esophagus – *smooth muscle

No serosa

Blood supply
- **Cervical** – inferior thyroid artery
- **Thoracic** – vessels directly off aorta (main supply to esophagus)
- **Abdominal** – left gastric artery (primary)

Innervation
- **Right vagus nerve**
  - Travels on *posterior portion of stomach as it exits chest
  - Becomes **celiac plexus**
  - Has **Criminal nerve of Grassi** → causes persistently high acid levels post-op if left undivided w/ vagotomy
- **Left vagus nerve**
  - On *anterior portion of stomach; goes to **liver + biliary tree**

Normal manometry
- **Pharyngeal contraction w/ food bolus**   70-120 mmHg
- **Upper esophageal sphincter** (*cricopharyngeus muscle*)
  - At **rest**   60 mmHg
  - W/ **food bolus**   15 mmHg
  - No pressure drop w/ food indicates failure of cricopharyngeus to relax
- **Lower esophageal sphincter**
  - At **rest**   15 mmHg
  - W/ **food bolus**   0 mmHg
  - Resting LES pressure frequently ≤ 5 w/ GERD
- **Esophageal contraction w/ swallow**   30-120 mmHg
  - Ineffective if < 10 mmHg throughout (ie burned out esophagus)

Normal Distances (anatomic areas of narrowing listed below, measurements are from incisors, esophagus is **30 cm** total length):
- **Cricopharyngeus**   15 cm
- **Aortic arch indentation**   25 cm
- **Diaphragmatic hiatus**   45 cm
- **LES is not visible – is a manometric finding**

Upper esophageal sphincter – *cricopharyngeus* muscle (circular muscle)
- Prevents air swallowing; recurrent laryngeal nerve innervation
- **MC site of esophageal perforation** - near cricopharyngeus (MCC - EGD)
- **MC site for foreign body** - near cricopharyngeus

Lower esophageal sphincter (40 cm from incisors) – relaxation mediated by inhibitory neurons; normally contracted at rest → prevents reflux
- 1) LES is not an anatomical sphincter *and*;
- 2) LES is not seen on EGD
- Is a physiologic zone (3-5 cm) of high pressure found on **manometry**

Swallowing stages (CNS initiates swallow)
- **Primary peristalsis** - occurs w/ food bolus and swallow initiation
- **Secondary peristalsis** - occurs w/ incomplete emptying and esophageal distention, consists of propagating waves
- **Tertiary peristalsis**- non-propagating, non-peristalsing, *dysfunctional*
- UES + LES normally contracted between meals to avoid reflux + air swallowing

Swallowing mechanism
- Soft palate occludes nasopharynx
- Larynx rises and airway opening is blocked by epiglottis
- Cricopharyngeus relaxes
- Pharyngeal contraction moves food into esophagus
- **LES relaxes soon after initiation of swallow** (vagus induced relaxation)

Surgical approach to esophagus

Cervical esophagus	left neck (left sided course here)
Upper thoracic	right (avoids the aorta)
Lower thoracic	left (left-sided course here)

Esophageal dysfunction
    Primary esophageal D/O's - achalasia, nutcracker, diffuse spasm
    Secondary esophageal D/Os - GERD (MC), scleroderma
  Endoscopy
    Procedure of choice for **heartburn**
    Procedure of choice for **foreign body** (Dx and Tx)
  Esophagogram (gastrografin, then barium)
    Procedure of choice for **dysphagia** and **odynophagia**
    Procedure of choice for **suspected perforation** (gastrografin, then
        thin barium)
  Esophageal Foreign Bodies
    Adults MC - food impaction (meat)
    Children: MC - coins
    Dx and Tx: **rigid EGD** in OR (need to intubate 1st)

**Achalasia
  1)   **Failure of LES to relax** and 2) **Absence of peristalsis**
  Sx's: *dysphagia (solids + liquids; in nearly all pts)* and **regurgitation**
  **Autoimmune destruction of neuronal ganglion cells *(Auerbach's*
    myenteric plexus)
  Dx: **Esophagogram** (initial test for dysphagia)
        Esophageal dilatation w/ tapering distally (bird's beak)
        **Manometry Studies (*best test* for Dx of Achalasia)
          1) *LES fails to relax* w/ swallowing (usually high, > 25 mmHg)
          2) *Loss of peristalsis* (low amplitude and fails to progress)
      EGD – needed for all pts to R/O esophageal **CA** (especially at EGJ)
  SCCA of esophagus - increased w/ achalasia (15 x); Sx's - weight loss
  Medical Tx: primary goal is relief of **obstruction at LES**
    Try **balloon dilatation** x 2 (80% effective), calcium channel blocker
  Surgical Tx *(definitive):* lower esophagus longitudinal **esophagomyotomy**
    (Heller Myotomy)

Diffuse esophageal spasm
  Sx's: **dysphagia** and **chest pain;** possible psych history
  Dx: *Manometry (best test for Dx DES)*
        High amplitude, repetitive, non-peristaltic, contractions (long
          duration); > 30% non-peristaltic
        *LES relaxes **normally***
      Barium swallow – corkscrew esophagus; may see diverticulum
  Medical Tx *(best Tx):* *calcium channel blocker* (diltiazem), Trazodone
    Decrease anxiety – psych assessment
  Indications for surgery: reserved for pts w/ refractory incapacitating
    episodes of dysphagia (last resort)
  Surgery Tx – long esophageal myotomy (length of thoracic esophagus)
    Right thoracotomy or thoracoscopic approach; include partial wrap
    Surgery better at resolving dysphagia than pain
    Surgery usually less effective than for achalasia

Nutcracker esophagus (MC primary esophageal D/O)
  Sx's: **chest pain** (MCC of non-cardiac chest pain); ± dysphagia
  Dx: *Manometry (best test for Dx of nutcracker)*
        Very high amplitude peristaltic waves (> 180 mmHg)
        *LES relaxes **normally***
      EKG, CXR, Troponins, and CK-MB ➔ R/O myocardial ischemia
  Medical Tx *(best Tx):* *calcium channel blocker* (diltiazem), Trazodone
    Decrease anxiety – psych assessment
  Indications for surgery: reserved for pts w/ refractory incapacitating
    episodes of chest pain (last resort)
  Surgery Tx – long esophageal myotomy (length of thoracic esophagus)
    Right thoracotomy or thoracoscopic approach include partial wrap
    Surgery usually less effective than for achalasia

**_Scleroderma_
Sx's: **heartburn** *(**_massive reflux_*, no LES tone) and **dysphagia**
Complete loss of LES tone w/ **fibrous replacement of smooth muscle**
throughout esophagus (**distal 2/3 of esophagus** most affected)
Esophagus MC affected organ by scleroderma
Risk of esophageal adenocarcinoma
**Manometry *(best test for Dx)* - **low LES pressure and aperistalsis
Medial Tx: PPI, reflux Tx, metoclopramide (Reglan)
Indications for operation - refractory GERD or cx's (eg ulcers, strictures)
Surgery – esophagectomy usual

**Caustic esophageal injury
Alkali – deep liquefaction necrosis, especially liquid (eg Drano, lye)
Worse injury than acid; also more likely to cause subsequent CA
Acid – coagulation necrosis; mostly causes gastric injury
Complications - esophageal / stomach perforation, necrosis, stricture
Risk of esophageal **squamous cell CA** later in life
Do not place NG tube; Do not induce vomiting (keep pt NPO)
Avoid neutralizing agents
Dx: Endoscopy – *best test* to assess **severity of injury**
Do NOT go past the point of severe injuries
Tx: **Perforation** – esophagectomy (right thoracotomy, allows removal of
entire esophagus) ****Do not repair caustic perforations**
If no perforation - serial **X-rays** and **exams**, IVFs, spitting, abx's, swallow
study HD #3, NPO until able to swallow own secretions, then clears
Indications for surgery – sepsis, peritonitis, worsening metabolic
acidosis, mediastinitis, free or soft tissue air, contrast extravasation,
PTX, large pleural effusion

**_Pharyngoesophageal Diverticulum_ *(Zenker's)*
Due to **ineffective relaxation of cricopharyngeus**
Pharyngeal constrictors push against this, creating high pressure
Diverticulum found posteriorly (MC) between **cricopharyngeus** and
pharyngeal constrictors (Killian's triangle)
Is a *false diverticulum* (not all layers; no muscle; pulsion diverticulum)
Sx's: **cervical dysphagia + regurgitation** of non-digested food (classic)
Dx: **Barium swallow** – posterior midline protrusion above UES
**NO EGD → *avoided* due to risk of perforation
Manometry studies – show lack of UES relaxation
Tx:****Cricopharyngeal myotomy** *(Key Point of Tx);* left cervical incision
**Removal of diverticula *not* necessary
Can remove or suspend the diverticulum

**Gastroesophageal reflux disease (GERD)
Sx's **heartburn** (worse 30-60 min after meal), worse lying down or stooping
Heartburn is from exposure of **esophagus** to **gastric acid**
Many pts just treated **empirically** w/ PPI w/o testing (99% effective)
Dx: need following before wrap - ****24 hr pH test** *(best test for Dx),*
manometry (R/O dysmotility problem), **EGD** w/ Bx's, and consider
barium Swallow (if unusual sx's, eg dysphagia)
*MCC of GERD - *incompetent LES (from low pressure)*
Cx's from GERD
Esophagitis – almost always gets better w/ PPI
MCC of **esophageal bleeding** – esophagitis from GERD
Peptic Stricture - GERD is MCC of **benign esophageal stricture**
Tx: **medical Tx** (PPI + periodic EGD dilatation), 95% effective
Esophageal Shortening
RFs - peptic stricture, giant hernia, previously failed wraps
Esophagus should lie (freely) 2 cm below hiatus after dissection
for wrap (otherwise need **Collis gastroplasty**)

**Barrett's
Present in 10% of pts w/ GERD; from long standing reflux
Squamous to *columnar metaplasia* (raised, pink lesion)
Specialized ****intestinal** type metaplasia highest RF for **CA**
*Barrett's CA risk <u>NOT</u> reversed w/ PPI or fundoplication
    Need continued **annual surveillance** even after wrap
Barrett's is <u>NOT</u> an indication for wrap
Surveillance for CA - 4 quadrant Bx at 1 cm intervals (3-6
    month after initial Dx, annually after that)
    Risk of **adenocarcinoma** w/ Barrett's – 0.5% per year
    50 x increased risk of esophageal CA compared to
        general population (**relative risk = 50**)
    **High grade dysplasia (HGD, or carcinoma in situ) is an
        indication for **esophagectomy** → 20% harbor **occult CA**
    *Make sure Dx of high grade dysplasia is confirmed by **2***
        experienced pathologists
**Lower Esophageal <u>Rings</u> (Schatzki's Ring)
Associated w/ GERD (almost all pts have <u>hiatal hernia</u>)
Lies at **squamo-columnar junction**; is a submucosal **fibrosis**
Sx's: dysphagia, food impaction can occur
    **Dx: barium esophagogram (<u>*best test*</u>; *often can't see w/*
        EGD)
Tx: **Asymptomatic** – nothing
     Symptomatic – ****dilatation + PPI** (sufficient in majority)
        Surgery if refractory (partial wrap, dilatation of ring)
**Resection of ring is <u>NEVER</u> indicated
Indications for wrap: avoid lifelong medication in young pt,
    refractory GERD or refractory cx's (esophagitis, stricture, bleeding)
Hiatal Hernias
    Type I (99%) – GE junction above diaphragm
    Type II – para-esophageal hernia; GE junction in normal position
    Type III – combined Type I and II
    Type IV – type II or III but also other organ (eg colon, spleen)

Paraesophageal Hernias (Types II. III and IV)
Sx's: trouble swallowing food, chest pain
    Incarcerated Hernias (Borchardt's triad) – chest pain, inability to
        vomit, and can't pass NGT; retching <u>*without*</u> vomiting (*classic*)
Risk of incarceration, strangulation, necrosis
Best test for Dx of paraesophageal hernia – **barium esophagogram*
CXR - air-fluid level in chest (incarcerated stomach)
Tx: repair w/ fundoplication to **anchor stomach** unless elderly, infirmed

Nissen Fundoplication
Key to hiatal dissection is finding **right crura*
Key to wrap is finding **left crura*
Divide **short gastric arteries**
Pull esophagus into abdomen
    Mobilize at least **5 cm** of intra-thoracic esophagus
    Need at least **2 cm** of <u>free esophagus</u> in abdomen
Wrap over **54 Fr** Bougie to prevent making it too tight
Want fundus wrap **2 cm** in length (loose but secure, 360-complete)
Approximate crura - repairs defect in phrenoesophageal membrane (an
    extension of **transversalis fascia*), prevents wrap herniation
Anchor wrap to **right crura**
Partial fundoplication wraps (Toupet, partial Nissen) – posterior 180
    wrap; used for GERD w/ poor esophageal contraction
Collis gastroplasty – used for **shortened esophagus**
    Used when not enough esophagus exists to pull into abdomen
    Staple stomach along cardia to lengthen esophagus tube (neo-
        esophagus) – the wrap ends up going around neo-esophagus

Difficult delivery of viscera from above diaphragm – incise hiatus, reduce the contents, and repair hiatus later

**Cx's from Nissen Fundoplication
    MC intra-op injury – esophageal perforation (Tx: repair)
    **MC Cx following Nissen – *dysphagia*
    1) ****Dysphagia**
        **Dx: Barium esophagogram *(best test)* – figures out problem
        Wrap too tight (dysphagia **early** post-op)
            **MCC of dysphagia following Nissen
            May be due to **edema**
            > 95% resolve w/ **conservative Tx**
            Tx: **clears** for 1 week, can try to **dilate** after 1 week
            Inability to **swallow liquids** or **foamy salvia** → re-op
            This Cx avoided by performing wrap over a 54 Fr bougie
        Late Dysphagia
            Dx: **barium esophagogram** *best study* to figure out problem;
              worry about CA and above Cx's
    2) ****Recurrent Reflux** - ****Dx: barium esophagogram** (best test), look for
        wrap disruption, Cx's
    3) **Gas, bloating** or **delayed gastric emptying**
        Simethicone for bloating or gas
        Reglan for bloating and delayed emptying
        May need **pyloroplasty** if from **injured vagal nerves**
    4) **Injury to vagus** (Cx's)
        Gallstones (cholecystectomy if symptomatic)
        Delayed gastric emptying (Reglan)
        Gas bloat syndrome in air swallowers (Tx Reglan + simethicone
            usually self-limiting)
    5) **Both vagus nerves injured** – Tx: pyloroplasty likely needed

**Boerhaave's Syndrome
    MC results in perforation in **lower left esophagus** (4 cm above EGJ; 80%)
    Sx's: **large meal + ETOH** → **forceful vomiting** episode → **chest pain**
        (classic); late SOB + fever ****Almost are *never* contained perforations**
    Dx: **CXR + AXR** – free / subcutaneous air, PTX, pleural effusion (MC left)
        **Esophagogram *(Best test*; gastrografin swallow, then thin barium) –
            finds perforation; chest CT w/ oral contrast is alternative
    Tx **(left thoracotomy usual):*

< 24 hrs	*repair* unless esophagus too damaged or mediastinitis
24-48 hrs	assess damage - if OK, repair, if not esophagectomy
> 48 hrs	**esophagectomy**

    Boerhaave's have **highest mortality for esophageal perforations – 40%*

*Esophageal Perforations
    MCC overall – EGD *(50% iatrogenic)*
    MC site overall – near cricopharyngeus (UES, narrowest point)
        Other sites – indentation of aortic arch, LES
    Sx's: **chest pain** and **dysphagia**
        Subcutaneous air, resp distress, fever - all suggest **free perforation**
    Dx: **CXR, AXR** and **neck films** (initial studies) – look for subcutaneous air
        *Esophagogram (best test, gastrografin followed by thin barium); get
            even w/ known perforation, identify location and multiple perforations*
        *No EGD for Dx
    Surgical approach to esophagus

Cervical	left neck (left sided course here)
Upper thoracic	right (avoids the aorta)
Lower thoracic	left (left-sided course here)

    Contained Perforation (unusual, most need repair)
        Needs to be self-draining back into esophagus, no systemic effects,
            no distal obstruction (eg no achalasia, stricture, or CA)

Conservative Tx: NPO x 7 days, spit, broad-spectrum abx's
Repeat esophagogram after 7 days, start clears if OK
Free perforation
1) **< 24 hours** (minimal contamination, no mediastinitis, not septic) →
Primary repair - longitudinal esophageal <u>myotomy</u> to see
length of injury, repair, cover w/ <u>viable tissue</u> (eg
intercostal muscle);
2) **24-48 hours** – assess esophagus and mediastinum → if favorable,
primary repair, if not, esophagectomy and diversion below
3) **> 48 hours, mediastinitis, gross contamination**, or **septic** pts
→*Esophagectomy* and *diversion* (cervical esophagostomy
for spit diversion); late gastric pull-up (6-8 wks)

**Leiomyoma
MC **benign tumor** of esophagus; **smooth muscle** cells (gray-white swirls)
MC found in **distal 2/3** of esophagus (where smooth muscle cells are)
In **muscularis propria** (submucosal)
Sx's: dysphagia, odynophagia (painful swallowing), pressure, lump throat
Dx: *Barium swallow (best test)* - smooth, convex filling defect
EGD w/ EUS - homogenous, hypo-echoic, overlying mucosa **intact**
**Do not biopsy - can form scar and make subsequent
resection difficult w/ high risk of disrupting the mucosa
Chest CT – hypo-dense tumor
Indications for surgery: **> 5 cm** (worry about CA) or **symptomatic**
Tx: thoracotomy and **extra-mucosal enucleation (***do not resect
esophagus); **Leave the mucosa intact*
Leiomyosarcoma → esophagectomy

**Esophageal Cancer
RFs: achalasia, caustic injury, ETOH, tobacco, nitrosamines, Barrett's
Sx's: *dysphagia and weight loss*; <u>jaundice</u> worrisome for liver spread
Dx: 1) **Esophagogram** (*best initial test for dysphagia*) - apple core lesion
2) **EGD w/ EUS** (*best test for T status* - <u>depth</u>) and **Bx**
3) *Chest/abd CT scan* - * *single best test for overall resectability*
Path
Most important prognostic factor – <u>nodal spread</u>
Spreads quickly along **submucosal lymphatics** (longitudinal)
Adenocarcinoma – *MC esophageal CA* (↑ in Caucasians, 50-60s)
MC in **lower 1/3** of esophagus; MC in background of **Barrett's**
MC mets – <u>liver</u>
Squamous cell CA (SCCA, ↑ in African-Americans, 60-70s)
MC in **middle 1/3** of esophagus
MC mets – <u>lung</u>
GE junction tumors are treated like **esophageal CA
Pre-op chemo-XRT (neoadjuvant) - **Cisplatin and **5-FU**
**For tumors > T1 (> submucosal invasion, eg GE junction CA > T1)
May **downstage** larger tumors and make them resectable
Surgery
1)   Need to be able to **tolerate surgery**
2)   Need to have **resectable CA** (No distant mets; no celiac or
supraclavicular nodal DZ, not invading another structure)
Esophagectomy (*most recommend at least *6-8 cm margins*)
**Right gastroepiploic artery - *primary blood supply to stomach
after replacing esophagus* (is a branch off GDA)
Chylothorax post-op - ensure adequate drainage, NPO, TPN, *short to
medium chain FA's*, octreotide – conservative Tx for 1-3 weeks
Failure of medical Tx or > 2 L/d - **ligate** thoracic duct (right side low)

Stomach

383. **All of the following are true except
    a. The right gastric artery is a branch of the common hepatic artery
    b. The left gastric artery is a branch off the celiac axis.
    c. A bleeding ulcer from the posterior 1st portion of the duodenum is likely bleeding from the proper hepatic artery
    d. The short gastrics are branches of the splenic artery

Answer c. **The **gastroduodenal artery** (GDA) is involved in ulcer bleeding in the 1st portion of the posterior duodenum. The **GDA** is a branch of the **common hepatic artery** and comes off after the right gastric artery.*

The **right gastric artery** is a branch off **common hepatic artery
The **left gastric artery** is a branch off the **celiac axis.
The **short gastrics** are branches of the **splenic artery

384. *Which of the following are true:
    a. Parietal cells are located primarily in the antrum
    b. G cells are located primarily in the antrum
    c. Complete vagotomy results in increased liquid emptying and decreased solid emptying
    d. Diarrhea following vagotomy is due to sustained motor myenteric complexes

Answer a. *Parietal cells* are located primarily in the body and fundus.
G cells are located primarily in the **antrum**
Complete vagotomy results in increased liquid emptying and decreased solid emptying
The MC Cx following vagotomy is **diarrhea is due to **sustained motor myenteric complexes** leading to non-conjugated **bile salts in the colon** and subsequent **diarrhea**; Tx - **cholestyramine** + **loperamide**.*
***Incomplete vagotomy** is the MCC of **recurrent peptic ulcer** after ulcer surgery. It is MC due to a missed Criminal Nerve of Grassi off the right vagus nerve posteriorly.*

385. **The best test for the diagnosis of H. pylori is:
    a. histiologic examination of endoscopic biopsies of the antrum
    b. urease test of biopsies of the fundus
    c. urease breath test
    d. ELISA

Answer a. The best test for the diagnosis h. pylori is ***histiologic examination of endoscopic biopsies of the antrum***. If H. pylori is present, Tx with 3 prong therapy should be started (amoxicillin, clarithromycin, proton pump inhibitor).

386. *A 45 yo man has been vomiting copious amounts of fluid for several hours due to gastric outlet blockage from a large gastric or possible duodenal ulcer. You place a naso-gastric tube. All of the following are true for this patient's volume replacement except:
    a. He likely has a hypochloremic, hypokalemic metabolic alkalosis
    b. The key is to replace the chloride deficit
    c. Initial volume replacement should be normal saline
    d. Maintenance therapy after resuscitation should be lactated ringers

Answer d. This pt has **gastric outlet obstruction**. This can result in *hypochloremic, hypokalemic metabolic alkalosis*. Adults w/ severe gastric fluid loss should have their volume replaced initially w/ **normal saline**. The key is to replace the *chloride deficit*. After volume resuscitation is started, potassium should be given as a separate infusion. Maintenance fluid for ongoing gastric losses is D5 1/2 NS w/ 20 meq K.

In **children w/ pyloric stenosis and severe dehydration, it is important to _hold the potassium_ until adequate urine output is established. Initially, volume resuscitation for severe dehydration is a bolus of **normal saline** (10 cc/kg) and then normal saline 2 x maintenance until the child makes urine. Then change to D5 1/2 NS w/ 10 meq of K. It may take up to 48 hours to fully resuscitate severely dehydrated children.

Tx for obstructing gastric or duodenal ulcer is NG tube suction, PPI, and TPN for up to a week. These usually open up

387. **A 61 yo man undergoes partial gastrectomy for adenocarcinoma and has a Billroth II anastomosis (gastro-jejunostomy). Two months after the procedure he develops severe abdominal pain and non-bilious vomiting. Eventually he has a bilious emesis and the pain is relieved. Which of the following tests is most diagnostic of this patient's symptoms:
   a. Abdominal CT
   b. EGD
   c. Angiography
   d. HIDA scan

   Answer a. **This pt is suffering from **afferent loop syndrome** (or afferent loop obstruction). **The best test for **afferent loop syndrome** is an **abd CT scan** (shows dilated fluid filled limb that does not fill with contrast).

388. **A pt w/ a PMHx of pancreatitis develops severe bleeding from gastric varices. You do not see any esophageal varices on EGD. U/S shows splenic vein thrombosis. The best treatment for this patient's most likely condition is:
   a. Splenectomy
   b. TIPS procedure
   c. Spleno-renal shunt
   d. Porto-caval shunt

   Answer a. **Gastric varices** without esophageal varices are most likely from **splenic vein thrombosis** related to pancreatitis and not cirrhosis. U/S or CT scan are used to demonstrate splenic vein thrombosis. Tx for symptomatic isolated gastric varices related to splenic vein thrombosis is **splenectomy**. _Asymptomatic_ splenic vein thrombosis should be _left alone._

389. **All of the following are improved after gastric bypass except:
   a. Diabetes
   b. Hypertension
   c. GERD
   d. Marginal ulcers

   Answer d. ***Marginal ulcers** are a complication of gastric bypass.
   Cx's from gastric bypass – marginal ulcers (Tx: PPI), Ca deficiency, Iron deficiency, B-12 deficiency.
   DM, HTN and GERD are all _improved_ w/ gastric bypass.

390. **A 50 yo man presents with epigastric pain unrelieved with PPIs. You perform EGD and a mass is found in the stomach mucosa _only_. You biopsy it and it comes back lymphoproliferative tissue lymphoma. The next appropriate Tx is:
   a. Total gastrectomy
   b. Partial gastrectomy
   c. Chemo-XRT therapy
   d. Tx for H pylori

Answer d. **Mucosa associated lymphoproliferative tissue lymphoma** (MALT lymphoma) is related to H pylori infection and is considered a low grade B cell NHL. **Initial Tx w/ 3 pronged Tx for **H. pylori (amoxicillin, clarithromycin and PPI)** cures 90%.

391. **A 50 yo man presents w/ epigastric pain unrelieved w/ PPIs. EGD shows a 6 cm intra-mural mass in the stomach. Bx comes back malignant stromal tumor (gastro-intestinal stromal tumor, GIST). The pt undergoes resection but post-op path shows liver mets. The next appropriate Tx is:
    a. Radiation therapy
    b. 5 fluorouracil and cisplatin
    c. Gleevec
    d. Do nothing

    Answer c. Surgical excision w/ clear margins is the best Tx for **GIST tumors** (75 % benign, 25% malignant). **Imatinib** (Gleevec) a tyrosine kinase inhibitor, has been extremely effective for malignant GIST tumors.

Normal Anatomy and Physiology
Blood supply
Celiac trunk – left gastric, common hepatic, and splenic arteries
  Right gastric artery is a branch off the common hepatic artery
  Gastroduodenal artery (GDA) is branch off common hepatic artery (comes off after the right gastric artery branch)
  Right gastroepiploic is a branch off GDA
  Left gastroepiploic and **short gastric** are branches of splenic artery
Greater curvature – right and left gastroepiploic's and short gastrics
Lesser curvature – right and left gastric arteries
Pylorus – gastroduodenal artery
Mucosa – simple columnar epithelium
Peristalsis only occurs in the <u>distal stomach</u>

Glands
Cardia glands – mucus secreting
Fundus and **body glands**
  1) **Chief cells** release **pepsinogen** *(1st enzyme in proteolysis)*
     Increase release – acetylcholine (vagus) and gastrin
  2) **Parietal cells** release H^+ and **intrinsic factor**
     Increase HCL release-gastrin, histamine, acetylcholine (vagus)
     Inhibit HCL release – **somatostatin**, secretin, CCK
     Intrinsic factor – binds B-12; complex absorbed in **terminal ileum**
     Pernicious anemia – lose parietal cells, decreased B-12 absorption, low HCl (elevated gastrin)
Antrum and **pylorus glands**
  1) **G cells** release **gastrin** - reason antrectomy helps w/ ulcer surgery
     Stimulated by **protein, acetylcholine** (vagus)
     Inhibited by H^+ in duodenum
  2) **D cells** secrete **somatostatin** – inhibits gastrin and acid release; inhibits many other GI functions (great inhibitor)
  3) **Mucus** and **HCO_3^- secreting glands** – protects stomach
Duodenum glands
  1) **Brunner's glands** – <u>alkaline mucus</u> (protects duodenum from acid; **jejunum does <u>not</u> have these**, can get **marginal ulcers** after roux-en-Y gastro-jejunostomy w/ long afferent limb)
  2) **Somatostatin, CCK,** and **secretin** – released w/ antral and duodenal acidification

Billroth I – antrectomy w/ gastro-duodenal anastomosis
Billroth II – antrectomy w/ gastro-jejunal anastomosis

Vagotomies

Vagal denervation
Vagal-mediated receptive **relaxation** of stomach is *removed*
Results in **increased gastric pressure** and **pyloric constriction**
Truncal Vagotomy alone - increases liquid emptying and decreases
solid emptying
Truncal Vagotomy and pyloroplasty - increases liquid emptying
and increases solid emptying
Gastric effects of vagotomy – decreases acid output by 90%, increases
gastrin, gastrin cell hyperplasia
**Non-gastric _truncal_ vagotomy effects
Diarrhea *(40%)* - ****_MC Cx_ *following truncal vagotomy*, caused by
**sustained motor-myenteric complexes (MMC's) forcing
bile acids into the colon; Tx: **cholestyramine, loperamide**
Cholelithiasis (gallstones)

**Gastric ulcers

RFs: males, tobacco, ETOH, NSAIDs, *H. pylori*, uremia, burns, sepsis
Most have *normal* **acid secretion** and **decreased mucosal defense**
MC location – **lesser curve** along **body** of stomach (85%)
H. pylori – found in 90% of duodenal and 70% of gastric ulcers
**Best test for Dx of H pylori – *histologic examination* of
endoscopic Bx's of *antrum*
Sx's: epigastric pain radiating to back; **relieved w/ eating**, recurs in 30 min
Cushing's Gastric Ulcer – associated w/ head trauma
Curling's Duodenal Ulcer – associated w/ burns

Medical Tx for Ulcers (duodenal and stomach)

*Proton pump inhibitor (PPI) plus H. Pylori Tx:
1) **Clarithromycin + amoxicillin** *(14 days)*
2) Refractory ulcer – metronidazole, tetracycline, and bismuth salts
D/C NSAIDS – consider exchanging for **COX-2 selective inhibitor** (eg
celecoxib) if no cardiovascular disease or add misoprostol (PGE)
D/C smoking and ETOH
Ulcer surgery rare since **PPIs** (99% of ulcers are Tx'd w/ PPI + H. pylori Tx)

*Duodenal ulcers

More common than gastric ulcers; **RFs** - same as gastric ulcers
From **increased acid production** and **decreased defense**
H. pylori – found in 90% of duodenal and 70% of gastric ulcers (↑s acid)
**Best test for Dx of H pylori – *histologic examination* of
endoscopic biopsies of *antrum*
Sx's: epigastric pain radiating to back; may worsen w/ eating (duodenal acid)
MC location – 1st portion of duodenum (MC location – anterior)
Anterior ulcers usually perforate (Tx - **omental patch*)
Posterior ulcers usually bleed from **gastroduodenal artery** (Tx -
*EGD clip, open artery ligation if that fails)
MC Cx of duodenal ulcers - bleeding (often minor, life-threatening if GDA)
EGD *(best test + best Tx for bleeding duodenal ulcer)*, Tx: Epi, clips,
cautery; vasopressin, octreotide and IV PPI to temporize until EGD
RFs for duodenal ulcer re-bleeding after EGD is performed:
#1 *spurting, bleeding blood vessel at time of EGD (60% re-bleed)
#2 visible blood vessel at time of EGD (40% re-bleed)
#3 diffuse oozing at time of EGD (30% re-bleed)
Criteria for surgery following EGD Tx for bleeding duodenal ulcer (any
of the following):
1) **> 4 units of blood** and **still bleeding**
2) In **shock** despite multiple blood transfusions
3) **Recurrent bleed** after maximal EGD Tx
→ all indications for OR

Upper GI but can't find bleeding source (eg too much blood, food) →
Angiography
Having trouble localizing bleeding source despite angiography (eg
small bleed) → Tagged RBC scan

Surgical options for refractory ulcers
1) Truncal vagotomy and pyloroplasty (**VP**, 5% recurrence)
2) Truncal vagotomy, antrectomy + Roux en-Y gastro-jejunostomy
(**VAR**, < 1% recurrence)
3) Highly selective vagotomy - hard to do (estimated 40% recurrence)
Advantages of Roux en-Y gastro-jejunostomy over Billroth I or Billroth II
1) Significantly reduced **bile reflux gastritis**
2) Decreased incidence of **dumping syndrome** w/ Roux limb
Billroth I and Billroth II rarely performed anymore

Obstruction from Duodenal and Gastric Ulcer
Get **metabolic alkalosis** (*hypokalemic, hypochloremic metabolic alkalosis*)
Tx: IVFs; NGT to decompress, PPI (majority open up w/ conservative Tx)

Post-gastrectomy complications
Post-vagotomy diarrhea
MC complication *following vagotomy or gastrectomy*
Caused by **sustained postprandial organized MMCs** (myenteric
motor complexes) leading to non-conjugated **bile salts** in
colon; usually resolves on its own
Tx: **cholestyramine, anti-motility agents** (loperamide)
Surgical option (very rare): reversed interposition jejunal graft
Dumping syndrome
Can occur after either gastrectomy or vagotomy and pyloroplasty
From rapid entrance of **carbohydrates** into **jejunum**
95% resolve w/ medical Tx
2 phases 1. Hyperosmotic load causes fluid shift into bowel (N/V,
diarrhea, dizziness, **hypotension**)
2. Reactive increase in insulin and **hypoglycemia** (2nd part
rarely occurs); 1-3 hours after 1st part
Dx: **Gastric emptying study** (*best test,* radionuclide colloid
scintigraphy); stomach dumps colloid quickly
Tx: **small, high protein, low-fat, low-carbohydrate meals**
No liquids with meals; No lying down after meals
Octreotide effective (given before meals)
Surgical options (*rarely* necessary)
Convert Billroth I or Billroth II to Roux-en-Y gastro-jejunostomy
Operations that either increase the gastric reservoir (jejunal
pouch) or slow emptying (eg reversed jejunal limb)
Alkaline reflux gastritis
Sx's: postprandial epigastric pain associated with N/V, bilious emesis
*Pain **not** relieved with vomiting*
Dx: **EGD** *(best test)* → evidence of bile reflux in stomach, histiologic
evidence of gastritis
Tx: **PPI, cholestyramine, metoclopramide**
Surgical option: conversion of Billroth I or II to Roux-en-Y gastro-
jejunostomy w/ afferent limb 60 cm distal to gastro-jejunostomy
Afferent loop Syndrome (afferent-limb obstruction, ie biliary limb)
Found w/ Billroth II or Roux-en-Y
Obstruction of afferent limb (RFs – long afferent limb)
Can be caused by stenosis, kinking, volvulus, or adhesions
Sx's: non-bilious vomiting + abd pain → **Pain relieved w/ bilious**
emesis *(classic)*
Can cause closed loop obstruction w/ fever, shock, and perforation
Dx: **CT scan *(best test for Dx)* - see a big loop of fluid filled bowel
Does not fill w/ contrast

EGD to look for recurrent tumor, fibrosis, food obstruction, tight
or twisted anastomosis – best test to figure out problem
Tx: **balloon dilation w/ EGD** may be possible
Surgical option: re-anastomosis w/ shorter (40-cm) afferent limb and
relieve cause of obstruction (may require conversion of B-II to
Roux en-Y gastro-jejunostomy)
Blind Loop Syndrome (biliary limb) – found w/ Billroth II or Roux-en-Y
From **stasis** leading to **bacterial overgrowth** (*E. coli*, GNRs) in
afferent limb
Sx's: pain, malabsorption w/ **B-12 deficiency** (bacteria use it up,
megaloblastic anemia), **steatorrhea** (bacteria deconjugate bile)
Dx: **EGD w/ afferent limb aspirate + culture** (*best test*)
Tx: **Tetracycline + Flagyl; metoclopramide** or **erythromycin** to
improve motility in afferent limb
Surgical option: re-anastomosis with shorter (40-cm) afferent limb
Delayed gastric emptying - Tx: **metoclopramide, erythromycin**

Gastric varices
90% of gastric varices are associated w/ esophageal varices
10% of gastric varices are isolated
Isolated gastric varices →
MC from **splenic vein thrombosis** (secondary to **pancreatitis**)
Very uncommonly from portal HTN or portal vein thrombosis
Dx: U/S (check to make sure splenic vein is the problem)
Splenic vein thrombosis (MCC – pancreatitis) *and* **gastric varices**
Leads to **isolated** gastric varices *without* elevation of pressure in
rest of portal system → **can bleed**
Tx: splenectomy; if asymptomatic – leave alone

Morbid obesity
All improved w/ gastric bypass – *diabetes, GERD, sleep apnea, venous*
stasis ulcers, hypertension, hyperlipidemia, life quality
Operative mortality 1%
Surgical indication - BMI > 40 or BMI > 35 with co-morbidities (HTN, DM,
CAD, pulmonary HTN, obstructive sleep apnea, severe GERD)
Roux-en-Y gastric bypass
Need **75-100 cm of jejunum** Roux limb if performing roux-en-Y
gastric bypass
Perform **cholecystectomy** during operation if stones present.
10-15% failure rate due to high carbohydrate snacking
Jejuno-ileal bypass - are no longer done
Associated with liver cirrhosis, kidney stones, osteoporosis (↓ Ca)
Need to correct these pts w/ Roux-en-Y gastric bypass if encountered

Complications from Roux en-Y gastric bypass
Leak: MCC leak overall – ischemia
MCC early leak – technical error; MCC late leak – ischemia
B-12 deficiency (intrinsic factor need acidic environment to bind B-12)
Sx's – Pernicious anemia, peripheral neuropathy, glossitis
Tx: B-12 shots every month
Fe deficient anemia (bypasses duodenum where Fe absorbed) – Tx: Fe
Calcium deficiency - bypasses duodenum where Ca is mainly absorbed
Sx's – hyper-reflexia, peri-oral tingling
Tx: calcium and Vitamin D (helps with absorption)
Gallstones (from rapid weight loss) Tx: cholecystectomy if sx's
Pulmonary Embolism (MCC of death); prevent, enoxaparin 0.5 mg/kg BID
Marginal ulcers (10%) – occur on jejunal side of anastomosis; Tx PPI
Stenosis: Sx's - hiccoughs, large stomach bubble, N/V (obstruction sx's)
Tx: **Early** – re-operate (technical problem)
Late (from ischemia) – usually responds to **balloon dilation**

**MALT Lymphoma (Mucosal-Associated Lymphoid Tissue Lymphoma)
- **Low grade B cell NHL** from mucosa lymphoid tissue
- **MC site** – stomach (80%)
  - ****Usually *confined to stomach* (90% of pts, stage IE)*
  - Related to *H. pylori* infection (90%)
  - Other sites – other GI tract, lung, Waldeyer's ring (oral tonsils)
- Sx's: **pain** (similar to ulcer) and **weight loss**
- Dx: **EUS w/ Bx** (mass or large folds; look for **H pylori**)
- Tx: 1) **Confined** to stomach (stage IE) or limited to peri-gastric nodes
    - ****1st line - H. pylori Tx** (4 prong - PPI, bismuth salts, amoxicillin, metronidazole) + **surveillance** → *cures 90%*
    - **2nd line - XRT** If MALT does not regress after above or if H pylori not present *(cures another 90%)*
    - Possible resection if above fails
  - 2) **Advanced DZ** (unusual; nodes other than peri-gastric, Stage III, or Stage IV) *or* if all above fail → **Chemo** $\pm$ XRT (CHOP-R)
- **Overall 5-YS** – 90%

**Gastrointestinal stromal tumors *(GIST tumors)*
- ***MC benign gastric neoplasm,** although can be malignant
- Sx: usually **asymptomatic**; obstruction and bleeding can occur
- Dx: **EGD w/ Bx** *(best test)* - these are ***c-kit positive*** (immuno-staining)
- Path - **spindle cells,** connective tissue
  - **MC location –** stomach (70%)
  - 25% **malignant** *(**behave like **sarcomas**)*
    - ****Rare nodal spread** (< 10%); **MC mets** – liver
    - **Malignant GIST Dx:**
      - 1) **> 5-10 mitoses / 50 HPFs** *or;*
      - 2) **Size > 5 cm**
  - **c-Kit –** receptor tyrosine kinase (stem cell growth factor receptor)
- Tx: ****Wedge resection** (1 cm margins) – ****no nodal dissection**
  - **Chemo** indications – *all malignant GIST tumors* (defined above)
    - ****1st line - **Imatinib** *(Gleevec),* receptor tyrosine kinase inhibitor; Sunitinib in pts refractory or intolerant of Imatinib

**Gastric Cancer
- Sx's: **epigastric pain** (unrelieved by eating) and **weight loss**
  - **Highest risk area** – Japan (50% of cancer-related deaths)
- Path 1) **Intestinal gastric CA** (ie adenocarcinoma)
    - Histology – shows **glands**
    - Overall 5-YS – 25%
  - 2) **Diffuse gastric CA** (ie linitis plastica)
    - Histology - diffuse proliferation of **connective tissue** throughout stomach; lymphatic invasion; no glands
    - Less favorable prognosis than intestinal
    - Overall 5-YS – 15%
- Tx: Mets outside resection area – surgery contraindication unless palliation
  - Splenectomy is generally not performed.
  - **Splenic invasion** – resect stomach + splenectomy en bloc
  - ****Intestinal gastric cancer**
    - ****GE junction tumor** → *Tx like esophageal tumor w/ esophagectomy* and 6-8 cm stomach margin
    - **Upper 1/3** of stomach → total gastrectomy and **esophago-jejunal anastomosis** (roux limb)
    - **Middle or lower 1/3** of stomach → distal gastrectomy and gastro-jejunostomy
  - ****Diffuse gastric cancer** (linitis plastica) Tx: total gastrectomy *for all* and ****esophago- jejunal anastomosis**
  - Chemo: 5-FU, doxorubicin, mitomycin C (poor response)

Liver

392. *All of the following are true of liver anatomy except:
     a.   The falciform ligament separates the left and right lobes of the liver
     b.   The hepato-duodenal ligament is where the common bile duct, portal vein and proper hepatic artery meet
     c.   The ligamentum teres carries the obliterated umbilical vein to the undersurface of the liver
     d.   The foramen of Winslow enters the lesser sac

     Answer a. The **falciform ligament** separates the medial and lateral aspects of the left lobe.

393. **All of the following are true except::
     a.   The caudate lobe receives separate right and left portal and arterial blood supply.
     b.   Most primary and secondary tumors are supplied by the portal vein
     c.   The MC left hepatic artery variant comes off the left gastric artery
     d.   The MC right hepatic artery variant is comes off the SMA

     Answer b. Most primary and secondary tumors are supplied by hepatic artery branches. **The MC **right hepatic artery variant** (replaced right hepatic artery) comes off the **SMA.** **The MC **left hepatic artery variant** (replaced left hepatic artery) comes off the **left gastric artery.**

394. **All of the following are true of bile acids except:
     a.   Primary bile acids include cholic and chenodeoxycholic
     b.   Secondary bile acids include deoxycholic and lithocholic
     c.   Tertiary bile acids includes urobilinogen
     d.   Bile acids are conjugated to taurine or glycine to improve water solubility

     Answer c. **Urobilinogen** is a breakdown product of conjugated bilirubin in the gut. It is reabsorbed, converted to **urobilin**, and released in urine (reason for urine *yellow color*).

395. *All of the following are true of spleno-renal shunts except:
     a.   Are indicated for Child's A cirrhosis with bleeding as the only problem
     b.   These can make ascites worse
     c.   These require ligation of the inferior mesenteric vein
     d.   These require splenectomy

     Answer d. *Spleno-renal shunts** do <u>not</u> require splenectomy.

396. *All of the following are indications for TIPS procedure except:
     a.   Worsening encephalopathy
     b.   Protracted variceal bleeding
     c.   Refractory ascites
     d.   Progressive ascites

     Answer a. *TIPS* (trans-jugular intra-hepatic porto-systemic shunt) does <u>not</u> improve encephalopathy and may worsen it. TIPS allows antegrade flow from the portal vein to the IVC and decompresses the portal system.

397. **All of the following are true of cirrhosis with ascites except:
     a.   PRN large volume paracentesis is Tx of choice for symptomatic ascites
     b.   Ascites from cirrhosis is due to leakage of splanchnic and hepatic lymph into peritoneum
     c.   Pleural effusions with ascites improve with control of the ascites
     d.   Umbilical hernias in pts w/ ascites should be left alone

Answer d. **Umbilical hernias w/ ascites** should be repaired (if there is overlying skin necrosis, do this emergently to prevent perforation). If skin necrosis is present at surgery, it should be resected. **Primary closure** should be performed if the skin is infected or perforated. Use **prolene mesh** if not infected or ruptured.

Ascites from cirrhosis is due to leakage of splanchnic and hepatic **lymph** into peritoneum

398. *All of the following are true of liver failure except:
    a.   Lactulose serves as a cathartic to remove ammonia forming bacteria and to prevent NH_3 uptake by converting it to NH_4
    b.   Neomycin gets rid of ammonia producing bacteria
    c.   Increasing total protein intake is important in liver failure
    d.   Development of asterixis is a sign that liver failure is progressing and is an early sign of encephalopathy

Answer c. Decreasing protein intake is important in liver failure to reduce the amount of ammonia in the body, which contributes to encephalopathy.

399. *Which of the following tests is most prognostic of liver function reserve:
    a.   Aminopyrine breath test
    b.   MEGX
    c.   Caffeine clearance test
    d.   Galactose elimination capacity

Answer b. *MEGX test* (monoethylglycineexylidide) test measures MEGX after the administration of lidocaine, which depends on the P-450 enzyme system and is 80% sensitive and specific in determining cirrhosis. It is the best test for *liver function reserve*.

The best indicator of *liver synthetic function* is *prothrombin time* (PT)

400. *A 25 yo woman develops RUQ pain, jaundice and ascites 2 weeks after child-birth. This is most likely related to which of the following:
    a.   Retained placenta
    b.   Hepatocellular carcinoma
    c.   Portal vein thrombosis
    d.   Hepatic vein thrombosis

Answer d. Post-partum hepatic vein thrombosis (Post-partum Budd Chiari Syndrome) is rare and related to ovarian vein thrombophlebitis that leads to IVC and hepatic vein thrombosis. **SMA arteriogram w/ venous phase contrast** will identify the lesion.

401. **A 40 yo woman from Greece presents to the ED with abd pain. Abd CT scan shows a calcified cyst in liver that has a double cyst wall. She has a positive Casoni skin test sent by fax from Greece. The most appropriate next step is:
    a.   Percutaneous drainage
    b.   Albendazole
    c.   Liver resection
    d.   Flagyl

Answer b. **You should never perform percutaneous drainage for echinococcal cysts** as spillage of the cyst can cause a severe anaphylactic reaction. Tx consists of **pre-op albendazole followed by resection of cyst.**

402. **A 45 yo man w/ recent travel to middle east develops RUQ pain and a maculopapular rash. Abd CT scan shows an abscess that is best treated with:
   a. Percutaneous drainage and antibiotics
   b. Flagyl
   c. Levofloxacin
   d. Praziquantel

Answer d. **Tx of *schistosomiasis liver abscess is***Praziquantel*.

403. **A 45 yo man on a mission trip to Mexico develops severe diarrhea and fever, from which he recovers. Stool cultures were positive for protozoa. Two weeks later he develops fever, chills, RUQ abd pain, and jaundice. Abd CT scan shows an abscess that is best treated with:
   a. Percutaneous drainage and antibiotics
   b. Flagyl
   c. Levofloxacin
   d. Praziquantel

Answer b. **An *amoebic abscess* is best treated w/ **flagyl*. Amoebic colitis is primary infection (entamoeba histolytica) that leads to abscess*

404. **A 45 yo man develops <u>LLQ pain</u>, fever and change in bowel habits from which he recovers w/ Abx's. Two weeks later he develops <u>RUQ pain</u>, fever and chills. An abd CT scan shows a large abscess which is likely best treated with
   a. Percutaneous drainage and antibiotics for E. coli
   b. Flagyl
   c. Levofloxacin
   d. Praziquantel

Answer a. A *pyogenic abscess* is best treated w/ **percutaneous drainage** and broad spectrum abx's These pts usually present w/ fever and RUQ pain. **GNRs are the MC organism in a pyogenic abscess (MC overall - **E. coli*). You should also cover for anaerobes. These pts can also present w/ multiple abscesses.

*Liver abscesses can arise weeks after an episode of **diverticulitis*, *appendicitis, endocarditis or other infectious process.* They can also arise following biliary tract manipulation (eg biliary stent placement, ERCP) and in many series this is the MCC of pyogenic abscess.

405. **All of the following are true of liver lesions except
   a. A 4 cm hyper-vascular lesion that is sulfur colloid negative, has no peripheral to central enhancement and has a normal AFP suggests adenoma and resection is usually indicated
   b. An asymptomatic 4 cm hyper-vascular liver lesion that displays obvious peripheral to central enhancement suggests hemangioma and no further Tx is necessary
   c. A 4 cm lesion w/ a central stellate scar and a positive sulfur colloid scan suggests focal nodular hyperplasia and no further Tx is necessary
   d. A 4 cm hyper-vascular lesion w/ multiple areas of necrosis associated w/ an AFP of 500 is likely benign and no further Tx is needed

Answer d. A liver mass that is hyper-vascular with necrotic areas and is associated with a significantly high AFP is **hepatocellular carcinoma (HCC)**. Tx is resection if resectable.

**A hyper-vascular lesion that is sulfur colloid negative, has no peripheral to central enhancement and has a normal AFP suggests *adenoma* and resection is usually indicated. These lesion are at high risk for rupture and hemorrhage.*

An asymptomatic hyper-vascular liver lesion that displays obvious peripheral to central enhancement suggests **hemangioma and <u>no further Tx is necessary</u> in majority. If the lesion is significantly symptomatic, <u>enucleation</u> is preferred over lobectomy.*

A 4 cm lesion w/ a central stellate scar and a positive sulfur colloid scan suggests **focal nodular hyperplasia and <u>no further Tx is necessary</u>*

Normal Anatomy and Physiology
**Blood supply
- **Arterial blood supply**
  - Right, left + middle hepatic arteries (follows hepatic vein system)
  - Most **primary** and **secondary tumors** of liver supplied by <u>hepatic artery</u> (can embolize unresectable tumors)
  - ****Hepatic artery variants** *(replaced arteries)*
    - ****Right hepatic artery off <u>superior mesenteric artery</u>** *(20%)*
      - MC hepatic artery variant
      - Behind **neck of pancreas** *(is **posterior** to portal vein)*
      - Posterolateral to CBD
    - ****Left hepatic artery off <u>left gastric artery</u>**
      - Found in gastro-hepatic ligament (lesser omentum) medially
- **Portal vein** - from superior mesenteric vein joining splenic vein
  - <u>No</u> valves
  - **Inferior mesenteric vein** – enters splenic vein
  - **Portal vein** – splits in 2 in liver; 2/3 of total hepatic blood flow
    - <u>Left supplies</u> – II, III, and IV
    - <u>Right supplies</u> – V, VI, VII, and VIII
- **Hepatic veins** – 3 hepatic veins join the IVC
  - <u>Left</u> – segments II, III, and superior IV
  - <u>Middle</u> – segments V and inferior IV
  - <u>Right</u> – segments VI, VII, and VIII
  - **Middle hepatic vein** joins left hepatic vein in 80% before IVC
  - **Accessory right hepatic veins** – drain medial aspect of right lobe directly into IVC
  - **Inferior phrenic veins** – also drain directly into the IVC
- **Caudate lobe** – receives separate right and left portal and arterial blood flow; drains directly into IVC via separate hepatic veins
- **Hepato-duodenal ligament** – where common bile duct, portal vein, and proper hepatic artery meet (portal triad)
- ***Portal triad** (ie porta hepatis): <u>portal vein</u> posterior, <u>common bile duct</u> lateral, <u>proper hepatic artery</u> medial; portal triad enters liver at segments **IV and V; Pringle maneuver** - porta hepatis clamping; will not stop hepatic vein bleeding
- ***Falciform ligament**
  - Separates medial and lateral segments of the **left lobe**
  - Attaches liver to anterior abdominal wall
  - Extends to **umbilicus** and carries remnant of umbilical vein
- ***Ligamentum teres**
  - Carries the obliterated umbilical vein to undersurface of liver
  - Extends from the falciform ligament
- Line drawn from the middle of the **gallbladder fossa** to IVC (ie portal fissure or **Cantlie's line**) separates right and left liver lobes
- **Foramen of Winslow** – goes into lesser sac; Anterior – portal triad; Posterior – IVC; Inferior – duodenum; Superior – liver
- **Glisson's capsule** – the peritoneum that covers the liver
- **Bare area** - posterior-superior surface not covered by Glisson's capsule
- **Gallbladder** – underneath segments **IV and V**
  - These areas may need resection w/ Gallbladder CA
- ***Kupffer cells** – liver macrophages; reticulo-endothelial system
- **Alkaline phosphatase** – normally located in canalicular membrane

<u>Not</u> made in liver → <u>von Willebrand's factor + factor VIII</u> (made in endothelium)

Hepatocytes most sensitive to ischemia - central lobular (acinar zone III)

75% of normal liver (tri-segmentectomy) can be safely resected w/o liver failure – remaining liver will regenerate as well

**Bilirubin

Breakdown product of Hemoglobin (Hgb → heme → biliverdin → bilirubin)

Conjugated to ***glucuronic acid* (enzyme glucuronyl transferase) in liver → improves water solubility

Conjugated bilirubin is then actively secreted into bile

**Bile acids (bile salts)

Bile contains <u>bile acids</u> (85%), <u>phospholipids</u> (MC - lecithin), <u>cholesterol</u>, <u>bilirubin</u>, and <u>proteins</u>

Cholesterol is used to make **bile acids**

HMG CoA → (*HMG CoA reductase*) → **cholesterol** → (*7-alpha-hydroxylase*) → **bile acids** (*statins inhibit HMG CoA reductase*)

HMG CoA reductase – rate-limiting step for cholesterol synthesis

*Bile acids are conjugated to **taurine** or **glycine*** (<u>improves water solubility</u>)

***Primary bile acids** (C's) – cholic and chenodeoxycholic

***Secondary bile acids** – deoxycholic and lithocholic (dehydoxylated primary bile acids by bacteria in gut)

Lecithin – main biliary phospholipid; solubilizes cholesterol and emulsifies fats in the intestine

Bile salts serve as mechanism for;

1) excreting **cholesterol** <u>and</u>

2) **emulsifying lipids** and **fat-soluble vitamins** in the intestine

Acute Liver Failure

Definition - **acute hepatic disease + coagulopathy + encephalopathy**

Sx's: malaise, jaundice; *Outcome determined by **encephalopathy***

Liver failure leads to inability metabolize **ammonia, mercaptanes,** and **false neurotransmitters** → get **encephalopathy**

Tx: **Lactulose - cathartic** gets rid of ammonia producing bacteria; also prevents NH_3 uptake by converting it to ammonium (NH_4)

Limit protein intake (< 70 g/day); give **branched chain amino acids** - metabolized by skeletal muscle (becomes impt energy source)

Neomycin – gets rid of bacteria that produce ammonia

**Cirrhosis

Fibrosis and nodular regeneration from hepatocellular injury

***Mechanism of cirrhosis**

Hepatocyte destruction** → fibrosis and scarring of liver → ↑ hepatic pressure → portal venous congestion → lymphatic overload → **leakage of splanchnic and hepatic <u>lymph</u> into peritoneum → ascites

Normal portal vein pressure < 12 mmHg

Coronary veins act as collaterals between portal vein and systemic venous system of lower esophagus (azygos veins)

Shunts can decompress portal system

Sx's: jaundice, ascites, spider angiomata, palmar erythema, steatorrhea

***Development of **asterixis** is a sign that liver failure is progressing*

Best indicator of synthetic function w/ cirrhosis – prothrombin time

Child's Class uses albumin, bilirubin, encephalopathy, ascites, nutrition

General Tx of cirrhosis:

Decrease **salt intake** (1 gm/d) and **fluid intake** (1-1.5 L/d)

Diuretics - spironolactone (counter-acts ↑aldosterone seen w/ liver impaired hepatic metabolism) and **furosemide**

Norfloxacin SBP prophylaxis (for pts w/ **previous** SBP or if admitted for **UGI bleeding**)

Propranolol prophylaxis against UGI bleed (only pts w/ **varices** or **previous** UGI bleed)

Pre-op preparation *(elective cases, eg* ****umbilical hernia *repair):*
   1st **removal of ascites** (<u>paracentesis</u>; relieves pressure off umbilical hernia) - replace w/ IV salt-poor albumin (1 g for every 100 cc removed; use 25% albumin in 50 cc bottle)
   2nd **correct coagulopathy** – all have abnormal PT; Tx – Vit K ± FFP
   3rd **umbilical hernia repair** - resect necrotic skin area if present, **primary closure** if infected or perforated; **prolene mesh** if not infected or ruptured
   4th **control ascites** after repair
   If overlying skin w/ umbilical hernia is **perforated or necrotic, *need* **emergent repair**
   **<u>No</u> hemorrhoidectomies or elective cholecystectomy in cirrhotic pts
   **<u>No</u> epidural or spinal anesthesia → risk of bleeding
   Umbilical hernia w/ ascites - Do **<u>not</u> *wait until hernia sac has ruptured to fix – should fix these electively*

Ascites
   General Tx of cirrhosis above controls ascites in 90%; if refractory →
   1) **Paracentesis** - PRN for **symptomatic ascites** (<u>*Tx of choice*</u> *for large volume ascites*; remove 4-6 L); replace w/ IV salt-poor **albumin** (1 gm for every 100cc taken off)
   2) **TIPS** (see below)
   Ascites from cirrhosis is due to leakage of splanchnic and hepatic **<u>lymph</u> *into peritoneum*

Bleeding Esophageal Varices
   Tx: **EGD w/* **banding, clips or sclerotherapy** *(95% effective)*
      Vasopressin and **Octreotide** to temporize until EGD
      TIPS – needed for *refractory* **emergent variceal bleeding**
   Late cx's - **strictures** from sclerotherapy, Tx - dilatation
   Bleeding varices have 30% mortality w/ 1st episode (50% **re-bleed**)

*TIPS (transjugular, intrahepatic, portosystemic shunt)
   *Makes encephalopathy <u>*worse*</u> *(shunted blood bypasses liver metabolism)*
   Decompresses portal system; allows antegrade flow from portal vein to IVC
   TIPS indicated for **Child's A or B** *with:*
      1) Refractory **variceal bleeding** (despite attempted EGD therapy)
      2) Refractory **ascites** (despite paracentesis attempts)
      3) Progressive **coagulopathy**
      4) Visceral **hypoperfusion**
   S/Es: development of **encephalopathy**; clotting of the shunt; bleeding
   Contra-indications to TIPS – encephalopathy; polycystic liver disease and Caroli's disease (intra-hepatic tract can traverse a cyst or the biliary system respectively, causing massive hemorrhage)
   Pre-hepatic portal hypertension is <u>not</u> relieved with TIPS.
   Open porta-caval shunt – same improvements as above but increased encephalopathy and increased mortality related to procedure (rarely used anymore <u>*unless*</u> TIPS unavailable)

Splenorenal shunt
   Low rate of encephalopathy; can leave the spleen
   Need to ligate: left adrenal vein, left gonadal vein, inferior mesenteric vein, coronary vein, pancreatic branches of splenic vein
   Used <u>only</u> for **Child's A** w/ **bleeding** (unusually used anymore)
   *Can make **ascites** <u>*worse*</u>
   *These are **<u>contraindicated</u>** *w/* **refractory ascites**
   *You do **<u>not</u>** *need* **splenectomy w/ procedure**
   Also, you do <u>not</u> decompress the portal system w/ this shunt – you <u>do</u> decompress esophageal and gastric varices

Child's A or B w/ indication for shunt → TIPS
Child's A that just has **bleeding** as symptom → *consider splenorenal shunt (more durable); otherwise TIPS*

*Post-partum hepatic vein thrombosis *(post-partum Budd Chiari)*
Sx's: postpartum liver failure w/ ascites
Ovarian vein thrombosis (often infected → **thrombophlebitis**) → leads to IVC thrombus formation → leads to **hepatic vein thrombosis**
Related to relative **hypercoaguable state** following pregnancy
Pts w/ **hypercoaguable syndromes** more susceptible
Infectious **pelvic thrombophlebitis** also involved (fever)
Dx: ***SMA arteriogram** *w/ **venous phase** contrast (usual)*
Tx: **heparin + abx's** (usually have **thrombophlebitis** of ovarian vein)

*Budd-Chiari Syndrome (occlusion of **hepatic veins** and/or **IVC**)
MCC - **polycythemia vera (MCC)*, other hypercoaguable states
Sx's: **RUQ pain, ascites** (MC Sx), **hepatomegaly, jaundice**
Dx:***SMA arteriogram** *w/ **venous phase** contrast (usual)*
Liver Bx shows **sinusoidal dilatation** and **centrilobular congestion**
Tx: **Heparin**, consider catheter-directed thrombolysis if acute
TIPS if refractory (needs to connect to IVC <u>above</u> obstruction)

*Portal vein thrombosis (can cause portal hypertension)
Usually caused by **extra-hepatic** thrombosis of portal vein
Sx's: **Ascites** <u>without</u> **liver failure** can occur if not due to cirrhosis
Esophageal varices can occur - **MCC of **massive hematemesis in children***
Etiologies – hypercoaguable state, CA, cirrhosis, trauma, pancreatitis
Dx: U/S or abd CT
Tx:**Heparin** for acute thrombosis to prevent clot propagation (avoid if UGIB)
Control **UGI bleed** from esophageal varices if present *(<u>no</u> heparin)*

**Liver Abscess
**Pyogenic abscess (need to make sure this is not CA)
MC hepatic abscess (80%)
MC organism – **<u>E. coli</u>** *(GNRs MC class)*
MCC overall – biliary tract disease w/ ascending infection (related to CBD stones, stricture, CA, stents, manipulation), **multiple** abscesses usual w/ biliary source
**Distant infection can cause liver abscess (eg appendicitis or diverticulitis → bacteremia → liver abscess)
Sx's: fever, chills, weight loss, RUQ pain, sepsis
Dx: **Abd CT** (usually <u>right</u> lobe), high **LFTs + WBCs**, + blood cultures
Tx: ****Percutaneous drainage + abx's** (GPCs, GNRs + anaerobes)
**Amoebic abscess (entamoeba histolytica)
Travel to Mexico or Latin America (fecal-oral transmission)
1° infection in **colon→amoebic colitis** (reaches liver via **portal vein**)
Sx's: fever, chills, RUQ pain, jaundice, hepatomegaly
Dx: Agglutinin + immuno-electrophoresis **Ab tests** (positive in 90%)
High **LFTs** and **WBCs**; Abd CT – <u>right</u> lobe usual
Tx: ****Flagyl** 1st *line (<u>not</u> drainage)* – most do <u>not</u> require aspiration
*Schistosomiasis abscess
Travel to middle east (Egypt); in water (penetrates skin)
Usually in <u>right</u> lobe of liver
Sx's: maculopapular **rash**, RUQ pain, can cause **variceal bleeding**
Dx: Agglutinin + immuno-electrophoresis **Ab tests**
High eosinophils; **stool** and **urine O and P**
Diffuse **petechiae** in rectum (lives in **mesenteric venules**)
Tx: ****Praziquantel** 1st line *(<u>not</u> drainage)* – <u>no</u> aspiration for majority

**Echinococcus Cyst (hydatid cyst)
>> Usually **right** lobe; **Sheep** – carriers; **dogs** – human exposure
>> Dx: ELISA for **IgG Ab's** (best test)
>>> Abd CT – ectocyst (**calcified**) + endocyst (****double cyst wall**)
>>
>> ****Do not aspirate** → can leak out and cause **anaphylactic shock**
>> Tx: ****Pre-op albendazole** (2 weeks) and then ****resection**
>>> ****Need to remove all of the cyst wall** (ectocyst) off liver
>>> ****Avoid rupture** of cyst and spillage of contents (anaphylaxis)

**Hepatic adenomas
> 80% symptomatic (MC RUQ pain)
> ****50% risk of significant bleeding** (rupture) – main reason for resection
> 5% risk of **malignancy**
> MC in **right lobe** of liver
> RFs – **women on OCPs**, autoimmune disease, steroids
> Sx's: RUQ pain, palpable mass, up to 20% w/ hypotension (hemorrhage)
> Dx: **Abd CT / MRI** – hyper-vascular, homogenous tumor
>> Sulfur colloid scan – no uptake (cold); no Kupffer cells in adenoma
>> Tagged RBC scan – negative
>> AFP – normal
>> ****No FNA** – bleeding risk
> ****Tx: Asymptomatic** (or very mildly symptomatic) _and_ on **OCPs / steroids**
>> _and_ **≤ 4 cm** →
>>> 1) **Stop OCPs / steroids** and;
>>> 2) **Serial CT scans** (every 4-6 weeks)
>>> Make sure mass **decreases** in size and eventually completely
>>>> goes away (takes 6-12 months) → if not, resection
>> **Significantly symptomatic** → resection
>> **> 4 cm** → resection
>> **Increase** in size or worsening **CT findings** (eg hemorrhage areas)
>>> while following → resection
>> **Worsening sx's** → resection
>> **Not on OCP's or steroids** → resection
>> Consider **embolization** if multiple and unresectable

**Focal nodular hyperplasia (FNH)
> No malignancy risk, very rare rupture
> Dx: **Abd CT / MRI** – hyper-vascular; homogenous; have a characteristic
>>> ****central stellate scar** (70%)→Not seen w/ adenoma or HCC
>> **Sulfur colloid scan** – positive in 70% (hot scan)
>>> ****Have Kupffer cells** that uptake colloid
>> Tagged RBC scan – negative, AFP – normal
>> FNA – not sensitive enough to DDx FNH vs. adenoma
> Tx: ****No resection** → **conservative Tx** usual

**Hemangiomas
> ****MC benign liver tumor**
> **Rupture rare**, women, most asymptomatic
> Dx: **Abd CT / MRI** – ****peripheral to central enhancement** (diagnostic)
>> **Tagged RBC scan** – positive (best test,; can confirm Dx)
>> ****No FNA** → risk of **hemorrhage**
> Tx: ****No resection** – conservative Tx unless very symptomatic,
> **Very symptomatic** - ****enucleation** preferred over formal resection) ± pre-
> op embolization (if child → steroids, see Pediatric Surgery Chp)

Hepatocellular CA (HCC, *Hepatoma); MC cancer worldwide (MCC – HepB)
> **Liver mets** to primary **hepatocellular CA** ratio **= 20:1**
>> Liver mets from other tumors far outnumber primary tumors
> Sx's: abd pain, weight loss, ascites, jaundice In US, 80% occur w **cirrhosis**
> Path:***Best prognosis** - fibrolamellar (young pts)
>> **Worst prognosis** - diffuse nodular
>> **AFP level** correlates w/ tumor size
> Tx: **Only 15% can be resected** (eg cirrhosis, porta hepatic lymph node
>> involvement, mets, or not enough liver would be left for survival)

Biliary System

406. *All of the following are true except:
    a. The highest concentration of CCK and secretin secreting cells is in the duodenum
    b. The common hepatic duct becomes CBD after joining the cystic duct
    c. The cystic artery is a branch of the right hepatic artery
    d. The cystic veins drain into the IVC

    Answer d. The cystic veins drain into the right branch of the portal vein.

407. **All of the following are true except:
    a. CCK and neural stimulation _relax_ the normally contracted sphincter of Oddi following meals
    b. Active reabsorption of conjugated bile acids occurs in the jejunum
    c. The gallbladder concentrates bile by active absorption of water
    d. Urobilinogen is a breakdown product of gut bilirubin that is reabsorbed and released in urine, causing the yellow color

    Answer b. Active reabsorption of conjugated bile acids occurs in terminal ileum. **The gallbladder concentrates bile by **active absorption of water**

408. **All of the following are true except
    a. Discovery of a 2 mm stone on intra-op cholangiography requires common bile duct (CBD) exploration and extraction
    b. ERCP w/ sphincterotomy and stone extraction is the best Tx for retained CBD stones after cholecystectomy
    c. Initial diarrhea after cholecystectomy is from excess bile salts in colon
    d. Glucagon _relaxes_ the sphincter of Oddi and can be used intra-op for choledocholithiasis to help flush gallstones out of the CBD

    Answer a. A CBD stone 2 mm or less will pass on its own. These should be left alone. **Glucagon _relaxes_ the sphincter of Oddi and can be used intra-op for choledocholithiasis to help flush gallstones out of the CBD.*

409. *A 50 yo woman presents to your office w/ RUQ pain after eating. The pain occurs about 2 hours after eating and is worse w/ fatty meals. The pain radiates to her right shoulder. You perform an U/S which shows normal biliary anatomy and no stones. The most appropriate next step in this patient's management is:
    a. CCK-CS test
    b. MR-cholangiopancreaticogram (MRCP)
    c. Abdominal CT
    d. Laparoscopic cholecystectomy

    Answer a. Cholecystitis sx's and lack of gallstones on U/S is suspicious for either chronic cholecystitis or biliary dyskinesia. *Cholecystokinin cholescintigraphy (CCK-CS) is the **most sensitive test** for cholecystitis.

410. **All of the following are true except:
    a. The MCC of shock following elective laparoscopic cholecystectomy within the 1st 24 hours is sepsis
    b. The best initial test for RUQ pain or jaundice is a RUQ U/S
    c. Elective cholecystectomy should be avoided in patients with cirrhosis
    d. Ceftriaxone can cause sludging and cholestatic jaundice

    Answer a. The MCC of shock following elective laparoscopic cholecystectomy within the 1st 24 hours is **hemorrhage**, MC related to **clips** falling off the **cystic artery**.

    **Elective cholecystectomy should be _avoided_ in patients w/ **cirrhosis.*

411. **All of the following are true except:
   a. The MC organism in emphysematous cholecystitis is E. Coli
   b. For unstable pts w/ acalculous cholecystitis, percutaneous cholecystostomy is an option
   c. Biliary colic in a pt w/ HepC cirrhosis is best treated w/ **ursodiol** (Actigal)
   d. Gangrenous cholecystitis is an indication for emergent cholecystectomy

   Answer a. The MC organism in **emphysematous cholecystitis** is *clostridium perfringens*.

   ***Elective cholecystectomy should be <u>avoided</u> in pts w/ **cirrhosis**. Biliary colic w/ HepC cirrhosis is best treated w/ **ursodiol** (Actigal).*

412. **During a very difficult laparoscopic cholecystectomy, you perform an intra-op cholangiogram through the cystic duct remnant and notice good distal filling of the CBD, but no filling of the proximal common hepatic duct despite changes in patient position. You convert to open procedure and there are 2 clips on the proximal hepatic duct, a divided hepatic duct, and one clip on the distal common bile duct. The most appropriate next step is:
   a. Whipple
   b. End to end anastomosis with absorbable suture
   c. Hepatico-jejunostomy
   d. Choledocho-jejunostomy

   Answer c. ***The most appropriate step is to perform a **hepatico-jejunostomy**. End to end hepatic duct anastomosis will result in anastomotic **stricture** with these injuries so it is not indicated. Choledocho-jejunostomy would be indicated w/ CBD transaction*

413. **The MCC of bile duct injury w/ laparoscopic cholecystectomy is:
   a. Excess caudal traction of the gallbladder fundus
   b. Excess cephalad retraction of the gallbladder fundus
   c. Misinterpreting intra-op cholangiogram
   d. Mistakenly dividing the hepatic duct.

   Answer b. ***Excess **cephalad retraction** of the gallbladder fundus*

414. **A 30 yo woman presents to your office 7 days after a laparoscopic cholecystectomy and complains of moderate abd pain in the RUQ, nausea and vomiting, and very mild jaundice. The most appropriate next step is:
   a. RUQ ultrasound
   b. Change pain medications
   c. ERCP
   d. Broad spectrum antibiotics

   Answer a. Pain, vomiting and jaundice after laparoscopic cholecystectomy are unusual. Work-up starts w/ RUQ U/S (initial study of choice for RUQ pain) and getting LFTs and a CBC.

415. **Ultrasound in the above woman reveals an 8 x 8 cm fluid collection in the gall bladder fossa. The bile ducts are normal size. The most appropriate next step is:
   a. Broad spectrum antibiotics
   b. Re-exploration
   c. ERCP
   d. Percutaneous drainage

   Answer d. Given sx's + fluid collection, percutaneous drainage is indicated

416. **You place a drain in the above pt and it reveals bile fluid. The most appropriate next step in this patient's management is:
   a. ERCP
   b. Exploratory laparotomy
   c. Abdominal CT scan
   d. Broad spectrum antibiotics

   Answer a. Bile fluid is worrisome biliary system injury. Need ERCP.

417. **ERCP on the above patient shows free extravasation of contrast from the cystic duct remnant. The most appropriate next step is:
   a. Exploratory laparotomy
   b. Broad spectrum antibiotics
   c. PTC tube
   d. ERCP, sphincterotomy, and stent

   Answer d. **The clip fell off the cystic duct remnant** and is causing the leakage of bile into the abdomen. This problem is effectively treated 95% of the time with ERCP, sphincterotomy, and a temporary stent. Eventually, the cystic duct remnant will scar down.

418. **All of the following are true of ERCP complications except:
   a. Retroperitoneal perforations are generally treated conservatively (NPO, abx's)
   b. Bile duct perforations are treated w/ a temporary stent across the perforation
   c. Free perforations of the duodenum are treated w/ stents
   d. Pancreatitis is the MC Cx following ERCP

   Answer c. ***Free perforations*** of the duodenum require open repair. **Contained** retroperitoneal perforations are treated conservatively

419. *All of the following are indications for ERCP for gallstone pancreatitis except:
   a. Elevated alkaline phosphatase
   b. Elevated Bilirubin after 24 hours of observation
   c. Jaundice
   d. Cholangitis

   Answer a. Elevated alkaline phosphatase is not an indication for ERCP.

420. *A 60 yo woman with no past medical problems presents to the emergency room with jaundice, right upper quadrant pain, and fever. Her blood pressure is 80/40 and her heart rate is 135. The most appropriate next step is:
   a. Emergent cholecystectomy
   b. Emergent ERCP
   c. Emergent PTC placement
   d. Volume resuscitation and IV antibiotics

   Answer d. This pt needs fluid resuscitation and antibiotics started before any diagnostic studies are performed. From the clinical scenario presented, this patient most likely has **cholangitis**. *Charcot's triad consists of fever, RUQ pain, and jaundice. Reynolds pentad includes Charcot's triad plus hypotension and mental status changes.*

421. *The above pt now has a blood pressure of 110/60 and a HR of 100 after aggressive IVFs. You obtain a RUQ U/S while giving IVF's which shows a dilated CBD (12 mm) and pneumobilia. The most appropriate next step is:
   a. Emergent cholecystectomy
   b. Emergent ERCP and sphincterotomy
   c. Emergent PTC placement
   d. Hepatico-jejunostomy

Answer b. The most effective treatment for **cholangitis** is decompression of the biliary system. This is most easily done with **ERCP and sphincterotomy**, which not only can decompress the biliary system but can also remove or treat any obstructive lesion (stone most commonly).

422. **A 75 yo woman from a nursing home presents to the emergency room with crampy abd pain. On AXR, you notice multiple air-fluid levels and distension of her small bowel. Her colon appears decompressed. She also has pneumobilia despite never having surgery before or manipulation of her biliary system. The most appropriate next step is:
    a.   Start broad spectrum antibiotics
    b.   Exploratory laparotomy
    c.   Percutaneous cholecystostomy tube
    d.   Endoscopic retrograde cholangiography

Answer b. ****Pneumobilia** *(in a pt who has never had manipulation of her biliary system) associated with small bowel obstruction is most consistent with **gallstone ileus**. The gallbladder in this pt has eroded into the duodenum and a large gallstone is now causing a small bowel obstruction.*

423. **The *primary surgery* for pts with gallstone ileus consists of:
    a.   Open the ileum and removing the obstruction
    b.   Whipple
    c.   Cholecystectomy
    d.   Hepatico-jejunostomy

Answer a. ***The primary surgery in this pt is to **relieve the small bowel obstruction**. That involves feeling for the gallstone, opening the proximal ileum (longitudinal **enterotomy**, transverse closure), and removing stone.*

The secondary procedure, *if the patient can tolerate it*, is cholecystectomy and closure of the hole in the duodenum. Elderly, infirmed patients should just have the stone removed without cholecystectomy.

424. **A 50 yo woman w/ chronic pancreatitis presents with jaundice. U/S shows dilated proximal bile ducts and a focal mid duct stenosis. The most appropriate next step in this pts work-up is:
    a.   ERCP
    b.   MRCP
    c.   Chemo-XRT
    d.   Exploration

Answer b. Discovery of a **biliary stenosis** is suggestive of **CA** (either bile duct, gallbladder or pancreatic), a common bile duct stone or benign stricture Of the items listed, ****MRCP** *is the most appropriate next step* as this picks up any masses in the gallbladder or pancreas and also provides good reconstruction of the biliary system. MRCP is also good at picking up stones. It is not invasive like ERCP (risk of pancreatitis and perforation) and ERCP will not pick up obvious masses.

425. **The most appropriate surgery for a resectable lower 1/3 bile duct CA would be:
    a.   Whipple
    b.   Hepatic lobectomy
    c.   Local bile duct resection with hepatico-jejunostomy
    d.   Wide local excision

Answer a. Resectable lower 1/3 bile duct CA should undergo Whipple.
*Upper ⅓ (Klatskin tumor) - Tx****hepatic lobectomy** if localized to one side
*Middle ⅓ - Tx: ****resect duct w/ hepatico-jejunostomy**
*Lower ⅓ - Tx: ****Whipple**

426. **A 50 yo woman undergoes routine laparoscopic cholecystectomy and gallbladder adenocarcinoma is found extending into the muscular layer. All of the following are true except:
   a.   Gallbladder adenocarcinoma is the MC CA of the biliary tract
   b.   The 1st nodes involved are the cystic duct nodes
   c.   This pt should undergo wedge resection of segment 4 and 5
   d.   This pt should undergo wedge resection of segment 7 and 8

   Answer d. **Gallbladder adenocarcinoma confined to the mucosa and lamina propria (stage Ia) can be treated with just **cholecystectomy**.

   If it **invades the **muscularis propria** (stage Ib), you need **wedge resection** of **segments 4 and 5** with 2-3 cm margins and stripping of the portal triad lymph nodes

   For tumors that go **beyond the **muscularis propria** and are resectable (Stage IIa or greater, T3 or T4 tumors), **formal resection** of segments IVb and V is necessary (possible right lobectomy)

   The 1st nodes involved are the **cystic duct nodes

Normal Anatomy and Physiology

   Gallbladder lies underneath **segments IV** and **V**
   Cystic artery is a branch off right hepatic artery, located in triangle of Calot
   Triangle of Calot (cystohepatic triangle) - cystic duct (lateral), common hepatic duct (medial), liver (superior)
   ***Cystic veins** – drain into **right branch** of **portal vein**, then liver
   Lymphatics – found on **right side** of common bile duct
   Innervation
      Parasympathetic – left vagus (anterior trunk)
      Sympathetic – splanchnic and celiac ganglions (T7-T10)
   Gallbladder
      Mucosa is **columnar epithelium**; does not have **submucosa**
      Common bile duct (CBD) and hepatic duct do not have **peristalsis**
      Fills by contraction of **sphincter of Oddi** at Ampulla of Vater
      ***Morphine** contracts and **Glucagon** relaxes the sphincter of Oddi
   Normal sizes
      CBD < 8 mm, (< 10 mm after cholecystectomy)
      Gallbladder wall < 4 mm
      Pancreatic duct < 4 mm
   ***Highest concentration of CCK and secretin releasing cells –
      duodenum
   ***Aberrant posterior right hepatic artery** (segments VI and VII)
      1% of the population
      At risk of injury w/ cholecystectomy (found in Triangle of Calot)
      Injury can result in **ischemia** to segments **VI** and **VII**
         (Sx's – fevers, pain, ↑LFT's, liver abscess)
   ***Aberrant posterior right hepatic duct** (from **segments VI or VII**)
      1% of the population
      Enters common bile duct **separately** from right hepatic duct
      Lies in gallbladder fossa and at **risk of injury** w/ cholecystectomy
   Bile excretion
      Cause **increase** in bile excretion - CCK, vagal input
      Cause **decrease** in bile excretion - somatostatin, sympathetic input
      Gallbladder contraction – CCK (constant, tonic contraction)

Composition and Essential Functions of bile
      1) Fat-soluble vitamin and essential fatty acid absorption
      2) Bilirubin and cholesterol excretion

	Hepatic Bile	Gallbladder Bile
Na (mEq/L)	140-180	225-375
CL (mEq/L)	50-100	1-10
Bile Salts (mEq/L)	1-50	250-350
Cholesterol (mEq/dl)	50-150	300-700

**Final bile composition determined by ***active reabsorption of water* (Na/K ATPase) in gallbladder (concentrates bile)

Bile Salts - bile salt pool (6 g)

- 90% of excreted bile salts are reabsorbed (**enterohepatic circulation**):
  1) *Active resorption* of <u>conjugated</u> bile acids in **terminal ileum** conjugated bile salts absorbed <u>only</u> in term. ileum (45%)
  2) *Passive resorption* of <u>non-conjugated</u> bile acids in **small intestine** (40%) **and colon** (5%)

Postprandial emptying of gallbladder max. at 2 hrs (80% emptied)

Bile secreted by **bile canalicular cells** (20%) + **hepatocytes** (80%)

Color of bile from **conjugated bilirubin**

*Stercobilin – breakdown product of conjugated bilirubin in gut; is what gives stool **brown** color

Urobilinogen – breakdown product of conjugated bilirubin in gut; is reabsorbed and released in urine (urobilin**), turns it **yellow**

Gallstones can form after terminal ileum resection from malabsorption of bile salts

10% of US has gallstones (10% radiopaque on X-ray), most asymptomatic.

Cholecystitis

Obstruction of **cystic duct** (MCC - gallstone) results in gallbladder wall distention and inflammation

Sx's: **RUQ pain** worse 1-2 hrs after meal (esp fatty meals), N/V, anorexia

Referred pain to shoulder or scapula

Persistent pain (unlike biliary colic, which is transient)

Biliary Colic - transient cystic duct obstruction caused by passage of a gallstone; resolves in 4-6 hrs

Murphy's Sign – pt resists deep inspiration w/ deep palpation to RUQ secondary to pain

*MC organism w/ cholecystitis – <u>E. Coli</u>; others - klebsiella, enterococcus

Dx: High **alkaline phosphatase** and high **WBCs** usual

Amylase and lipase can be mildly elevated w/ cholecystitis

Significant elevations in **AST/ALT** or **amylase/lipase** – need to worry about <u>cholangitis</u> and gallstone <u>pancreatitis</u>

U/S - Best initial test for either **jaundice or RUQ pain

95% sensitive for picking up **stones**

Acute cholecystitis findings – gallstones, GB wall thickening (> 4 mm), peri-cholecystic fluid, sonographic Murphy's

Stones – hyper-echoic focus, posterior shadowing, movement of focus w/ change in position

Dilated CBD (> 8 mm if gallbladder present) suggests CBD stone (or benign / malignant stricture if no stones)

Dilated pancreatic duct (> 4 mm) suggests Ampulla of Vater stone (or benign / malignant stricture if no stones)

**CCK-CS Test (cholecystokinin cholescintigraphy)

**Most sensitive test for cholecystitis

Used if U/S is non-diagnostic; checks for **chronic cholecystitis** and **biliary dyskinesia**

*Technetium (Tc) is given, taken up by liver, and then excreted in biliary tract (99mTc-HIDA cholescintigraphy, CS)

*Cholecystokinin (CCK) is given to stimulate gallbladder contraction

234

Results
1) If gallbladder **cannot be seen** → **cystic duct obstruction** by stone; Tx: cholecystectomy
2) If **> 60 minutes to empty** after meal → *chronic cholecystitis*; Tx: cholecystectomy
3) If gallbladder **ejection fraction < 40%** after 1 hr → *biliary dyskinesia*; Tx: cholecystectomy (95% get relief)

Cholecystostomy tube (percutaneous, CT or U/S guided)
For pts who are **very ill** and **cannot tolerate cholecystectomy**
When pt stable, perform cholecystectomy

CBD stone ≤ 2 mm discovered **intra-op** - leave alone, will pass on its own
Best Tx for late CBD stone after cholecystectomy - ERCP w/ sphincterotomy
Bile duct injury intra-op – open and repair
   Partial transection (< 50%) – primary repair over stent
      Complete transection – hepatico-jejunostomy or choledocho-jejunostomy over stent
      Do not try primary repair (will get stenosis or leak)
      Do not try to attach to duodenum (won't reach)
Diarrhea after cholecystectomy – excess **bile salts** in colon (not stored in gallbladder anymore); **MC Cx following cholecystectomy**
MCC of late post-op stricture after cholecystectomy – ischemia
Shock following laparoscopic cholecystectomy
   Early (1st 24 hours) – hemorrhagic shock, clip fell off cystic artery
   Late (after 24 hours) – septic shock from accidental clip on CBD w/ subsequent cholangitis (usually occurs at median of **7 days**)
Ceftriaxone – can cause gallbladder sludging and cholestatic jaundice
Air in biliary system – MCC is previous ERCP and sphincterotomy
   Can also occur w/ **cholangitis** or **erosion** of biliary system into duodenum (eg gallstone ileus)
Bacterial infection of bile
   MC route (w/o previous biliary tract manipulation) – dissemination from **portal system**
   Retrograde infection from bacteria in duodenum very rare unless previous sphincterotomy
Highest incidence of positive bile cultures - post-op strictures (MC – E. coli, often polymicrobial)
Porcelain gallbladder – diffuse calcification of gallbladder wall; high risk for gallbladder CA; Tx - cholecystectomy
Ursodiol (Actigall) – dissolves gallstones < 2cm; indicated for either:
   1) pts w/ cholecystectomy indications who are too high risk for surgery (eg ** cirrhosis) or 2) prevention of stone formation in pts w/ rapid weight loss
Cirrhosis w/ gallstones – no elective cholecystectomy (high mortality) – give Ursodiol
Acalculous cholecystitis
   MC after severe burns, prolonged TPN, trauma, major surgery
   Sx's: RUQ pain, N/V
   Primary pathology – **bile stasis** leading to distention and ischemia
   RFs – narcotics, fasting, increased viscosity (eg dehydration, ileus, transfusions)
   Dx:
      U/S – dilated GB, sludge, gallbladder wall thickening, peri-cholecystic fluid, **No stones**
      Labs – high WBCs, high alkaline phosphatase
      HIDA scan (CCK-CS) – is positive (ie no gallbladder filling)
   Tx: **cholecystectomy** or percutaneous **cholecystostomy tube** if pt is too unstable (tube stays in for 6-8 weeks to form tract); Abx's

235

**MCC of common bile duct injury w/ laparoscopic cholecystectomy →
**Excess cephalad retraction of gallbladder fundus *(70%)*
  You think it's the cystic duct but really it is the CBD brought up from
   excess traction (considered a **Class III injury**)
  Minimize risk of injury by visualizing the triangle of Calot (want to see
   the cystic duct going into the gallbladder)
**Cystic duct remnant bile leak *after cholecystectomy (clips fell off cystic*
 duct) ****Tx: ERCP, sphincterotomy, temporary stent** *(also need*
 percutaneous drainage of fluid collection)
*ERCP prior to cholecystectomy (signs CBD stone might be present):
  1) **Jaundice** – *immediate* ERCP
  2) **Cholangitis** (RUQ pain, fever, jaundice) – *immediate* ERCP
  3) **U/S** showing dilated CBD or stone in CBD – *immediate* ERCP

  4) Persistently high **amylase** (> 1000 U/L) or **lipase** after 24 hrs
  5) Persistently high **bilirubin** (> 4 mg/dL) after 24 hrs
  6) Persistently high **AST** or **ALT** (> 200) after 24 hrs

**Pts w/ gallstone pancreatitis should have cholecystectomy after
recovery from pancreatitis but on same admission (ie prior to discharge)

Routine ERCP for gallstone pancreatitis *is discouraged* since the
probability of finding residual stones is low and there is a 1-2% Cx rate

**ERCP Cx's – pancreatitis (MC Cx, 5%), bleeding, cholangitis, perforation
Retroperitoneal perforation (contained) - conservative Tx (NPO, abx's)
Bile duct perforation – place temp stent across perforation; will heal
Free perforation of duodenum (intra-peritoneal extravasation of contrast)
  – open repair

****Cholangitis**
Sx's *Charcot's triad* - **RUQ pain**, **fever**, and **jaundice** *(classic)*
   Reynolds' pentad - Charcot's triad plus **mental status changes** and
    shock (ie sepsis)
   MCC – gallstones; ****MC organism – *E. coli*

Dx:
   U/S (usual initial test) – CBD will be dilated (**> 8 mm**, > 10 mm after
    cholecystectomy) if due to obstruction of biliary system
   ERCP *(best test)* – can remove stone if present or place stents
   Labs – high LFTs, high WBCs, positive blood cultures

Tx:
   **Initial Tx → fluid resuscitation + start abx's
    Optimize hemodynamics if **septic shock** (Reynold's Pentad)
     **Do this before ERCP (stabilize pt before ERCP)
   **ERCP w/ sphincterotomy →
    Decompresses biliary system (most effective Tx for
     cholangitis) - remove stone if present or stent if stricture
    If that fails, place a **PTC tube** to decompress
    If that fails, go to OR for intra-op **T-tube** to decompress
   *If due to gallstones, should have cholecystectomy after recovery
    from cholangitis (before hospital discharge)
   Cholangitis due to infected PTC tube → change PTC tube

****Gallstone ileus**
Fistula between **gallbladder** and 2nd portion of **duodenum**
Gallbladder releases stone, causing **small bowel obstruction** (SBO)
Usually occurs in **elderly**
MC site of obstruction – terminal ileum
Sx's: N/V, distension, abdominal pain (**SBO sx's*) and **pneumobilia*
Dx: **AXR** and **CXR →** **air in biliary tree** (pneumobilia) + **SBO** (*Classic*)

Tx: ****Remove stone** *w/ longitudinal enterotomy proximal to obstruction (milk it out); transverse closure*
    **Can leave gallbladder and fistula if pt frail and old
    If not to sick → cholecystectomy, resect fistula, and close duodenum

**Bile Duct CA (cholangiocarcinoma)
RFs: ulcerative colitis, choledochal cysts, sclerosing cholangitis, cirrhosis
Sx's: **painless jaundice** (early), then **weight loss** (late, *classic*)
Dx: U/S *(best initial test for RUQ pain or jaundice)* – shows dilated ducts
    **MRCP – defines duct anatomy and looks for a mass (less invasive than ERCP and can pick up a mass)
Path: Invades contiguous structures early – only 10% resectable
Tx: staging laparoscopy - often resectability determined at time of surgery.

    Upper ⅓ (Klatskin tumors) **– MC type (75%), worst prognosis
        Tx: ****hepatic lobectomy** (often w/ extended resection) and
            stenting of contra-lateral bile duct if mostly localized to a lobe
    Middle ⅓ – Tx: resect duct w/ ****hepatico-jejunostomy
    Lower ⅓ – Tx: ****Whipple

    Overall 5-YS: 5% (after resection for cure 25%)
    Palliative stenting is used for unresectable DZ

**Gallbladder adenocarcinoma
MC cancer of biliary tract (although still rare)
4 x more common the bile duct CA
RFs   **Gallstones** (#1, *most important* risk factor), **porcelain gallbladder, primary sclerosing cholangitis** (PSC), gallbladder **adenomas**
Sx's: **jaundice** initially, followed by **RUQ pain**
Dx: U/S *(best initial test for RUQ pain or jaundice)*
    **MRCP - **Mid-bile duct obstruction not caused by gallstones is gallbladder CA (or bile duct CA) until proven o/w
Path
    1st spreads to **segments IVb and V
    1st nodes involved are **cystic duct nodes (right side of portal triad)
    MC site of mets – liver
    High incidence of **tumor implants** in **trocar sites** when discovered after laparoscopic cholecystectomy
    *Laparoscopic approach contraindicated for gallbladder CA
    80% present w/ **stage IV** disease – only 20% resectable
    Best prognosis – papillary sub-type
    *Can be found incidentally after cholecystectomy
Tx:
    1) ****Confined to mucosa + lamina propria** (T1, stage I-a, **no muscle invasion**) **– **cholecystectomy** sufficient
    2) ****Muscle invasion only** (T2 Stage Ib, invades muscularis propria)
        a) ****Wedge resection of segments IVb and V** w/ 2-3 cm margin and **portal triad lymph node dissection** (regional lymphadenectomy)
    3) ***Beyond muscle** and **resectable** (Stage IIa or greater, T3 or T4 tumors)
        a) Formal **resection of segments IVb and V** (possible right hepatectomy + IVb resection) w/ 2-3 cm margins *and;*
        b) Stripping **portal triad lymph nodes**
        c) Depending on invasion, may need **CBD resection w/ hepatico-jejunostomy**
    Some recommend excision of previous laparoscopic port sites ≥ T2

Overall 5-YS: 5% (after resection for cure 30%)

Pancreas

427. *Which of the following pancreatic enzymes is secreted in active form?
    a. Amylase
    b. Trypsin
    c. Chymotrypsin
    d. Pepsin

    Answer a. **Amylase** and **lipase** are secreted in active form.

428. *All of the following are true exocrine functions of the pancreas except:
    a. Secretin primarily causes HCO3- release
    b. CCK primarily causes enzyme release and is the most potent pancreatic acinar cell stimulant
    c. Acetylcholine (vagus) increases HCO3- and enzyme release
    d. Somatostatin increases pancreatic endocrine and exocrine function

    Answer d. **Somatostatin** decreases both pancreatic endocrine and exocrine function.

429. **All of the following are true of the pancreas except
    a. Annular pancreas is treated w/ pancreatic resection
    b. Pancreas divisum associated with pancreatitis is usually first treated w/ ERCP and sphincterotomy
    c. Refractory chronic pancreatitis with dilated ducts is treated w/ pancreatico-jejunostomy (Puestow or Frey procedure)
    d. MRCP is the best test for common bile duct stricture complicating chronic pancreatitis (to assess for CA and define anatomy)

    Answer a. Annular pancreas is treated with duodeno-jejunostomy (MC) or duodeno-duodenostomy. ****MRCP** *is the best test for* **CBD stricture** *complicating chronic pancreatitis (to assess for CA and define anatomy).*

430. *All of the following are true of acute pancreatitis except:
    a. Occurs from impaired extrusion of zymogen granules and activation of degradation enzymes in the pancreas, leading to auto-digestion
    b. ARDS and pancreatic necrosis are from release of phospholipases
    c. MCC of death from pancreatitis is hemorrhage
    d. Coagulopathy and DIC are from release of proteases

    Answer c. *The MCC of death in* **acute pancreatitis** *is* **infection and sepsis** *(MC GNRs).*

431. *A 56 yo woman presents to the ED with severe abd pain. She has no other PMHx. She occasionally drinks. You get routine labs which are significant for an amylase of 24,000 and lipase of 7000. AXR is unremarkable. Her WBC is 17,000. Her blood pressure is 80/40 and HR is 120. She is afebrile. On exam she is fairly tender in the epigastric area. The most appropriate next step is:
    a. Start IVF's and get an U/S
    b. Start IVF's and get a CT scan
    c. Start IVF's and go to OR
    d. Start IVF's and go to MRI

    Answer a. The initial steps for pancreatitis are to start giving **IV hydration** (lose a lot of volume w/ pancreatitis), keep the pt NPO and **R/O gallstones** *(MCC of acute pancreatitis).* If there was a dilated CBD or an obvious CBD stone on U/S, you would go with ERCP, sphincterotomy, and stone extraction *after* resuscitation. ***Prophylactic abx's*** *are indicated for severe pancreatitis or if worsening clinically.*

432. *The above pt worsens clinically so you start abx's. Abd CT scan shows that 80% of the pancreas does not light up w/ IV contrast and there is no abscess or air bubbles. The appropriate next step is:
   a.   Whipple
   b.   Necrotic debridement
   c.   Percutaneous drain
   d.   Continue current management

   Answer d. *Sterile pancreatic necrosis* is left alone. Removing sterile necrotic material does not improve outcomes and may worsen prognosis (80% mortality w/ debridement of sterile necrosis).

433. **A 55 yo man with significant ETOH abuse has an acute episode of pancreatitis that resolves. Four weeks later he presents with epigastric pain, emesis and fullness after eating. You order a CT scan and there is a <u>new</u> 6 cm pancreatic pseudocyst. The next appropriate action is:
   a.   Percutaneous drainage
   b.   Resection
   c.   Conservative management with TPN or feeding tube past the ligament of Treitz
   d.   Cysto-gastrostomy

   Answer c. **Conservative Tx** *(NPO, TPN) is indicated for pts with a new onset symptomatic* **pancreatic pseudocyst**. **Spontaneous resolution** *occurs in 50%.* **You should not operate on pancreatic pseudocysts unless they are mature (> 3 months) <u>and</u> are either 1) persistently symptomatic or 2) are growing.*

   The 3 month waiting period is required to allow the cyst wall to mature so you can sew to it (**open cysto-gastrostomy**). The 3 months also allows the cyst to attach to the stomach posterior wall for **percutaneous cysto-gastrostomy.**

   Pseudocysts are generally not just drained percutaneously due to high recurrence (90%) and the potential for seeding infection. You certainly would <u>not</u> want to leave an indwelling drain in a pseudocyst. Pseudocysts are *non-epithelialized* sacs and are high in amylase.

434. **The above pt returns to clinic in 6 weeks. CT scan shows the cyst is the same size. He is tolerating a regular diet and does not have any sx's. The next appropriate action is:
   a.   Percutaneous drainage
   b.   Resection
   c.   Follow conservatively
   d.   Cysto-gastrostomy

   Answer c. Because the cyst is not causing any symptoms and is not growing, the treatment of choice is to follow the lesion. You should not operate on stable (ie no change in size) asymptomatic pseudocysts.

435. *You are performing a Whipple for a pancreatic head mass. You attempt to pass your finger behind the pancreas from below and get a large amount of blood return when you remove it. You place pressure on the neck of the pancreas and tamponade the bleeding. You have most likely injured the:
   a.   Aorta
   b.   Inferior vena cava
   c.   Celiac artery
   d.   Superior mesenteric vein

Answer d. The superior mesenteric vein (SMV) lies directly behind the neck of the pancreas and is the structure MC injured when trying to free this area. Divide the pancreas neck to get to the bleeding.

436. *Most significant risk factor for pancreatic adenocarcinoma is:
    a. Tobacco
    b. Alcohol
    c. High fat diet
    d. Nitrosamines

    Answer a. The most significant risk factor for the development of pancreatic cancer is tobacco use.

437. *A 55 yo woman undergoes Whipple for pancreatic CA. Post-op day 7 she complains of N/V. U/S shows a large fluid collection anterior to the pancreas (9 x 9 cm). The most appropriate next step in management is:
    a. Percutaneous drain placement and send the fluid for amylase, lipase, bilirubin and cytology
    b. Reglan
    c. Octreotide
    d. Re-operation

    Answer a. The 1st test in a pt w/ post-op N/V after pancreas surgery is an **U/S**. You should place a percutaneous drain if a fluid collection is present and send the fluid off. This is suspicious for **duct leak**.

438. *The fluid above has an amylase of 10,000. The most appropriate next step is::
    a. NPO, octreotide and follow drainage output
    b. Re-operation with revision of the pancreatic anastomosis
    c. Triple antibiotics
    d. Nothing

    Answer a. Now with a percutaneous drain, you have a controlled **pancreatic fistula**. The vast majority will resolve w/ conservative Tx.

439. **All of the following are true for palliation of metastatic pancreatic adenocarcinoma except:
    a. Biliary stent is the first line Tx for symptomatic obstructive jaundice
    b. Celiac axis block can provide effective pain relief
    c. Whipple is the best option for obstruction
    d. Gastro-jejunostomy is the best option for duodenal obstruction

    Answer c. Whipple should rarely be used as a palliative maneuver.

440. **All of the following are true except:
    a. The MC mets for pancreatic endocrine tumors is the liver
    b. Octreotide scan is effective for locating insulinomas
    c. Functional endocrine tumors generally respond to debulking
    d. Pancreatic endocrine tumors that are most commonly located in the pancreatic head are gastrinoma and somatostatinoma

    Answer b. Unlike other pancreatic endocrine tumors, octreotide is not effective for locating insulinoma. **Selective arterial calcium stimulation w/ hepatic venous insulin sampling** is the best localizing study for insulinomas not on CT scan (Ca^{++} stimulates insulin release from tumor)

441. *All of the following are true of insulinomas except:
    a. C peptide should be elevated
    b. Diazoxide can be used for metastatic disease
    c. Blind Whipple may be necessary for tumor that is not localized
    d. These tumors are evenly distributed throughout the pancreas

Answer c. Blind pancreatic resections should be avoided.

442. *All of the following are true of gastrinoma except:
   a.   Gastrin > 200 pg/ml _and_ BAO > 15 mEq/hr are diagnostic of gastrinoma
   b.   Octreotide scan is the best test for localizing the tumor
   c.   Vagotomy and antrectomy is indicated for severe symptoms with metastatic disease that has failed maximal medical therapy
   d.   Approximately 50% have multiple tumors

   Answer c. If medical therapy has failed, total gastrectomy is usually the best therapy for severe symptoms (**vagotomy + antrectomy _won't work_** – HCl secreting cells are in the body of stomach)

443. *A 50 yo woman with a pancreatic mass in the tail of the pancreas develops watery diarrhea and hypokalemia. The most likely diagnosis is:
   a.   Glucagonoma
   b.   Gastrinoma
   c.   Somatostatinoma
   d.   VIPoma (VIP – vasoactive intestinal peptide)

   Answer d. Watery diarrhea and hypokalemia (without concomitant gastric ulcer disease) is most consistent with **VIPoma**. The diarrhea associated with VIPoma will _not_ get better with proton pump inhibitors whereas the diarrhea found with gastrinoma will get better with proton pump inhibitors.

   *The combination of **5-FU** and **alpha interferon** is very effective for metastatic VIPoma.*

444. *A 50 yo woman with a pancreatic mass develops diabetes, gallstones and steatorrhea. The most likely diagnosis is:
   a.   Glucagonoma
   b.   Gastrinoma
   c.   Somatostatinoma
   d.   VIPoma

   Answer c. The above is consistent with **somatostatinoma**.

445. *A 50 yo woman w/ a pancreatic mass develops diabetes and migrating skin lesions w/ central clearing, erythema, blisters and crusting. The most likely diagnosis is:
   a.   Glucagonoma
   b.   Gastrinoma
   c.   Somatostatinoma
   d.   VIPoma (VIP – vasoactive intestinal peptide)

   Answer a. Development of diabetes and necrolytic migratory erythema is most consistent w/ **glucagonoma**.

446. *The previous pt is noted to have a 5 cm liver met on pre-op CT scan (confirmed with Bx) that looks resectable and a 1 cm deep liver met that is not resectable. The pancreatic mass in the head of the pancreas looks resectable. The most appropriate Tx is:
   a.   Nothing
   b.   5-fluorouracil and XRT
   c.   Morphine drip
   d.   Resection of the pancreatic mass and the large liver met

Answer d. Debulking surgery is effective palliative treatment for functional endocrine tumors so resecting the large liver mass is indicated if the primary could also be resected.

Non-endocrine tumors (ie adenocarcinoma) of the pancreas with a liver met would be considered unresectable and you would not perform a resection.

If the liver mass cannot be resected safely, **radiofrequency** ablation *(coagulation necrosis)* and **cryoablation** (protein and cell membrane *denaturation*) are options.

Normal Anatomy and Physiology

Head (including uncinate and neck) **body,** and **tail**
Uncinate process – rests on aorta, behind SMV and SMA
Blood supply
  Head - **superior** (off <u>GDA</u>) and **inferior** (off <u>SMA</u>) pancreatico-duodenal arteries; each has **anterior** and **posterior** branches
    *Inferior pancreaticoduodenal artery is <u>1st branch</u> off <u>SMA</u>
    *Middle colic is first branch going only to bowel
  Body - great, inferior and caudal pancreatic arteries (all splenic artery branches)
  Tail – splenic and dorsal pancreatic arteries
  Venous drainage into the **portal system**
  SMA and **SMV** – **behind** neck of pancreas (*SMV is to right of SMA*)
  SMA and **SMV** – lie **anterior** to the 3rd and 4th portions of duodenum
  Portal vein – forms behind neck of pancreas (SMV and splenic vein)
Lymphatics – celiac and SMA nodes
Exocrine function of pancreas
  Ductal cells – secrete $HCO3^-$ (have **carbonic anhydrase**)
    ↑ flow leads to ↑HCO_3^- and ↓ Cl^-
  Acinar cells – secrete pancreatic **digestive enzymes** and Cl^-
    Enzymes – amylase, lipase, trypsinogen, chymotrypsinogen, carboxypeptidase
    Amylase and **lipase – *only pancreatic enzymes secreted in active form*
    Amylase – hydrolyzes alpha 1-4 linkages of glucose chains
    Lipase – converts TAGs to FFAs and mono-acylglycerides
    Enterokinase – released by <u>duodenum</u>, converts trypsinogen to trypsin; **trypsin** then activates other pancreatic enzymes including trypsinogen
    ***Trypsin can <u>auto-activate</u> in acidic environments* (pH < 6)
Endocrine function of pancreas (islet cells)
  Alpha cells – glucagon
  Beta cells (center of islets) – insulin
  Delta cells – somatostatin
  PP cells – pancreatic polypeptide
  Islet cells w/ VIP, serotonin, neuropeptide Y, and GRP also
  Islet cells receive **majority of blood supply** compared to size
  Blood travels to islet cells first, then travels to acinar cells
Hormonal control of pancreatic **exocrine function**
  Secretin – ↑s HCO_3^- release mostly (**ductal** cells)
  CCK – ↑s enzyme release mostly (most potent **acinar** cell stimulant)
  Acetylcholine (vagus) – ↑s HCO^- and enzyme release
  Somatostatin – ↓s exocrine and endocrine function
  CCK and **secretin** released mostly by cells in **duodenum**
Development
  Ventral pancreatic bud - forms uncinate and inferior portion of pancreas head; contains **duct of Wirsung** (major duct)
  Dorsal pancreatic bud - tail, body, and superior aspect of pancreatic head; contains **duct of Santorini** (minor duct)

Duct of Wirsung – major pancreatic duct, merges w/ CBD before
entering duodenum
Duct of Santorini – small accessory pancreatic duct that drains
directly into duodenum
Ampulla of Vater – fusion of pancreatic duct and CBD, opens into
duodenum
***Sphincter of Oddi** - muscle band at Ampulla entrance to duodenum
Controls flow of bile and pancreatic secretions into duodenum
Marks transition from **foregut** to **midgut** (where celiac stops
supplying gut and SMA takes over)
ERCP w/ sphincterotomy opens this
****CCK and IV glucagon** _relax_ *the sphincter of Oddi*
Morphine contracts the sphincter of Oddi

*Annular pancreas
From **failure of clockwise rotation** of the **ventral pancreatic bud**
2nd portion of duodenum is trapped in pancreas – get duodenal obstruction
Sx's: **feeding intolerance** (N/V; duodenal obstruction); pancreatitis (adults)
RFs: Down's syndrome
Dx: **AXR** – double bubble sign (duodenum and stomach distension)
UGI – will show stenosis
Tx: ***duodeno-jejunostomy** (MC; or duodeno-duodenostomy)
****Pancreas is _not_ resected**
If **pancreatitis** is the problem → ERCP w/ sphincteroplasty

*Pancreas divisum
Failed fusion of pancreatic ducts; most are asymptomatic
Can result in **pancreatitis** from Duct of Santorini (Accessory Duct) stenosis
Dx: **ERCP**
Minor papilla will show long and large duct of Santorini
Major papilla will show short duct of Wirsung
Tx: ***ERCP w/ sphincteroplasty** if sx's, open sphincteroplasty if that fails

**Heterotopic pancreas
****MC location** – duodenum, usually asymptomatic; resection if sx's

**Chronic pancreatitis
Corresponds to irreversible parenchymal fibrosis
Islet cells (endocrine) usually preserved, **exocrine function** decreased
MCC – ETOH (80%); 2nd – idiopathic
Sx's: **pain** (MC), **weight loss**, **steatorrhea**, malabsorption (fat soluble vit's)
Dx: **Abd CT** – shrunken fibrotic pancreas w/ **calcifications**; **chain of lakes**
(advanced DZ) → alternating dilation and stenosis in pancreatic duct
Tx: 1st line - **analgesics + pancreas enzyme replacement** (pancrealipase);
TPN w acute episodes; celiac splanchnicectomy can relieve pain
Surgical indications: incapacitating refractory pain, failure to R/O CA,
biliary obstruction (need to R/O CA), abscess
Surgical options:
***Lateral pancreatico-jejunostomy** (Puestow or Frey)
For **ducts $\geq$ 8 mm**; pancreatic duct to jejunum anastomosis
***Distal pancreatic resection** – for normal duct size and only distal
portion of gland is affected
Whipple – for pts w/ isolated **pancreatic head** DZ w/ normal ducts
80% get pain relief w/ surgery; Diabetes often a Cx long after surgery
***Common bile duct (CBD) stricture w/ proximal dilatation*
Sx's; pain, jaundice, cholangitis
*Dx **MRCP (best test)** – finds masses (worry about CA here),
delineates anatomy, finds stones (non-invasive, avoids ERCP
Cx's)*
Tx: choledocho-jejunostomy (if benign stricture)

**Splenic vein thrombosis
> Can lead to **isolated gastric varices** w/o portal HTN (<u>no esophageal</u>
> > <u>varices</u>)
> MCC - chronic pancreatitis
> Sx's: **bleeding** from **gastric varices** that form as collaterals
> Tx: ****splenectomy**; if asymptomatic, leave alone

<u>Pancreatic ascites</u> (or pancreatic pleural effusion)
> MC from leaking **pancreatic pseudocyst** or leak in **pancreatic duct**
> > (can leak retroperitoneal, gets above diaphragm → **pleural effusion**)
> MC with **chronic pancreatitis**
> *Majority resolve spontaneously w/ conservative Tx*
> Tx (similar to pancreatic fistula – do <u>not</u> rush to operate on these pts):
> > **Drain ascites or pleural effusion** (fluid high in **amylase** > 1000)
> > **Octreotide** (to ↓ pancreatic output)
> > **NPO and TPN**

*Acute pancreatitis
> **MCC** – **Stones** (35%) and **ETOH** (30%)
> > Other causes – ERCP, hyperlipidemia, hypercalcemia, viral infection
> > RF for **necrotizing pancreatitis** – obesity
> **Mortality rate** – 10% (hemorrhagic pancreatitis – 40%, more severe form)
> Sx's: abd pain radiating to back; N/V, fever, anorexia, jaundice
> **Ecchymosis** (retroperitoneal signs hemorrhagic pancreatitis) - <u>Fox's</u>
> > (inguinal ligament), <u>Cullen</u> (peri-umbilical), and <u>Grey Turner</u> (flank) sign's
> Dx:
> > **RUQ U/S** - look for **stones** and biliary **obstruction**; if obstructed, get
> > > **ERCP** (sphincterotomy + stone extraction) *after* resuscitation
> > **Abd CT** – if really sick to check for **infected necrotic pancreatitis** or
> > > **abscess** (necrotic pancreas will <u>not</u> light up w/ IV contrast)
> > **Labs** – ↑WBCs, ↑amylase, ↑lipase
> > Mildly increased amylase can be found w/ sialoadenitis, cholecystitis,
> > > perforated ulcer, bowel obstruction, intestinal infarction
> Path
> > From impaired extrusion of zymogen granules and activation of
> > > degradation enzymes in pancreas → leads to **auto-digestion**
> > **MCC death** – infection, usually GNRs
> > **ARDS* – from release of phospholipases
> > **Coagulopathy and DIC* – from release of proteases
> > **Pancreatic fat necrosis** – from release of phospholipases
> > Other cx's – shock, renal failure
> > **Ranson's:** Age >55, WBC >16, Glucose >200, AST >250, LDH >350
> > > **After 48 hrs** – Hct decrease of 10, BUN increase of 5, Ca < 8,
> > > > PaO2 < 60, Base deficit > 4, Fluid sequestration > 6 L
> > > **> 8 criteria** – near 100% mortality
> Tx:
> > **NPO,** *aggressive* **fluid resuscitation** (up to <u>10</u> L/d)
> > **Abx's** for stones, severe pancreatitis or necrosis, failure to improve,
> > > fever, or infection
> > **Enteral feeds** (jejunal if possible) decreases **infectious cx's** and
> > > improves **survival** compared to TPN (start after acute period)
> > **ERCP w/ sphincterotomy** and **CBD stone** extraction if present (*after*
> > > resuscitation)
> > **Pts w/ gallstone pancreatitis should undergo **cholecystectomy**
> > > *when recovered from pancreatitis but **during <u>same admission</u>***
> > <u>Avoid Morphine</u> → contracts sphincter of Oddi, worsens attack
> > **Surgery** (open debridement) only indicated for **infected necrosis** or
> > > **abscess **Leave sterile necrosis alone**
> > **Abscess* - need **open debridement**; percutaneous drainage not
> > > effective for pancreatic abscess *(classic teaching)*

**Pancreatic pseudocysts
Sx's: **pain** (MC Sx), **weight loss**, and **bowel obstruction** (compression)
  MCC – chronic pancreatitis (can occur w/ acute pancreatitis)
Dx: Abd CT (*best test*); signs of **acute** (edema, fluid) or **chronic**
  pancreatitis (shrunken pancreas, calcification, dilated ducts) in most
Path – non-epithelialized sac, MC in **head** of pancreas, **small** cysts (< 5
  cm) usually resolve spontaneously; can be large; are high in **amylase**
Pseudocyst Criteria:
  1) Need PMHx of **pancreatitis, pancreatic surgery,** or **trauma** *and:*
  2) **Not** **a complex cyst** (no fronds or septae; no mass) *and:*
  3) **Not** growing on serial CT scan
  *If above not met, worry about **CA** (eg pancreatic cyst -cystadenoma*
    or -cystadenocarcinoma; Dx EUS aspiration for fluid + cytology)
    Serous fluid – likely cyst-adenoma (can follow)
    Mucin in fluid – cyst-adenocarcinoma, need resection
    Amylase – likely pseudocyst
Tx:
  Only need to Tx pseudocysts that are either:
    1) continually **symptomatic** *or*
    2) are **growing** (worry about CA) – need to resect
    **Asymptomatic stable pseudocysts - *leave alone*
  Continued sx's - *expectant management for **3 months (TPN or*
    feeding tube past ligament of Treitz if unable to eat)
    **50% resolve on their own
    ***If above fails will need* **cysto-gastrostomy *(endoscopic or*
      open) **after 3 months of sx's** *(cysto-gastrostomy is felt to*
      be the most effective Tx for symptomatic pseudocysts)
    *****Need 3 months of conservative Tx before cysto-gastrostomy*
      to allow pseudocyst to mature. The **cyst wall** needs to
      be thick and **mature** to be able to sew to it with open
      cysto-gastrostomy; also, for endoscopic cysto-
      gastrostomy to work, the pancreatic pseudocyst needs to
      be attached (scarred) to **posterior stomach wall**
  Open cysto-gastrostomy – posterior stomach sewn to cyst wall

**Pancreatic adenocarcinoma (ductal)
RFs – **smoking** (#1), obesity, chronic pancreatitis; *Not* RF – ETOH
Sx's: ***painless jaundice** (tumor in head), then **weight loss**
  *Pain as a Sx *still potentially resectable*
Path
  > 95% from **exocrine pancreas** (*ductal adenocarcinoma*)
  Majority in **head** (70%), **lymphatic** spread 1st
  CA 19-9 – serum marker for pancreatic CA
  15% resectable; 5-YS survival with resection – 25%
Tx:
  Resection if resectable (eg no distant mets, not invading any major
    structure)
  Diagnostic laparoscopy before Whipple – if mets to peritoneum,
    omentum, or liver → close and palliate
  Whipple (pancreatico-duodenectomy) removes pancreatic head,
    duodenum, CBD, and gallbladder, ± gastrectomy →
    1) pancreatico-jejunostomy, 2) choledocho-jejunostomy, and 3)
    gastro-jejunostomy then performed to Roux limb of jejunum
  Distal pancreatectomy – *does not* require roux limb (just over-sew
    pancreas)
  Prognosis based on vascular + nodal invasion *(ability to get clear
    margin)*
  *Bleeding behind neck of pancreas after blunt dissection – SMV;
    divide pancreas to control bleeding
  Post-op chemo-XRT → 5-FU + gemcitabine
    Gemcitabine – nucleoside analogue anti-metabolite

Palliation – *biliary stents (or PTC tube) for symptomatic jaundice, ***gastro-jejunostomy for duodenal obstruction; ***celiac plexus block** (50% effective) or ***XRT** for pain; ***pancrealipase** for steatorrhea

Cx's from Whipple:
- ***MC Cx** – delayed gastric emptying; Tx – metoclopramide
- ****Pancreatic duct or bile duct leak** *(treat like <u>fistula</u>)*
  - Usually presents w/ increased drainage from pancreatic drain (fluid high in **amylase**)
  - Tx: ensure **appropriate drainage, octreotide, NPO, TPN**
  - ****Vast majority of fistulas resolve w/ conservative Tx**
  - **Do not re-operate early on these pts** – *tissue very friable and will do more harm than good*
- **Nausea and vomiting** – get U/S *(best test)* or CT
  - DDx – delayed gastric emptying, anastamotic leak
- **Marginal ulceration** – from acid; on **jejunal** side; have pain;Tx: PPI
- ***Bleeding after Whipple or other pancreatic surgery** – go to angio for **embolization** as 1st move *(Not re-operation); <u>avoid surgery</u>* as the tissue planes are very friable early and pancreatic bleeding is extremely hard to control operatively
- ***High volume centers** (> 12/year) have ↓ed peri-operative mortality

5-YS after resection – 25%

Functional endocrine pancreatic tumors

Octreotide for treating mets – effective for all <u>except</u> somatostatinoma
Octreotide scan for locating – effective for all <u>except</u> insulinoma
Tumors w/ predilection pancreatic head - gastrinoma, somatostatinoma
*All of these tumors respond to **debulking** *(decrease sx's)*
Liver mets – 1st for all
Streptozocin – toxic to islet cells of pancreas

**Insulinoma

MC islet cell tumor of pancreas; 90% benign; even distribution in pancreas

Sx's: **Whipple's triad**
1) **Fasting hypoglycemia** (< 50)
2) **Sx's of hypoglycemia**, (palpitations, ↑ed HR, diaphoresis)
3) **Relief w/ glucose**

Dx: Labs
1) **Insulin to glucose ratio > 0.4** after fasting (72 hours)
2) Fasting glucose **< 50** and Fasting insulin **> 24**
3) **↑ C peptide** and **pro-insulin** → if <u>not</u> elevated suspect Munchausen's syndrome (self-injection of insulin)
The above are **<u>diagnostic</u>**

Localization:
Abd CT (or MRI)
EUS (endoscopic U/S) – finds 80%
**Selective arterial calcium stimulation w/ hepatic venous insulin sampling (localizes tumor – Ca++ causes release of insulin from tumor); used if trouble localizing w/ above
*Notably, many of these will <u>not</u> light up on octreotide scan

Tx:
Enucleate if < 2 cm (has pseudo-capsule)
Can have multiple lesions (enucleate each if < 2 cm)
Formal resection if > 2 cm (Whipple or distal pancreatectomy)
Trouble finding tumor – Intra-op U/S to help
Still can't find tumor – *<u>avoid blind pancreatic resection</u>* and perform post-op **selective arterial calcium stimulation** w/ hepatic venous insulin sampling to localize the tumor
Metastases – **5-FU** and **Streptozocin**
Octreotide, diazoxide (inhibits release of insulin)

*Gastrinoma (Zollinger-Ellison syndrome; ZES)
    50% malignant, 50% multiple (esp w/ MEN)
    Majority (75%) in **gastrinoma triangle**
        1. Common bile duct
        2. Neck of pancreas
        3. Third portion of the duodenum
   Sx's:
        1)   **Refractory** or **complicated ulcers** (many, unusual locations)
        2)   **Diarrhea** (improved w/ PPI)
   Dx: Always need 1) fasting **serum gastrin level** <u>and</u>: 2) stomach **basal
        acid output** to make Dx:
        Gastrin > 200 pg/ml <u>and</u> **BAO > 15** mEq/hr → are diagnostic of
           gastrinoma
        Secretin stimulation test
           Pts w/ gastrinoma will have an ↑ in gastrin (> 200 increase)
           Normal pts have ↓ gastrin w/ secretin
        Abd CT (or MRI) to localize; look for multiple tumors
        Octreotide scan (*best test for localizing tumor*)
        EUS – also good at localizing tumors
   Tx:
        Duodenum
           < 2 cm - duodenotomy w/ resection + regional node dissection
           > 2 cm - formal resection (eg Whipple) + take regional nodes
           Be sure to check pancreas for separate primary (50% multiple)
        Pancreas
           < 2 cm - enucleation + regional node dissection
           > 2 cm - formal resection (eg Whipple) + take regional nodes
           Look around for multiple tumors (gastrinoma triangle)
        Can't find tumor →
           Perform duodenostomy and look inside duodenum for tumor
               (20% of micro-gastrinomas there)
           Blind pancreatic resections are generally <u>not</u> indicated

*VIPoma (Verner-Morrison Syndrome)
    Majority **malignant**; most in **distal** pancreas
    Sx's: **watery diarrhea, hypokalemia** and **achlorhydria** (WDHA syndrome)
        Hypokalemia from diarrhea
    Dx: fasting **VIP** levels
    Tx: resection
    Mets – **5-FU** and ***interferon*** *(work very well)*; debulking may also help

*Somatostatinoma
    Majority **malignant,** most in **head** of pancreas
    ****Worst prognosis** of pancreatic endocrine tumors (85% have mets at Dx)*
    Sx's: **diabetes, gallstones,** and **steatorrhea** *(classic triad)*
    Dx: fasting **somatostatin** level
    Tx: resection, **cholecystectomy** with resection
    Mets – **5-FU** and **Streptozocin**

*Glucagonoma
    Majority **malignant**, most in **distal** pancreas
    Sx's: **diabetes** and **dermatitis** (70%, **necrolytic migratory erythema**)
    Dx: fasting **glucagon** level (≥ 500-1000 pg/mL)
    Tx: resection
    Mets – **5-FU** and **Streptozocin**, octreotide

Spleen

447. All of the following are true of splenic red pulp except:
    a. Acts as a filter for aged or damaged RBCs
    b. Contains high concentrations of lymphocytes
    c. Pitting involves the removal of abnormalities in the RBC membrane
    d. Culling involves removal of less deformable RBCs

    Answer b. The **white pulp** contains high concentrations of lymphocytes.

448. *All of the following are true of white pulp except:
    a. IgG is the most common immunoglobulin in the spleen.
    b. Serves an immunologic function with high concentrations of lymphocytes and macrophages
    c. Is the major site of bacterial clearance that lacks pre-existing antibodies
    d. Is the largest producer of IgM

    Answer a. **IgM** is the MC immunoglobulin in the spleen.

449. *All of the following are true except:
    a. Tuftsin acts as an opsonin
    b. Properdin can activate complement
    c. The splenic artery is a branch off the superior mesenteric artery
    d. Spur cells and target cells increase after splenectomy

    Answer c. The **splenic artery** is a branch off the celiac axis.

450. A 18 yo girl undergoes splenectomy for ITP. Five days post-op she has a BP of 85/40, temp 101 F, lethargy, abdominal pain, nausea and vomiting. The pts blood pressure seems unresponsive to fluid challenge. All of the following are true of this condition except:
    a. The MCC is withdrawal of exogenous steroids
    b. ACTH is likely elevated in this patient
    c. Serum cortisol levels need to be drawn before treatment
    d. Serum cortisol is likely < 15 in this patient

    Answer c. You do not need a serum cortisol before treating **adrenal insufficiency**. Dexamethasone should be given. Note Dexamethasone does not interfere w/ the ACTH stimulation test for adrenal insufficiency.

451. *Certain genetic disorders may require splenectomy to prevent premature destruction of blood elements. The MC congenital DZ requiring splenectomy:
    a. Hereditary spherocytosis
    b. Hereditary elliptocytosis
    c. Protein kinase deficiency
    d. Beta thalassemia minor

    Answer a. The MC congenital abnormality requiring splenectomy is **hereditary spherocytosis**. Splenectomy is curative for this disease. Cholecystectomy should be performed at the same surgery.

452. *Excluding genetic disorders which involve membrane proteins, the most common congenital abnormality requiring splenectomy is:
    a. Hereditary elliptocytosis
    b. G6PD deficiency
    c. Pyruvate kinase deficiency
    d. Hereditary spherocytosis

    Answer c. The MC non-membrane protein congenital abnormality requiring splenectomy is **pyruvate kinase deficiency**.

453. *Continued destruction of blood elements following splenectomy can be related to an accessory spleen. The most common location of an accessory spleen is:
   a. Liver
   b. Kidney
   c. Adrenal gland
   d. Splenic hilum

Answer d. The MC location of an **accessory spleen** is the splenic hilum.

454. *The most common non-traumatic condition requiring splenectomy:
   a. Immune thrombocytopenic purpura (ITP)
   b. Thrombotic thrombocytopenic purpura (TTP)
   c. Hereditary spherocytosis
   d. Pyruvate kinase deficiency

Answer a. The MC non-traumatic indication for splenectomy is **ITP**.

455. **All of the following are characteristic of ITP except:
   a. Enlarged spleen
   b. With splenectomy, platelets are classically given after ligation of the splenic artery
   c. In children < 10, this often resolves without further treatment
   d. The primary therapy is steroids

Answer a. ***ITP patients have **normal spleens**.*

   With splenectomy, platelets are classically given <u>after</u> ligation of the **splenic artery
   **In children < 10, this often resolves without further treatment
   The primary therapy is **steroids

456. **All of the following are true of lymphoma except:
   a. FNA is all that is needed for the diagnosis of lymphoma
   b. Non-Hodgkin's lymphoma involving the mediastinum and spleen would be considered stage III disease
   c. The MCC of chylous ascites is lymphoma
   d. The MC 2nd malignancy following radiation therapy only for lymphoma is breast CA

Answer a. FNA is not adequate for the Dx of lymphoma as architecture is needed (need 1 cm^2 of tissue). Core needle Bx or open Bx are indicated.

   The MCC of **chylous ascites** is **lymphoma
   *** Non-Hodgkin's lymphoma involving the mediastinum and spleen would be considered **stage III disease***

457. **All of the following are common indications for splenectomy except:
   a. Splenic abscess
   b. Refractory isolated splenic lymphoma
   c. Myelofibrosis w/ myeloid metaplasia causing transfusion dependency
   d. Sickle cell anemia

Answer d. **The spleen usually infarcts with sickle cell anemia and splenectomy is rarely required.

   *****Splenic abscess** requires **splenectomy***
   *****Myelofibrosis** w/ myeloid metaplasia causing **transfusion dependency** requires splenectomy*

458. **A 3 yo undergoes splenectomy for hereditary spherocytosis. Six weeks later, the child returns to the ER with a fever of 104, chills, rigors, and a systolic blood pressure of 60. The child's WBCs are 20 All of the following are true of the child's most likely condition except:
   a. The condition is more common in patients who undergo splenectomy for malignancy or hematologic disease compared to trauma
   b. The MC organism involved is N. meningitides
   c. Children less then 5 years of age undergoing splenectomy are at higher risk
   d. The condition is due to a specific lack of immunity to capsulated organisms

Answer b. **The MC organism involved in *Post-Splenectomy Sepsis Syndrome (PSSS)* is strep pneumoniae.**

   **The condition is due to a specific lack of immunity to capsulated organisms*
   ***Thalassemia** specifically considered higher risk*
   ***Highest risk for PSSS** – Wiskott-Aldrich syndrome (immune deficiency resulting in ↓ed antibody production)*

Normal Anatomy and Physiology
   Vascular supply
   Splenic artery (off celiac trunk) and **short gastrics** (off splenic artery) are considered end arteries
   Splenic vein is posterior and inferior to splenic artery (behind spleen); splenic artery is just superior to the pancreas
   Red pulp (85%)
   Acts as a **filter for aged** or **damaged RBCs**
   Pitting – the removal of abnormalities in RBC membrane
   Howell-Jolly bodies – nuclear remnants
   Heinz bodies – hemoglobin (siderocytes)
   Pappenheimer bodies - iron
   Culling – removal of less deformable and old RBCs
   White pulp (15%)
   Immunologic function
   Contains **lymphocytes** and **macrophages**
   The major site of **bacterial clearance that lacks preexisting Ab's**
   Site of removal for **poorly opsonized bacteria, particles,** and other **cellular debris**
   Serves as antigen-processing center for **dendritic cells** and **macrophages; involves helper T cells** (adaptive immunity)
   *Largest producer of **IgM***
   ***MC immunoglobulin in spleen** – IgM*
   Tuftsin - an **opsonin**; produced in spleen
   Properdin - an **opsonin**; produced in spleen; activates **complement**
   Accessory spleen – most commonly found at splenic hilum (20% of pts)
   MC non-traumatic condition requiring splenectomy – ITP
   Indication for splenectomy – ITP far greater than for TTP
   Post-splenectomy changes
   ↑RBCs, ↑WBCs, ↑platelets
   Will see **Howell-Jolly, Heinz,** and **Pappenheimer bodies**
   Will see **spur cells** and **target cells**
   If platelets >1-1.5 x 10^6, need ASA (most of these changes transient)
   Liver picks up some splenic functions
   MC splenic tumor (and MC benign splenic tumor) - hemangioma
   Tx: splenectomy if symptomatic
   MC malignant splenic tumor – Non-Hodgkin's lymphoma
   MCC splenomegaly – Non-Hodgkin's lymphoma
   MC malignant non-blood cell tumor – angiosarcoma (Tx: splenectomy)
   Dermoid cysts (cystic teratomas): Tx - splenectomy (CA risk)

Splenic abscess: Tx - splenectomy (MC organism – streptococcus)
Echinococcus: Tx - splenectomy after initial Albendazole
Reticuloendothelial system – monocytes and macrophages;
   locations – spleen, liver, lymph nodes, (Kupffer cells), lung (alveolar
      macrophages)

Other spleen problems
Spontaneous splenic rupture – mononucleosis (MC), malaria, sepsis
Splenosis – splenic implants; MC after trauma
Hypo-splenism (eg splenectomy) – see Howell-Jolly bodies, Heinz bodies,
   Pappenheimer bodies, Target cells and Spur cells

Acute Adrenal Insufficiency (Addisonian crisis, adrenal crisis)
Sx's: **fever, N/V, abd pain** and **hypotension** (unresponsive to fluid/pressors)
   Causes – *withdrawal of exogenous steroids (MCC),* bilateral
      adrenal hemorrhage (MC related to sepsis), adrenalectomy
Dx: high **ACTH** and low **cortisol**
   Cosyntropin test (*best test,* ACTH given and cortisol measured)
   Baseline cortisol < 15 or **change < 9** ug/dl after stimulation test =
      adrenal insufficiency
Tx: 1) **Dexamethasone + fludrocortisone**
            Give prior to ACTH stimulation test (dexamethasone does NOT
               interfere w/ ACTH stimulation test)
            Do not wait on test results if clinically suspected
         2) **Volume** to temporize while waiting for steroids to take effect
            Hydrocortisone after above
   Relative potency of steroids
         1 x – cortisone, hydrocortisone
         5 x – prednisone, prednisolone, methyl-prednisolone
         30 x – dexamethasone
Prophylaxis – hydrocortisone 100 mg at start of case, then wean

*Congenital hemolytic anemias (membrane protein defects)
   *Hereditary Spherocytosis
      *MC congenital hemolytic anemia requiring splenectomy
      Spectrin deficit (membrane protein) deforms RBCs, get **splenic
         sequestration → splenomegaly**
      Sx's: pigmented stones, anemia, jaundice, splenomegaly
      Splenectomy after age 5-6 (get through **immunizations**)
      Tx: **splenectomy + cholecystectomy** (if gallstones); splenectomy is
         curative

*Congenital hemolytic anemias (non–membrane protein defects)
   *Pyruvate kinase deficiency
      *MC congenital hemolytic anemia not involving a membrane
         protein requiring splenectomy
      Congenital hemolytic anemia, altered glucose metabolism
      RBC survival increased w/ splenectomy (may be required in minority)
   Warm antibody autoimmune hemolytic anemia
      Is the MC **autoimmune hemolytic disease** (MC- IgG against RBCs)
      Indication for splenectomy: if refractory to steroids and IVIG
   Beta thalassemia
      MC thalassemia; persistent **Hgb F**
      Major – both chains affected; **Minor** – 1 chain, asymptomatic
      Sx's: pallor, poor body growth, head enlargement
      Most die in teens secondary to hemosiderosis
      Splenectomy may ↓ hemolysis and sx's
   Sickle cell anemia – Hgb A replaced w/ Hgb S
      Spleen usually auto-infarcts and *splenectomy rarely required*
   G6PD deficiency - precipitated by infection, certain drugs, fava beans
      Splenectomy rarely required

Immune thrombocytopenic purpura (ITP)

Etiologies – many (drugs, viruses, immuno-deficiencies, etc)

Sx's: Most asymptomatic; can get purpura, gingival bleeding, bruising

In children < 10 years → usually resolves **spontaneously** (90%)

Typically follows **infection** (usually viral) in children (peak age 5)

Path

Low platelets (< 100,000)

Spleen is normal

Caused by **anti-platelet Ab's** (IgG); platelets then get chewed up by macrophages in spleen, leading to **bleeding diatheses**

Tx:

Initial

Steroids (#1 primary therapy, hydrocortisone)

Immunoglobulin (Ig, gammaglobulin) used if steroid-resistant

Splenectomy indicated for those who **fail steroids** and **medical Tx**
1) Removes the source of IgG production (B cells in the spleen)
2) Removes the source of phagocytosis
3) 80% respond after splenectomy

Acute Bleeding – **steroids** and **immunoglobulin** (IV-IG)

Platelets may be required to stop profuse bleeding

Pre-splenectomy issues:

Steroids start at beginning of case

Immunoglobulin 1 week pre-op (prolongs life of platelets)

Immunizations – S pneumoniae, H. influenza, and N. meningitides (2 weeks before operation best)

With splenectomy, platelets are given after ligation of the splenic artery

Post-splenectomy issues:

Immunizations if not already given

ASA for platelets > 1-1.5 x 10⁶

Prophylactic Daily Augmentin for 6 months in children < 10 **helps** prevent IPSI (PSSS)

Persistent thrombocytopenia post-op

Look at smear for **asplenic changes** in RBCs (should see Howell-Jolly, Heinz and Pappenheimer bodies if no spleen is present)

If asplenic changes not present, consider **accessory spleen** (MC located at the **hilum**; Dx – CT scan)

Tx: **steroids** and **immunoglobulin**

reoperation if accessory spleen

Thrombotic thrombocytopenic purpura (TTP)

Loss of platelet inhibition – leads to thrombosis and infarction, profound thrombocytopenia (not Ab mediated)

Sx's (classic pentad)

Low platelets (profound)

Mental status changes

Kidney failure

Fever

Hemolytic Anemia (jaundice)

Majority (80%) arise from deficiency or inhibition of **enzyme ADAMTS13** (responsible for cleaving large **vWF molecules**); these large vWF molecules go un-cleaved and cause **thrombosis**

Deaths MC from **intracerebral hemorrhage** or **acute renal failure**

Tx: **Plasmapheresis** (#1 primary therapy) – gets rid of vWF molecules

Immunosuppression – steroids, vincristine, cyclophosphamide

Splenectomy rarely indicated

**Lymphoma

1) **Hodgkin's**

MC Sx – painless swollen lymph node in neck
Nodal DZ w/ orderly anatomic spread to adjacent nodes
Reed Sternberg cells
MC sub-type – nodular sclerosing
Lymphocyte predominant – better prognosis
Lymphocyte depleted – worst prognosis

2) **Non-Hodgkin's lymphoma** (includes 40+ types of lymphoma)
Sx's reflect involved sites (eg abdominal fullness, bone pain)
Diffuse; nodal and extra-nodal DZ usual; non-contiguous spread
MC type – B cell (90%)
Worse prognosis than Hodgkin's
Generally **systemic disease** by the time the diagnosis is made

B symptoms (constitutional, worse prognosis) – fever, night sweats, weight loss

Dx:

*Core needle or **excisional lymph node Bx** (need **architecture**, not just cells); *FNA not adequate for Dx*
Bone marrow Bx
Chest/abd/pelvic CT - does NOT reliably detect spleen or liver involvement; need 2nd modality (→ **gallium MRI** or **PET**)

**Staging

A – Asymptomatic

B – Symptomatic (eg night sweats, fever, weight loss) – unfavorable

I – 1 LN region

II – ≥ 2 LN regions (non-contiguous) same side of the diaphragm

III – LN regions on ****both sides** of the diaphragm

IV – disseminated involvement of 1 or more extra-lymphatic organs (eg liver, bone, lung, ect. *except* spleen)

Staging laparotomy *rarely* performed as it does not impact Tx

Tx 1) Hodgkin's: chemo **ABVD** (MC) – doxorubicin (Adriamycin), bleomycin, vinblastine, dacarbazine

2) NHL: **CHOP-R** (MC) – Cyclophosphamide, doxorubicin (Hydroxy-), vincristine (Oncovin), Prednisone, Rituximab (anti-CD20, kills B cells)

Overall 5-YS: HL – 85%; NHL– 65%

Surgery for lymphoma today involves:

Getting lymph node tissue for Dx
Tx of chylous effusion
Splenectomy for isolated splenic lymphoma (rare)
**MCC of chylous ascites – *lymphoma*

These pts are at high risk for **2nd malignancies** related to **therapy**:
MC from **prior XRT + chemo** – lung CA, leukemia
MC from **prior XRT only** – breast CA
Also at risk for earlier onset **coronary atherosclerosis**

Myelofibrosis w/ myeloid metaplasia of the spleen (spleen acts as bone marrow) – causes splenomegaly and consumption of blood products (anemia, thrombocytopenia)

**Almost always need splenectomy:

1) **Hereditary spherocytosis**
2) **Hereditary elliptocytosis**
3) ****Splenic vein thrombosis** w/ gastric variceal **bleeding**
4) **Echinococcal Cyst** (MC splenic cyst)
5) ****Splenic Abscess** (MC organism – streptococcus; followed by staph) – splenectomy Tx of choice

Usually need splenectomy
   1) <u>Refractory</u> **Warm antibody type autoimmune hemolytic anemia**
   2) <u>Refractory</u> **ITP in adult**
   3) **Isolated splenic lymphoma** (rare, marginal zone B cell lymphoma –
      causes splenomegaly)
   4) ****Myelofibrosis w/ myeloid metaplasia (MMM)** if transfusion
      dependent, is causing pain, or severe thrombocytopenia

**_Overwhelming post-splenectomy infection_ (OPSI)
   (Post-splenectomy sepsis syndrome, PSSS)
   Lifetime risk after splenectomy: 1-2%
   Increased risk for OPSI:
      MC in **children aged ≤ 5** *(the younger the pt, the higher the risk)*
      MC **< 2 years** after splenectomy (80% of all cases)
      MC w/ **non-traumatic** causes for splenectomy (eg malignancy,
         hemolytic disorders such as **thalassemia;** immunodeficiencies)
      **Thalassemia *specifically considered higher risk*
      **Highest risk for OPSI – *Wiskott-Aldrich syndrome (immune
         deficiency resulting in ↓ed antibody production)*
   Path
      **Condition is due to a specific lack of immunity to **capsulated
         organisms** *(lack of* ****IgM** *immunoglobulin)*
      *MC organism w/ OPSI – <u>strep pneumoniae</u> (pneumococcus)
         others - H influenza, N, meningitides, S. aureus, group A strep
   Mortality rate 50% (highest in **children**)
   Prevention
      One should try and delay splenectomy until **after 5 years of age**
         Allows Ab formation; child can get **fully immunized**
      Pts should be immunized against **pneumococcus, meningococcus,**
         and **H. influenzae** at least **2 weeks before** elective
         splenectomy or 2 weeks after a traumatic splenectomy
      Booster immunization every 3 years for **pneumococcal vaccine**
      They also need an annual **influenza virus immunization**
      Prophylactic Augmentin for children aged < 10 for 6 months (take
         every day)
      Explain to parents they need to bring child to ED for any **fever**.
      Early broad-spectrum I.V. abx's for suspected infection
      These pts need **abx prophylaxis** for **dental procedures**

Small bowel

459. All of the following are true except:
   a. The 1st branch off the superior mesenteric artery (SMA) is the inferior pancreatico-duodenal artery
   b. The division between the 3rd and 4th portions of duodenum is the SMA
   c. The 2nd and 3rd portions of the duodenum are retroperitoneal
   d. The 3rd portion of the duodenum contains the Ampulla of Vater

   Answer d. The 2nd portion of the duodenum contains the Ampulla of Vater.

460. **All of the following are true except:
   a. Brunner's glands secrete alkaline solution
   b. Goblet cells secrete mucus solution
   c. Diarrhea in Carcinoid Syndrome is from serotonin
   d. 5-HIAA is the most sensitive test for detecting carcinoid tumors

   Answer a. **Brunner's glands** *are found in the duodenum and secrete* *alkaline solution to serve as a protective barrier to acid coming from the stomach. The jejunum lacks Brunner's glands, which is reason **marginal ulcers** occur after roux-en-Y gastro-jejunostomy with a long afferent limb.*

   Goblet cells *secrete* **mucus**
   *Serotonin released from carcinoid tumors can cause **diarrhea**.*
   *Chromogranin A is the most sensitive test for **detection** of carcinoid tumors (almost 100% have it) but it would not give location*

461. *A pt undergoes resection of a small bowel carcinoid and an isolated liver met. Two years later she develops vague abdominal complaints but you cannot identify any new lesions on CT scan. The best study to *localize* recurrent carcinoid tumor is:
   a. HIDA scan
   b. MIBG scan
   c. Octreotide scan
   d. MRI

   Answer c. *Octreotide scan* is the most sensitive diagnostic test for localizing a **carcinoid tumor** not apparent on CT scan.

462. **All of the following are true of carcinoid tumors except:
   a. The site with the highest malignant potential is the ileum
   b. Octreotide is very effective Tx for metastatic carcinoid tumors
   c. Chromogranin A is the most sensitive test for detecting carcinoid tumors (essentially 100% have this)
   d. The 5-YS for carcinoid tumor w/ metastases is 5%

   Answer d. The 5-YS for **carcinoid tumor w/ mets** is 30%. Palliation is an important part of Tx for these pts (can survive a long time). **Octreotide** *is very effective for Tx of Carcinoid Syndrome Sx's*

463. *You perform an appendectomy on a 25 yo man for presumed appendicitis and find a 1 cm tumor at the tip of the appendix. Pathology comes back on the tumor as carcinoid. The most appropriate next step in management is:
   a. Right hemicolectomy
   b. Close
   c. XRT post-op
   d. Chemotherapy post-op

   Answer b. (see below)

464. *You operate on a 25 yo man for presumed appendicitis based on CT scan and find a 2.5 cm tumor at the tip of the appendix. Pathology comes back on the tumor as carcinoid. The most appropriate next step in management is:
   a. Right hemicolectomy
   b. Close
   c. XRT post-op
   d. Chemotherapy post-op

   Answer a. Appendectomy is adequate treatment for **carcinoid tumors** localized to the appendix as long as they are < 2 cm, not at the base, and there is no evidence of mesenteric lymph node invasion or metastatic disease. If above criteria not met, perform right hemi-colectomy. Carcinoid tumors have the best 5-YS (85%) of all appendiceal malignancies.

465. **All of the following are true of rectal carcinoid except:
   a. Carcinoid syndrome is common with rectal carcinoids
   b. For patients with rectal carcinoids > 2 cm, 70% have metastases
   c. Small (< 2 cm) low rectal carcinoids can undergo local excision
   d. Muscularis propria invasion requires formal resection

   Answer a. Carcinoid syndrome is infrequent w/ **rectal carcinoids.**

   ***Small** (< 2 cm) low rectal carcinoids can undergo local excision.*
   ***Large** (> 2 cm) low rectal carcinoids require formal resection (eg APR)*

466. **A pt has a localized adenocarcinoma confined to the junction of the 3rd and 4th portions of the duodenum. Which of the following is most appropriate for this pt:
   a. Pancreatico-duodenectomy
   b. Distal pancreatectomy and duodenal resection
   c. Duodenal resection with duodenal-jejunal anastomosis
   d. Duodenal resection and splenectomy

   Answer c. **The best option for **distal duodenal CA** is to remove the 3rd and 4th portions of the duodenum* and perform duodenal to jejunal anastomosis (not perform a Whipple). Take the duodenum all the way past the ligament of Treitz.

   Adenocarcinoma in the 1st and 2nd portions of the duodenum usually requires Whipple (high likelihood the Ampulla is involved)

467. *All of the following are true of small bowel tumors except:
   a. Adenocarcinoma is the MC malignant small bowel tumor, with a high proportion arising from the duodenum (40%)
   b. The duodenum is the MC location for small bowel adenomas
   c. Ampullary villous adenomas rarely harbor occult CA
   d. Obstructive jaundice with heme positive stools is classic for ampullary villous adenoma (or carcinoma)

   Answer c. Up to 70% of **ampullary villous adenomas** have CA in them.

468. *All of the following are true of lymphoma except:
   a. Isolated small bowel lymphoma _outside_ the 1st and 2nd portions of the duodenum is generally resected
   b. Isolated pancreatic lymphoma usually requires Whipple
   c. The MC small bowel site for lymphoma is the ileum
   d. B cell is the MC type of lymphoma

   Answer b. *Isolated **pancreatic lymphoma** should undergo chemo ± XRT*

469. *All of the following are true of a mucocele of the appendix except:
    a.   Benign lesions can be left alone
    b.   Pseudomyxoma perotonei is the most dreaded complication
    c.   These may have malignant or benign etiologies
    d.   MCC of death w/ pseudomyxoma peritonei is small bowel obstruction

    Answer a. Benign **mucoceles of the appendix** should undergo
    appendectomy. Mucoceles of the appendix can arise from either a
    retention cyst, mucosal hyperplasia, cystadenoma, or cystadenocarcinoma.
    The mucocele fills w/ mucoid material and can eventually rupture.

    The central issue here is that **endothelial cells** within the mucocele
    (regardless of benign or malignant etiology) can form implants on
    peritoneal surfaces. These implants can grow, release mucoid material,
    form more implants, ect. and eventually cause **bowel obstruction** in a
    process known as *pseudomyxoma peritonei.* **The MCC of death in
    these patients is **small bowel obstruction**.

    Because of this, all mucoceles should be resected. Most encourage open
    procedures with discovery of a mucocele. *You want to avoid spillage of
    the mucocele's contents to prevent implants.* If cystadenocarcinoma is
    found, **right hemi-colectomy** is indicated. Pseudomyxoma peritonei can
    be caused by other mucin secreting tumors (eg Ovarian Mucinous CA)

470. **All of the following are true of intussusception in adults except:
    a.   Most commonly there is a malignant lead point
    b.   Barium reduction should be performed
    c.   The MC scenario in adults is the ileum going into the right colon
    d.   Cecal adenocarcinoma is the MC lead point in adults

    Answer b. **Barium enema reduction is not indicated for **adult
    intussusception**. **The MC adult scenario is a **cecal adenocarcinoma**
    forms the lead point and peristalsis takes the tumor and ileum into right
    colon, forming intussusception.*

471. *Concerning short gut syndrome, all of the following are true except:
    a.   This is a clinical diagnosis of inability to absorb enough water and
          nutritional elements to be off TPN
    b.   The length of bowel in general needs to be at least 75 cm if there is
          no ileo-cecal valve
    c.   The length of bowel in general needs to be at least 50 cm if the ileo-
          cecal valve is present
    d.   High fat diets can help with the syndrome

    Answer d. Short gut syndrome is a clinical diagnosis of inability to
    maintain appropriate hydration and nutrition without the use of TPN. High
    fat diets will worsen short bowel syndrome.

472. *You perform laparoscopy on a 25 yo man for presumed appendicitis and find
    terminal ileitis with edematous mesentery, lymphadenopathy and mesenteric fat
    wrapping (creeping fat). The cecum is not involved. The ileitis area is non-
    obstructing. The most appropriate next step in management is:
    a.   Appendectomy
    b.   Close
    c.   Place a drain
    d.   Ileal resection

    Answer a. Pts w/ **presumed appendicitis** but instead have terminal ileitis
    not involving the cecum should undergo appendectomy so that confusion of
    ileitis with appendicitis will not occur in the future.

473. **A 70 yo man presents w/ a 7 day history of RLQ pain, WBCs 16 with a left shift, and a mild fever. He has mild localized tenderness in his RLQ but no gross peritonitis. Abd CT shows a phlegmon near the cecum and you cannot identify an appendix. All of the following are true in this pts management except:
    a. He should be started on IV antibiotics and bowel rest
    b. If an abscess is identified, it should be drained percutaneously
    c. This patient should undergo emergent surgery
    d. Symptoms can be minimal in this population

Answer c. **Perforated appendicitis** with *delayed presentation* and *subsequent phlegmon formation* is MC in the elderly who can have reduced sx's from appendicitis. **Surgery at this time point (well after the time of rupture) has a high Cx rate and should be avoided.

These pts should be placed on antibiotics and bowel rest. If an **abscess** is identified, **percutaneous drainage** should be performed. An **interval appendectomy** is performed in 6-8 weeks when the pt recovers. Occasionally, what was thought to be ruptured appendicitis turns out to be a **perforated cecal colon CA**.

Small Bowel Anatomy and Physiology
Duodenum
Bulb (1st portion) – 90% of ulcers here; more distal think gastrinoma
Descending (2nd) – contains Ampulla of Vater
Transverse (3rd) – overlies the SMA and SMV
Ascending (4th) – distal portion held in place by ligament of Treitz
Vascular supply
Superior pancreaticoduodenal artery (anterior and posterior branches) - off gastroduodenal artery
Inferior pancreaticoduodenal artery (anterior and posterior branches) - off SMA (***1st branch of the SMA***)
Many communications between these artery systems
SMA eventually becomes **ileocolic artery**
Anatomical features
2nd and 3rd portions of duodenum are **retroperitoneal**
3rd to 4th portions **transition point** is the acute angle between the aorta (posterior) and SMA (anterior)
Jejunum - apx 100 cm long, long vasa recta off SMA, circular muscle folds
Maximum site of all absorption except:
Iron (*duodenum*) – have both **heme** and **Fe transporters**
Calcium (*duodenum*)
Bile acids (*ileum* – non-conjugated; *terminal ileum* – conjugated)
B$_{12}$ (*terminal ileum*)
Folate (*terminal ileum*)
95% of all **NaCl + water** absorbed in **jejunum** (maximum site)
Ileum - apx 50 cm long, short vasa recta coming off SMA, flat appearance
Normal bowel sizes: Small bowel (3 cm), Transverse colon (6 cm), Cecum (9 cm)

Migrating motor complex (MMC, gut motility)
Phase I – rest
Phase II – acceleration and gallbladder contraction
Phase III – **peristalsis*
Phase IV – deceleration
Motilin is most important hormone in migrating motor complex *(initiates phase III peristalsis)*

Intestinal brush border – microvilli, **intra-membrane enzymes** break down **carbohydrates** (eg maltase, sucrase) and allow absorption

Cell types

Enterocytes (simple columnar cells) – absorptive cells
Goblet cells – secrete **mucus (Mucin); protective layer
Brunner's glands (in duodenum) – secrete **alkaline solution;
  protects duodenum from acid, lubricates, creates alkaline
  environment for **activation of enzymes**
  jejunum _lacks_ Brunner's glands – reason **marginal ulcers
    occur after gastro-jejunostomy
**Peyer's patches (GALT; gut associated lymphoid tissue)
IgA – produced from mucosal linings and released in lumen
Paneth cells – host defense against microbes
Enteroendocrine cells – many types; endocrine function on gut
Enterochromaffin cells (APUD, carcinoid precursor) – release
  serotonin (5-HT) impt. for gut secretion, peristalsis, nausea

Bowel Obstruction

Sx's: N/V, crampy abd pain, previous surgery or XRT
  If still **passing gas** – partial bowel obstruction
  Fever – need to worry about perforation
  Look for **hernias** and **rectal mass**; guaiac stools
Abd/pelvic CT scan - air-fluid levels, distended loops of bowel, distal
  decompression; if **previous CA** → need CT to R/O recurrence
Path - **3rd spacing of fluid** into bowel lumen (give volume resuscitation)
  Air w/ bowel obstruction is from **swallowed nitrogen**
MCC _without_ previous surgery
  Small bowel – hernia
  Large bowel – cancer
MCC w/ previous surgery
  Small bowel – adhesions (by far the MCC)
  Large bowel – cancer
Tx: NGT to decompress, IVF's (need volume resuscitation w/ obstruction),
  bowel rest, correct electrolytes (esp K and Mg); serial exams and X-
  rays → cures 80% of partial, 20% of complete SBO
Surgical indications: non-reducible hernia (inguinal or ventral),
  progressing pain, peritoneal signs, fever, high WBCs, failure to
  resolve (3-5 days)

**Carcinoid Tumors (AKA neuroendocrine tumor, NET)

Sx's:
  Abd pain (often mistaken for appendicitis), possible **SBO**
  Pain from **mass** or **vasoconstriction + fibrosis** (desmoplastic rxn)
  Carcinoid syndrome (10%) – intermittent **facial flushing** and
    diarrhea (_hallmark sx's,_ from **liver mets** that bypass
    metabolism) ± hypotension, bronchoconstriction
Dx: **Abd CT**
  *Octreotide scan (_best test_ for localization)
    *Highest sensitivity for *localizing tumor
  *Chromogranin A serum level (glycoprotein, _100%_ have this)
    *Highest sensitivity for *detecting tumor
  Urine 5-HIAA (from serotonin breakdown, _not all have it._)
    False positive 5-HIAA – fruits
Path
  Kulchitsky cells (neural crest cells, neuroendocrine)
    Part of amine precursor uptake decarboxylase system (APUD)
    Serotonin → diarrhea
    Kallikrein → facial flushing
    Bradykinin → hypotension, bronchoconstriction
  *MC site – appendix (50% of all carcinoids, only 2% malignant)
  *Site w/ highest mets + highest Carcinoid Syndrome rate – ileum
    (35% malignant, 20% Carcinoid Syndrome)
Tx: **Carcinoid in appendix**

> < 2 cm, base and meso-appendix not involved, <u>no</u> nodes / mets
> → **appendectomy**
>
> ≥ 2 cm, involved base or mesoappendix, positive nodes or mets
> → **right hemicolectomy**

Carcinoid elsewhere in GI tract (<u>except</u> rectal) – majority Tx like CA
(segmental resection w/ lymphadenectomy)

Debulking – good for palliation if suffering from carcinoid syndrome

If liver met resection is performed, also perform **cholecystectomy** for
future **hepatic arterial embolization** of symptomatic mets

**Octreotide – <u>very useful</u> for Tx of carcinoid syndrome sx's

Overall 5-YS – 85%

**5 -YS w/ mets – 30%; Palliation important part of Tx (can survive
long time). ****Octreotide** is very effective for sx's

**<u>Colon and Rectum Carcinoids</u>

15% of all carcinoids; infrequent carcinoid syndrome

Metastases related to tumor size:<1 cm (rare), 1-2 cm (10%), >2 cm (70%)

**Low rectal carcinoids

> < **2 cm** → WLE with negative margins
>
> > **2 cm** <u>or</u> invasion of **muscularis propria** → APR

Colon or higher rectal carcinoids – can't reach w/ trans-anal

> < **1 cm** → endoscopic removal
>
> ≥ **1 cm** <u>or</u> invasion of **muscularis propria** → appropriate
> segmental resection w/ adenectomy

<u>Rectal carcinoids</u> are more common than colon and have better prognosis

*<u>Benign small bowel tumors</u> (rare)

Benign are more common than malignant

MC benign small bowel tumor – adenoma (can become CA)

> MC in **Duodenum Ampulla**

**Ampullary villous adenoma (can become CA, pre-malignant)

> Villous adenoma in the Ampulla of Vater
>
> Sx's: ****obstructive jaundice and heme positive stools** (classic)
> can cause pancreatitis
>
> Dx: Get ERCP w/ Bx's to truly define lesion
> > High **false negative rate** w/ Bx (ie Bx misses CA harboring in
> > adenoma) – up to 70% have CA in them at path
>
> Tx: **WLE** - will likely end up doing **sphincteroplasty** or **ductoplasty**
> after resection of benign tumor
> > Send for frozen section to confirm benign (Whipple if malignant)
> > ****Do <u>not</u> perform Whipple if benign**

**<u>Malignant small bowel tumors</u> (all rare)

Adenocarcinoma (40%)

> **MC malignant small bowel tumor**
>
> High proportion in **duodenum** (40%) w/ 70% of those in 2nd portion
> > Usually originate in Ampulla (**ampullary adenocarcinoma**)
> > from previous villous adenoma
> >
> > RFs for Duodenal CA – FAP, Gardner's, polyps, adenomas
>
> Sx's: obstruction, jaundice, heme positive stools
>
> Tx: Resection and adenectomy if resectable
> > ****Duodenal adenocarcinoma**
> > > *If in **1st or 2nd portions** of duodenum – need **Whipple**
> > > (high likelihood **Ampulla** is involved)
> > >
> > > **If in **3rd or 4th portions** of duodenum – resection w/
> > > **duodeno-jejunal anastomosis** (<u>Not</u> Whipple)

*Lymphoma
> **Small bowel lymphoma**
>> ***MC site** – <u>ileum</u> (↑ed lymphoid tissue - Peyer's Patches)
>> ***MC type** – <u>B cell</u>
>> **Post-TXP lymphoma** – ↑ risk of bleeding, perforation
>> Sx's - obstruction
>> RFs - SLE, AIDS, Crohn's, post-TXP
>> Dx:: abd CT, UGI w/ SBFT, node sampling
>> Tx : **wide en bloc resection** w/ negative margins, mesenteric + para-
>>> aortic lymph node sampling outside zone of resection, liver Bx

> **Tx for lymphoma <u>isolated</u> to a specific area:**
>> 1) **1st and 2nd portions of duodenum** - chemo ± XRT *(No Whipple)*
>>> If 3rd or 4th portion of duodenum - resection
>> 2) **Ileum and Jejunum** – wide en bloc resection (include nodes), then
>>> chemo ± XRT
>> 3) **Colon lymphoma** (MC cecum) – wide en bloc resection (include
>>> nodes), then chemo ± XRT
>> 4) **Anal lymphoma** (↑ w/ AIDS) – chemo ± XRT
>> 5) **Pancreatic lymphoma** – chemo ± XRT
>> 6) **Gastric lymphoma** – surgery only for stage I, o/w chemo ± XRT
>> 7) **Splenic lymphoma** (marginal zone lymphoma) - splenectomy,
>>> chemo, or watchful waiting
>> 8) **Thyroid lymphoma** – chemo ± XRT

**_Intussusception in adults_
> Worrisome for **CA** in adults (70% have **malignant lead point**, eg cecal
>> CA); can occur w/ small bowel or cecal tumors
> ****MCC in adults** – *adenocarcinoma of the cecum*
> Do **not** reduce w/ barium enema in adults → go to OR for resection
> Tx: OR for manual reduction, resection of lead point + compromised bowel

<u>**Short Bowel Syndrome**</u> (short gut syndrome)
> Inability to absorb enough water and nutritional elements to be off TPN
> Dx is made on sx's, not length of bowel
> Sx's: diarrhea, steatorrhea, weight loss, nutritional deficiency (lose fat, B-
>> 12, electrolytes, water), abd pain
> Dx: **Sudan red stool stain** – checks for **fecal fat**
>> **Schilling test** – checks for B-12 absorption (**radio-labeled B-12**
>>> released in **urine** after absorption)
>> In general, probably need at least 75 cm without ileo-cecal valve and
>>> 50 cm with competent ileo-cecal valve to survive off TPN
> Tx: **H2 blockers** (to reduce gastric acid secretion)
>> **Octreotide** (to reduce GI secretions)
>> **Loperamide** (to slow gut motility)
>> **Pancrealipase** (helps fat absorption)
>> **Restrict fat** (prevent steatorrhea)
>> **Lactase** (improve carbohydrate absorption)
>> **TPN for acute episodes** (chronic TPN leads to cirrhosis)
>> Consider **small bowel transplant** for refractory cases
> **Hyper-secretion of acid** with short bowel → ↓ pH → ↑intestinal motility;
>> interferes w/ fat absorption → steatorrhea
> **Interruption of bile salt resorption** (if terminal ileum gone) interferes with
>> micelle formation and causes steatorrhea

Appendicitis

Sx's: **1st** anorexia, **2nd** abd pain (peri-umbilical), **3rd** vomiting
Pain gradually migrates to **RLQ** as peritonitis sets in.
CT scan – diameter **> 7 mm** or wall thickness **> 2 mm** (looks like a bull's eye), fat stranding, no contrast in appendiceal lumen
MC area to perforate – midpoint of anti-mesenteric border
MCC in children – lymph node hyperplasia (can follow a viral illness)
MCC in adults – fecalith
Luminal obstruction followed by (in order): distention of appendix, venous congestion and thrombosis, ischemia, gangrene necrosis, and rupture

Delayed presentation of perforated appendicitis
Days after initial pain episode
MC in the **elderly** who can have minimal sx's
CT scan shows **walled-off perforated appendix** (phlegmon)
Tx: Abx's and bowel rest (is a non-operative situation)
Percutaneous drainage if abscess present
Interval appendectomy electively (6-8 wks) as long as sx's improving
F/U colonoscopy to R/O perforated cecal CA

Children and elderly
Higher propensity to **rupture** secondary to delayed diagnosis
Children often have **higher fever** + more **vomiting / diarrhea**
Elderly – sx's can be minimal
Appendicitis is rare in infants
Pregnancy – uterus displaces appendix cephalad (can have RUQ pain)
Perforation – pt generally more ill; can have evidence of sepsis
Fever or abd pain after appendectomy - Abd CT, look for abscess
Abscess → percutaneous drainage

Regional Terminal Ileitis – mimics appendicitis (RLQ pain)
1) enlarged mesenteric LN's
2) symmetric inflammation and thickening of **terminal ileum** and **cecum**
Use above to differentiate regional ileitis vs. appendicitis
Infections causing ileitis – yersinia, campylobacter, salmonella
5% is actually early **Crohn's Disease**

Yersinia infection – mimics appendicitis
Sx's: fever, RLQ abd pain, N/V, diarrhea, no peritoneal signs
MC in **children**
Infection causes **mesenteric lymphadenitis**
Comes from contaminated food (feces/urine)
CT scan shows *enlarged lymph nodes and inflamed ileum* (differentiates from appendicitis)
Tx: tetracycline or Bactrim

Gastroenteritis – N/V, diarrhea
Presumed appendicitis but find ruptured ovarian cyst, endometriosis, *thrombosed ovarian vein*, or *regional terminal ileitis* not involving cecum → **still perform appendectomy** (as long as base of appendix at cecum is not involved)
Appendix cystadenoma – Tx appendectomy only if completely excised
Appendix cystadenocarcinoma – Tx right hemicolectomy

Colon and Rectum

474. *All of the following are true except:
   a.   The internal anal sphincter is under internal pudendal nerve control (voluntary)
   b.   The main nutrient to colonocytes is short chain fatty acids
   c.   The rectal lateral stalks contain the middle rectal arteries
   d.   The inferior rectal artery is supplied by branches of internal iliac artery

   Answer a. *The **internal anal sphincter** is supplied by the pelvic splanchnic nerves, not the pudendal nerve. There is no voluntary control of the internal anal sphincter.*

475. *For patients with UC, all of the following improve after colectomy except:
   a.   Ocular problems
   b.   Arthritis
   c.   Anemia
   d.   Ankylosing Spondylitis

   Answer d. Primary sclerosing cholangitis and ankylosing spondylitis do not get better after colectomy

476. *All of the following are true of ulcerative colitis (UC) except:
   a.   The MC extra-intestinal manifestation requiring colectomy is failure to thrive
   b.   The MC indication for pouch takedown with permanent ileostomy (ie APR) is incontinence
   c.   Steroids are the best therapy for acute exacerbations
   d.   Low grade dysplasia can be followed

   Answer d. *Any dysplasia w/ UC is indication for **procto-colectomy**.*

477. *All of the following are indications for procto-colectomy in pts w/ UC except:
   a.   Toxic megacolon worsening after 72 hours of IV steroids + antibiotics
   b.   Perforation
   c.   Isolated ulcerative proctitis for 20 years
   d.   Low grade dysplasia on biopsy

   Answer c. *Isolated ulcerative proctitis* does not have increased CA risk and should not undergo prophylactic colectomy.

478. **A 35 yo woman with Crohn's disease is started on Infliximab and flagyl for a peri-anal fistula. All of the following are true of Infliximab therapy except:
   a.   The MC serious infection in pts taking Infliximab is tuberculosis
   b.   Aggressive surgical resection is indicated for peri-anal fistulas from Crohn's disease
   c.   Isoniazid is indicated for patients with a positive PPD
   d.   Long term Flagyl is associated w/ peripheral neuropathy

   Answer b. Conservative Tx in indicated for Crohn's peri-anal fistulas.
   ***Tuberculosis** has been the MC serious infection in pts w/ **Infliximab** (anti-TNF Ab). Pts w/ a positive PPD should get Isoniazid while on Infliximab.
   Long term Flagyl is associated w/ **peripheral neuropathy.**

479. **All of the following are true of Crohn's disease except
   a.   Refractory strictures involving the 3rd and 4th portions of the duodenum would likely benefit best from resection and duodeno-jejunostomy
   b.   Short strictures in the jejunum and ileum can be treated w/ stricturoplasty to avoid resection and conserve bowel

c. A Whipple is likely the best treatment for strictures in the 1st and 2nd portions of the duodenum
d. Pts undergoing gastro-jejunostomy are susceptible to marginal ulcers

Answer c. Duodenal Crohn's disease is unusual. ***Tx for refractory strictures in the 1st and 2nd portions is **gastro-jejunostomy + vagotomy** (no Whipple; also can't really perform stricturoplasty here). Some type of vagotomy is needed to avoid **marginal ulcers.***

***For refractory strictures in the 3rd and 4th portions of the duodenum, resection and **duodeno-jejunostomy** is usually indicated.*
*****Short strictures** in the jejunum and ileum can be treated w/ **stricturoplasty** to avoid resection and conserve bowel*

480. ***A 60 yo man undergoes open cholecystectomy for cholecystitis and requires increased narcotics to control pain. Five days later, he develops abd distension and pain. Plain film shows a distended colon that is 10 cm at the cecum. You start IVF's, place an NGT, stop narcotics and keep the pt NPO, however the distension continues. The most appropriate next step in this pt is:
    a. Cecostomy
    b. Colectomy
    c. Neostigmine
    d. Nothing

    Answer c. *****Neostigmine** is effective for **Ogilvie's Syndrome**. If that fails or if the cecum is > 12 cm, **decompressive colonoscopy** is indicated.*

481. ***A 75 yo woman from a nursing home with long-term constipation requiring laxatives presents with abdominal pain and distension. You get a plain film and the colon is very distended and looks like an 'ace of spades' or 'bent inner tube' pointing to the RUQ. She does not have peritoneal signs. You start IV fluid hydration. The most appropriate next step in management is:
    a. Colonoscopy
    b. Low anterior resection (LAR)
    c. Abdominoperineal resection (APR)
    d. Do nothing

    Answer a. Given the scenario, this pt most likely has a **sigmoid volvulus**. Colonoscopy will decompress 80% of these patients. ***After decompression, a **bowel prep** should be given followed by **sigmoid resection** during the <u>same hospital admission</u>.*

482. ***In an average male patient, the most distal extent of a rectal cancer which still allows for a low anterior resection with an appropriate margin is:
    a. 8 cm from the proximal anal canal
    b. 6 cm from the proximal anal canal
    c. 4 cm from the proximal anal canal
    d. 2 cm from the proximal anal canal

    Answer d. ***The most distal rectal tumor extent which would still allow a 2 cm margin is about 2 **cm from the proximal anal canal**. You need a 2 cm rectal cuff above the anal canal which will be resected with the end to end stapler (send the donut in stapler to path as this is part of your margin). In general, it is easier to perform LAR in women compared to men because their pelvic bones are wider.*

    *****Rectal tumors** that are **T3** or **T4** or have **positive nodes** should undergo neoadjuvant **chemo-XRT** before resection.*
    T1 or T2 tumors w/ **negative nodes** can just undergo resection

483. **A 60 yo man undergoes LAR for sigmoid adenocarcinoma. The final path report states the tumor invaded the muscularis propria and there was tumor in 2 mesenteric lymph nodes. What is the pathologic TNM classification for this CA?
   a.   T1, N0, MO
   b.   T1, N1, MO
   c.   T2, N0, M0
   d.   T2, N1, M0

   Answer d. **Invasion of the *muscularis propria* makes it T2.
   Involvement of 2 nodes makes it N1. The pts CA is T2N1M0, stage III

484. **For the above question, following resection what is the appropriate next step:
   a.   5-FU, Leucovorin, and oxaliplatin
   b.   5-FU, Leucovorin, and oxaliplatin plus XRT
   c.   XRT
   d.   Nothing

   Answer a. **Because there was nodal involvement, this patient is stage III
   and needs chemotherapy (**leucovorin, 5-FU, and oxaliplatin** - FOLFOX).
   XRT is not indicated for colon CA (unlike some rectal CA's)

485. *Ten days after a LAR, your pt develops fever, a white blood cell count of 19,000, and mild abdominal tenderness. Your order a CT scan of the abdomen and pelvis which shows an 8 x 8 cm fluid collection near your anastomosis. The next appropriate step is:
   a.   Re-exploration and repair of the leak at the anastomosis
   b.   Percutaneous drainage
   c.   Abdominoperineal resection
   d.   Takedown of the anastomosis with placement of colostomy and Hartman's pouch

   Answer b. This pt most likely has a leak from his anastomosis and subsequent **abscess** formation. **Percutaneous drainage** is the most appropriate Tx.

486. *A 30 yo man w/ a thickened sigmoid and diverticula presents w/ recurrent urinary tract infections and pneumaturia. The best test for the likely diagnosis is:
   a.   CT scan
   b.   MRI
   c.   cystoscopy
   d.   colonoscopy

   Answer c. Cystoscopy is the best test for **colo-vesicle fistula.**

487. **All of the following are true of colo-rectal CA w/ mets to the liver except
   a.   The most accurate way of identifying liver mets intra-op is U/S
   b.   Mets to segments I and II likely requires left lobectomy and caudate resection
   c.   5 year survival for resectable liver mets is about 35%
   d.   Four liver mets is considered unresectable

   Answer d Number of mets does not influence resection as long as all of the lesions are completely resectable and you leave adequate liver reserve.

**Resectable liver mets pre-op
   Resect if completely resectable and leaves adequate liver function (need 1 cm margin) - number of tumors, size, and location are not factors if you can get complete resection (even bi-lobar lesions)
   Wedge vs. **formal resection** depends on location, number, liver reserve
   Mets to segments 1 and 2 → need **left hepatic lobectomy + caudate resection (if sufficient liver reserve)

265

The most accurate way of identifying **liver mets intra-op is U/S*

488. **A 55 yo man is undergoing a colectomy for adenocarcinoma. When you enter the abdomen, the tumor appears to be invading about 0.5 cm into the duodenum. The best management would be:
    a.   Right hemicolectomy only and leave the duodenal component
    b.   En bloc right hemicolectomy including the portion of the cancer invading the duodenum (even if Whipple is necessary)
    c.   Wedge the duodenum lesion out only
    d.   close

    Answer b. ***Direct invasion of another structure requires **en bloc** resection, even if you have to perform a Whipple to get en bloc resection.*

489. **All of the following are true except:
    a.   The MC location for colon cancer is the sigmoid colon
    b.   TRUS is the best method for assessing T and N status of rectal tumors
    c.   CEA is useful for screening for colon CA
    d.   CEA is useful to detect colon CA recurrence and for following response to Tx

    Answer c. ***CEA has not been useful for colon CA screening. **TRUS is the best method for assessing T and N status of rectal tumors. *The MC location for colon CA is the **sigmoid colon***

490. *A 55 yo man undergoes LAR for a low rectal CA now returns to clinic 6 months later w/ constipation. You perform anoscopy in the office and notice a mass at the previous suture line. Biopsies show adenocarcinoma. After a metastatic disease work-up, the next appropriate step is:
    a.   Local resection
    b.   Chemotherapy w/ Leucovorin
    c.   5000 rads of XRT
    d.   Abdominoperineal resection (APR)

    Answer d. **Recurrence at the suture line following LAR demands APR unless the pt has mets that would preclude surgery. You should re-stage pts w recurrences (Abd/Pelvic CT, CXR, LFT's, and CEA).*

491. **A 50 yo man undergoes neo-adjuvant chemo-XRT followed by LAR for rectal CA. Six months later he has severe bleeding from his rectum. He has required several transfusions. All of the following are true except:
    a.   Proctoscopy is the initial diagnostic method of choice in this pt
    b.   APR is likely needed for radiation proctitis
    c.   Formalin fixation of the rectum is for the best Tx radiation proctitis
    d.   Recurrent rectal CA should be considered

    Answer b. *You should avoid APR for bleeding from late radiation proctitis. **Formalin fixation of the rectum usually suffices.*

492. **An 85 yo man has an extensive rectal villous adenoma w/ atypia. All of the following are true except:
    a.   Trans-anal excision of the tumor is indicated
    b.   Abdominal perineal resection (APR) is indicated if the adenoma cannot be completely resected
    c.   A T1 CA area w/ 2-3 mm margins on pathology after resection requires no further Tx
    d.   Well differentiated T1 lesions have a better prognosis

Answer b. ***APR is <u>not</u> indicated for low rectal villous adenomas with atypia. Trans-anal excision of the tumor is indicated. **A T1 CA area w/ 2-3 mm margins on pathology after resection requires no further Tx.*

493. **All of the following are true of FAP except:
     a. Patients w/ FAP have polyps present at birth
     b. Late diagnosis of FAP in a 30 yo requires total colonoscopy, EGD to R/O adenocarcinoma and CT scan to look for desmoids tumors
     c. Desmoid tumors incorporating the mesentery should not be resected
     d. In pts who have undergone total procto-colectomy for FAP, the MCC of death is duodenal CA

     Answer a. Pts w/ **FAP** have polyps that develop in **puberty**. ***Total procto-colectomy is indicated at age 20.*

     **Late diagnosis of FAP requires total colonoscopy and EGD to R/O CA, followed by total procto-colectomy (also CT scan to R/O desmoid tumors).

     Patients with FAP can develop **duodenal polyps** (usually peri-ampullary) which should be removed as they have malignant potential. ***Following colectomy, **peri-ampullary duodenal CA** is the MCC of death with FAP.*

     ***Desmoid tumors (eg mesenteric mass) also occur in pts w/ FAP. If significantly involving the mesentery, resection is <u>not</u> indicated do to the high incidence of **short bowel syndrome** following resection and **high recurrence rate**. Tx: **Sulindac + Tamoxifen** if not easily resectable*

494. **All of the following are true of hereditary non-polyposis colon cancer syndrome (HNPCC, Lynch Syndrome) except (Amsterdam criteria):
     a. Needs to be in 3 primary relatives, over 2 generations, with one person being less than 50 at the time of diagnosis of cancer
     b. Colon cancers are right sided predominant
     c. Ovarian, breast and stomach cancer can also occur in these patients
     d. The patients have thousands of polyps

     Answer d. ***These pts do <u>not</u> form thousands of polyps like FAP. HNPCC involves a defect in **mismatch repair genes (hMSH2, hMLH1, hPMS1, hPMS2). **Colon CA's are **right sided predominant** (eg cecal) w/ HNPCC.*

495. **All of the following are true of Peutz-Jeghers except:
     a. Prophylactic colectomy in indicated
     b. These pts are at higher risk of extra-intestinal malignancies
     c. The MC CA in these pts is Breast CA
     d. These pts form GI tract hamartomatous polyps

     Answer a. ***Prophylactic colectomy is <u>not</u> indicated for Peutz-Jeghers.*
     These pts are at higher risk of **extra-intestinal malignancies
     The MC CA in these pts is **Breast CA
     These pts form **GI tract hamartomatous polyps

496. **After a sigmoid resection for diverticulitis, the colostomy stoma appears dark. The most appropriate next step is:
     a. Heparin
     b. tPA
     c. Reoperation and revise
     d. Nitropaste

     Answer c. ***Reoperation and revise.* It is very likely that the stoma is being compressed by fascia, has a twist, or has been too devascularized.

Anatomy and Physiology

Colon secretes **K⁺** and reabsorbs **Na⁺** and **water** (mostly right colon and cecum)

Layers - Mucosa (columnar epithelium), Submucosa, Muscularis propria, Serosa

Retroperitoneal portions – ascending, descending, sigmoid colon, and rectum

Peritoneum – covers anterior portions of upper and middle⅓ of rectum

Vascular supply

> **Ascending** and **2/3 of transverse colon** supplied by **superior mesenteric artery** (SMA; eg ileocolic, right colic and middle colic arteries)
>
> > **1/3 transverse, descending colon, sigmoid colon,** and **upper portion of rectum** supplied by **inferior mesenteric artery** (IMA; left colic, sigmoid branches, superior rectal artery)
>
> **Marginal artery** – travels along colon margin, connecting SMA to IMA (provides collateral flow)
>
> **Arc of Riolan** – a short direct connection between SMA and IMA
>
> *Superior rectal artery* – branch of **IMA**
>
> *Middle rectal artery* – branch of **internal iliac** (the *lateral stalks* during LAR or APR contain the middle rectal arteries)
>
> *Inferior rectal artery* – branch of **internal pudendal** (off **internal iliac**)
>
> Rectal arteries = hemorrhoidal arteries
>
> Internal iliac arteries = hypogastric arteries

Watershed areas

> **Splenic flexure** (Griffith's point) – SMA and IMA junction
>
> **Rectum** (Sudeck's point) – superior rectal and middle rectal artery junction
>
> Colon more sensitive to ischemia than small bowel due to **poor collaterals**

Venous drainage

> Generally follows arterial except IMV, which goes to the splenic vein
>
> Splenic vein joins SMV to form portal vein behind neck of pancreas
>
> **Superior** and **middle rectal veins** drain into **IMV** (then **portal vein)**
>
> **Inferior rectal veins** drain into **internal iliac veins** and eventually **inferior vena cava** (can get isolated lung mets w/ low rectal tumors)

Nodal supply

> **Ascending, transverse, descending,** and **sigmoid** follow arterial supply
>
> **Superior** and **middle rectum** – drain to IMA nodes
>
> **Lower rectum** – primarily to IMA nodes, also to internal iliac nodes

External anal sphincter – under _voluntary_ (CNS) control

> The continuation of **puborectalis muscle**
>
> **Inferior rectal** (anal) branch of **internal pudendal nerve** (sympathetic)
>
> The puborectalis is part of the **levator ani muscle group** (striated muscle)

Internal anal sphincter – _involuntary_ control

> The continuation of **muscularis propria** (circular layer, smooth muscle)
>
> Innervation by **pelvic splanchnic nerves** (S2-S4, parasympathetic)
>
> **No pudendal innervation** (No voluntary control, normally contracted)

Distances from anal verge (sigmoidoscopy):

Anal margin (between anal verge and dentate)	0-2 cm
Anal canal (proximal to dentate)	2-5 cm
Rectum	5-15 cm
Recto-sigmoid junction	15-18 cm

Levator ani – marks transition between anal canal and rectum

Short-chain fatty acids – main nutrient of colonocytes

Denonvilliers' fascia (anterior) – Recto-vesicular fascia in men

> Recto-vaginal fascia in women

Waldeyer's fascia (posterior) – recto-sacral fascia

Disuse pouchitis

> **Diversion or disuse proctitis** (eg Hartman's Pouch after sigmoidectomy)
>
> Sx's: grey mucus drainage from pouch (sloughed dead mucosa), urgency
>
> **Tx: short-chain fatty acid enema**

Infectious pouchitis (eg J-pouch or Kock pouch following total colectomy)

> Sx's: purulent drainage, can be bloody; fever
>
> Dx: colonoscopy – erythematous, friable pouch; inflammation
>
> Tx: **cipro + flagyl**; if refractory or severe sepsis may need APR

Ulcerative Colitis (UC)

Inflammation of **colonic mucosa**; involves **colon** and **rectum** only

Bimodal Age of onset – 20's and 60's; increased in **Ashkenazi Jews**

Sx's: **Bloody diarrhea, abd pain, fever,** and **weight loss** *(classic)*

    Toxic megacolon or **toxic colitis** → fever, tachycardia, hypotension, high WBCs, bloating, > 6 bloody BM's/day

    Almost universally involves the *rectum* (exam - bleeding universal)

    Spares anus (unlike Crohn's)

<u>No</u> colonoscopy w/ suspected toxic megacolon / colitis - risk of perforation

Stable UC Tx - <u>5-ASA</u> drugs (eg sulfasalazine), <u>loperamide</u>

    Low residue diet - avoid fiber in cereal, bread, nuts, vegetables

    Avoid chronic prednisone if possible, use for flares

Acute UC flares Tx - <u>Steroids</u> *(best Tx for acute exacerbation)*; Add <u>abx's</u> **(cipro + flagyl)** for fever, ↑ed WBC, or if worried about toxic megacolon or toxic colitis; <u>Infliximab</u>

Surgery - surgery is **curative** for UC, unlike Crohn's

*****Surgical indications:** significant <u>hemorrhage</u>, refractory <u>toxic megacolon</u> or toxic colitis (fails to improve after 72 hrs), persistent <u>obstruction or stricture</u>, *any <u>dysplasia</u> (including low grade)*, <u>CA</u>, <u>failed medical Tx</u> (> 10-12 bloody stools / d), *systemic Cx's* (MC is *****failure to thrive**), failure to wean high dose steroids, perforation (MC- transverse colon)

*****Emergent or urgent surgery** - total procto-colectomy and end ileostomy

    No ileo-anal anastomosis in acute setting

Elective surgery

    Total procto-colectomy, rectal mucosectomy, J-pouch (from ileum), and **ileo-anal anastomosis**; need temporary loop ileostomy (6-8 weeks while pouch heals)

    Pouch <u>not</u> used if severe rectal disease w/ incontinence

    Can also just perform **APR** and **place ileostomy** (want ileostomy output < 500-1000 cc/d; use **loperamide** to slow output)

Ileo-anal anastomosis - **15%** eventually need **takedown** (w/ APR + ileostomy) secondary to: 1) *incontinence (MC reason for takedown)* 2) **CA** or **dysplasia**, 3) refractory **proctitis / sepsis**

Colon CA

    CA risk w/ **pan-colitis** (highest UC risk)

        2% at 10 yrs, 8% at 20 yrs, 18% at 30 yrs from Dx

    CA more evenly distributed throughout colon

    RFs - Left sided colitis, co-existent **primary sclerosing cholangitis**

    *****CA risk is <u>not</u> elevated in pts w/ isolated ulcerative proctitis** (although it can occur and should still undergo surveillance).

    *****Any <u>dysplasia</u>** is an indication for total colectomy

Prophylactic Colectomy – classic teaching is at 10 yrs from Dx; at 20 years, especially in pts w/ *****family Hx** of colon CA, pts diagnosed at a *****young age**, and pts w/ *****primary sclerosing cholangitis**, the case is strong for prophylactic colectomy

Surveillance: start at 8 yrs w/ pan-colitis, 15 yrs w/ isolated left sided colitis

    Any dysplasia – 30% actually have colon CA

Extra-intestinal manifestations:

    *****MC extra-intestinal manifestation requiring total colectomy** – failure to thrive in children

    *****Does <u>not</u> get better w/ colectomy** → primary sclerosing cholangitis, ankylosing spondylitis

    *****Gets better with colectomy** → ocular problems, arthritis, anemia

    50% get better → pyoderma gangrenosum (spreading ulcers w/ violaceous edges), Tx: high dose steroids, Infliximab

    Can get thromboembolic cx's w/ UC (eg DVTs, PEs)

    Associated w/ **HLA B27** – sacroiliitis and ankylosing spondylitis

*****NSAIDs should be <u>avoided</u>** - are not effective treatment for Crohn's or UC and have been implicated in induction of a form of UC.

**Crohn's Disease (CD)
    Transmural inflammation of GI tract w/ **skip lesions**
    Bimodal age distribution - 20's and 60's; RFs - Ashkenazi Jews
    Sx's: Intermittent **abd pain, diarrhea** (not grossly bloody) and **weight loss**
        Toxic megacolon or toxic colitis - fever, tachycardia, ↑WBC, bloat
        Extra-intestinal manifestations - arthritis, pyoderma gangrenosum,
            ocular disease, growth failure, megaloblastic anemia (folate +
            B-12 malabsorption), gallstones, kidney stones
        Anal disease - MC Sx of Crohn's *(*large skin tags)*
        Can occur anywhere from **mouth to anus** (*MC site* - terminal ileum):

Small bowel only	30%
Small bowel and large bowel	50%
Large bowel only	20%
Isolated upper tract	rare

    Stable CD Tx - 5-ASA drugs (eg sulfasalazine), loperamide
        Low residue diet - avoid fiber in cereal, bread, nuts, vegetables
        Avoid chronic prednisone if possible, use for flares
    Fistulas (enterocutaneous, colovesicle, perianal or anorectal-vaginal) -
        Add **Infliximab + flagyl** (effective for healing); conservative Tx best
    Acute flares Tx - Steroids (*best Tx for acute exacerbation*); *Add* **abx's**
        (**cipro + flagyl**) if fever, ↑ WBCs, or if worried about toxic megacolon
        or toxic colitis; can also add **Infliximab**
    **Drug S/Es: **flagyl* – peripheral neuropathy w/ chronic use
                *Infliximab – TB reactivation
    Surgery – unlike UC, Crohn's is not curative
        Segmental resection usual; *exceptions* - refractory toxic megacolon
            / colitis or colon perforation will require **total abdominal**
            colectomy w/ ileostomy
        Surgical indications – obstruction, refractory toxic megacolon /
            colitis, perforation, refractory to medical Tx, CA or dysplasia
    *Fissures - **NO lateral internal sphincteroplasty w/ Crohn's (will not
        heal);* Tx: sitz baths, bulk, lidocaine jelly, stool softeners, NTG cream
    Hemorrhoids or perianal skin tags w/ Crohn's → **NO resection*
    Operative findings of CD - creeping mesenteric fat, strictures, skip lesions
        (segmental disease), transmural involvement, cobble-stoning, fistulas
    Crohn's usually **spares rectum** (unlike UC)
    **NO pouches or ileo-anal anastomosis w/ Crohn's
    **Duodenal Crohn's (get strictures, ulceration, or edema; rare)
        Medical Tx as above, surgery if refractory
        Tx: for **1st + 2nd** portions of duodenum
            1) ****Gastro-jejunostomy + vagotomy** (+ *pyloroplasty*)
                Vagotomy to avoid **marginal ulceration**
                Stricturoplasty not an option in 1st + 2nd portions of duodenum
        Tx: for **3rd + 4th** portions of duodenum
            1) **Resection w/ duodeno-jejunostomy* (usual)
            2) could also do a stricturoplasty if short stricture
        **Do not perform Whipple for duodenal Crohn's
    **Stricturoplasties
        **Used if pt has short strictures to save small bowel length
        Longitudinal incision on anti-mesenteric border; close transversely
        10% leakage / abscess / fistula rate w/ stricturoplasty
    W/ resection, do not need clear margins, just **2 cm from gross disease**
    Cx's after terminal ileum resection (or from **severe terminal ileum
        disease which has become non-functional for absorption)
        1) ↓ed **B-12** and **folate uptake** can result in **megaloblastic anemia**
        2) ↓ed **bile salt uptake** causes osmotic **diarrhea** (bile salts) and
            steatorrhea (↓ fat uptake) in colon
        3) ↓ed **bile salt uptake** can result in the formation of **gallstones**
        4) ↓ed **oxalate binding to Ca** secondary to increased intra-luminal
            fat → oxalate then gets absorbed in colon → released in urine
            → **Ca-oxalate kidney stones** (hyperoxaluria)

CA surveillance for Crohn's:
Pts w/ Crohn's pan-colitis are at same CA risk as UC
Surveillance for Crohn's pan-colitis same as for UC

Ogilvie's syndrome - pseudo-obstruction of the **colon.
RFs - opiates, bed-ridden pts, infections, surgery and trauma
Can get massively dilated colons; small bowel is not dilated *(unlike ileus)*
Rectal exam should reveal an **air-filled rectum**
CT scan should be used to R/O mechanical obstruction if not sure
Tx::
1) R/O true large bowel obstruction and perforation (peritoneal signs)
2) IVF's to replace volume deficit
3) Correct **electrolytes** (K and Mg)
4) **Stop drugs** that slow the gut (eg narcotics)
5) Place a **naso-gastric tube**
6) ****Neostigmine** 2.5 mg IV should be given if the above fails
7) ****Colonoscopy** to decompress the colon if size is **12 cm** or more
or for **failure of medical Tx over 24-48 hours**
8) If colonoscopy fails to decompress, proceed w/ **cecostomy** (or
right hemi-colectomy w/ colostomy and MF if bowel not viable)
Neostigmine (acetylcholinesterase inhibitor) **S/E's:**
Bradycardia - make sure **atropine** should is available.
Contraindicated if cardiac disease (especially bradycardia).
Contraindicated in pts w/ **renal failure**

Ileus
Etiologies - surgery (MC), electrolyte abnormalities (low **K** and low **Mg**),
peritonitis, ischemia, trauma, drugs, pancreatitis
AXR - dilatation is uniform throughout stomach, small bowel, colon, and
rectum w/o decompression
Tx - bowel rest, IVF's, NGT, correct electrolytes, ambulation, limit narcotics

**Sigmoid volvulus
Sigmoid colon folds over on itself, causing closed loop obstruction
RFs: nursing home pts; laxative abuse; high-fiber diets (Iran, Iraq)
Sx's: Pain, distention, obstipation – causes closed loop obstruction
Dx: **Abd/pelvic CT** *(best test)* – shows closed loop obstruction
AXR – Bent inner tube or Ace of Spades sign; point (or line) to RUQ
Gastrografin enema – may show bird's beak sign (tapered colon)
**Tx: **Decompress w/ colonoscopy (80% reduce, 50% recur), then
bowel prep and **resection on same hospital admission**

*Cecal volvulus
Less common than sigmoid volvulus; sx's similar to small bowel obstruction
Dx: **Abd/pelvic CT** *(best test)* – shows closed loop obstruction and dilated
proximal small bowel (can appear as a **small bowel obstruction** w/
dilated cecum in the RLQ)
Tx: **right hemicolectomy** best Tx w/ 1° anastomosis (very hard to detorse)
If frail pt and **incontinent** → consider just colectomy with ileostomy and
mucus fistula (MF) or Hartman's Pouch (HP)

*Diverticulitis
Diverticuli
Herniation of mucosa through sites where arteries enter colon
muscular wall, is a **false diverticula** caused by **straining**
(usually w/ low fiber diet; creates high intra-luminal pressure)
Majority on **left side** (90%) in the sigmoid colon
Diverticulitis is a result of **mucosa perforation** in the diverticulum w/
adjacent fecal contamination (infection and inflammation of colonic
wall and surrounding tissue)
Sx's: LLQ pain, fever, tenderness, constipation; elevated WBCs

Dx: **Abd and Pelvic CT** *(best test)* – bowel wall thickening, fat stranding
    Make sure you see diverticuli on CT scan, if not, most likely CA
    *Need F/U **colonoscopy** after acute phase to R/O **colon CA***
Tx: **Uncomplicated** - IVF's, Abx's (cipro + flagyl), bowel rest 5-7 d
    Complicated Diverticulitis
        Abscess → percutaneous drainage
        Free perforation → OR, resection, colostomy
        Obstruction – conservative Tx and see if it opens up
            If that fails (try 3-5 d) → OR, resection
    *Colo-vesical fistula (MC fistula in men w/ diverticulitis)
        Sx's: fecaluria, pneumaturia → get ***cystoscopy** *(best test)* to
            confirm problem; also get **UA** to look for enteric contents
        Tx: resection of involved bowel; repair defect in bladder,
            interpose omentum; re-connect bowel; diverting ileostomy
    *Colo-vaginal fistula (MC fistula in women w/ diverticulitis) – similar
        to above except you close defect in the vagina
    Inability to exclude CA → elective resection
    Late sigmoid strictures can form → resection if severe
  Right-sided diverticulitis – 80% discovered at time of incision for
    appendectomy; Tx: right hemicolectomy, primary anastomosis
  Immunosuppressed pts should undergo resection **after a <u>single</u> severe
    episode of diverticulitis.*
  When performing sigmoid resection for diverticulitis, the **distal margin of*
    *resection should be ***normal rectum**.*

**<u>Colorectal cancer</u>
  MC location – sigmoid colon
  Adenomas – villous, sessile, and large (> 2 cm) have ↑ed CA risk
  RFs – diet high in red meat
  Assoc. w/ **strep bovis** infection (endocarditis, bacteremia) - marker
  Sx's: change in bowel habits, constipation, small caliber stools, bleeding;
    iron deficient microcytic anemia, pain
  **CEA - useful for 1) prognosis (predicts worse prognosis), 2) to detect
    recurrence, and 3) to follow response to Tx; ****<u>not</u> useful as a screen**
  Path
    Most impt prognostic indicator – node status (nodal spread 1st)
    MC site for mets – liver (#1) and lung (#2)
        Isolated liver or **lung mets** should be resected
        Colon CA typically does <u>not</u> go to bone
    Better prognosis – lymphocytic penetration
    Worse prognosis – mucinous (Signet Ring Cell), mucoepidermoid,
        obstruction or perforation, high CEA, vascular / nerve /
        lymphatic invasion, rectal tumors, ulcerative tumors
    Main gene mutations: APC (tumor suppressor), **p53** (tumor
        suppressor), **k-ras** (oncogene **GTPase**), **DCC**
  **Staging
    T
        Tis: involves only the mucosa; has not grown beyond
            muscularis mucosa (inner muscle layer).
            carcinoma in situ or *intra-mucosal carcinoma*
        T1: through muscularis mucosa and into <u>submucosa</u>
        T2: through submucosa and into ****<u>muscularis propria</u>** (outer
            muscle layer).
        T3: through muscularis propria and into <u>subserosa</u> (or non-
            peritonealized peri-colic or peri-rectal tissue)
        T4: through the wall of the colon or rectum and into nearby
            organs or tissues (or perforates visceral peritoneum)
    N   **N0:** None; **N1:** 1-3, **N2:** 4 or more nearby lymph nodes.
    M   **M0:** No mets, **M1:** mets

Stage

Stage I:	T1, N0, M0 or T2, N0, M0
Stage IIA:	T3, N0, M0
Stage IIB:	T4, N0, M0
Stage IIIA:	T1, N1, M0 or T2, N1, M0
Stage IIIB:	T3, N1, M0 or T4, N1, M0
Stage IIIC:	Any T, N2, M0
Stage IV:	Any T, Any N, M1

TRUS (trans-rectal U/S) for **rectal CA (*best test* for **T + N** status)
  T3 or T4 rectal lesions get neoadjuvant chemo-XRT
  Best at assessing **depth** (sphincter involvement) and **nodes
**Tx:
  Ultimately resection for all unless stage IV
    (some stage IV disease may be resected, see below)
  En bloc resection includes: associated **mesocolon, regional
    lymph nodes (adenectomy), adequate **margins** ($\geq$ 2 cm); take
    Waldeyer's and Denonvilliers **fascia** for rectal tumors
  **Rectal tumors
    T3, T4 or positive nodes – neoadjuvant chemo-XRT 1st
    T1 or T2 w/ negative nodes – resection (<u>no</u> neoadjuvant Tx)
  **2-cm margins usual
    Exception: low rectal T1 lesions (or small T1 focus in rectal
      villous adenoma) can accept 2-3 mm margins
Standard resection techniques:
  Right hemi-colectomy – take right colic and ileo-colic arteries
  Transverse colectomy – take the middle colic artery
  Extended right hemicolectomy – for **hepatic flexure* tumors
    Take right colic, ileo-colic and middle colic arteries
    Will need to resect most of the transverse colon
  Left hemi-colectomy – take left colic artery
  Extended left hemicolectomy – for **splenic flexure* tumors
    Take left colic and middle colic arteries
**Low anterior resection (LAR)
  Sigmoid colon and portion of rectum are resected
  Take sigmoidal and rectal arteries
  For sigmoid and rectal tumors
  Leave main inferior mesenteric artery (and left colic) intact to supply
    left colon
  Need at least 2 cm margin - **needs to be at least **2 cm from
    levator ani muscles → **If not, perform APR**
  Preoperative chemo-XRT - preserves sphincter function in some
    due to tumor shrinkage
  Local recurrence after LAR → Tx: APR (re-stage pt 1st)
  Abscess following LAR – percutaneous drain
Low rectal T1 lesion (limited to submucosa) – assess w/ **TRUS
  Can be excised **trans-anally** if:
    1) **< 4 cm** in size
    2) **< 1/3 circumference**
    3) **Negative margins** (need at least **2 mm** margin)
    4) **Well differentiated**
    5) **No neuro / vascular / lymphatic invasion**
  Otherwise pt needs APR or LAR
Abdominoperineal resection (APR)
  Removes rectum and anus w/ permanent colostomy
  Rectal pain w/ rectal CA → need APR
  Can have post-op **impotence + bladder dysfunction** (nerves)
  For <u>malignant</u> lesions not amenable to LAR (<u>not</u> for benign tumors)
  Risk of local recurrence higher w/ rectal CA than colon CA
  Watch for **ureters** (travel over iliacs) and **iliac vessels**

Watch for **pudendal nerves** (in pelvic sidewall, risk of incontinence)
when taking down the **lateral stalks**
Lateral stalks contain **middle rectal arteries**

Post-op (chemo-XRT)
*****Stage III** and **IV colon CA** – adjuvant chemo (<u>no</u> XRT for colon CA)
*****Stage II** and **III rectal CA** – neoadjuvant chemo-XRT, surgery, then
adjuvant chemo
Stage IV rectal CA – chemo-XRT ± surgery (possibly just colostomy)
****Chemo*
5-FU, Leucovorin, and *oxaliplatin (FOLFOX, 6 cycles)*
If mets, add **Bevacizumab** (monoclonal Ab to vascular
endothelial growth factor, VEGF)
XRT (5000 rads)
Decreases local recurrence
XRT damage – rectum MC site of injury → vasculitis,
thrombosis, ulcers, strictures, bleeding
Pre-op chemo-XRT (neoadjuvant) may **downstage tumors** (can
have complete response) allowing LAR instead of APR

5-YS for Colorectal CA: Stage I - <u>95</u>%, II - <u>80</u>%, III - <u>65</u>%, IV - <u>10</u>%
F/U colonoscopy - perform after **1 year**; *mainly to check for new*
colon CA's (metachronous lesions); 5% get **another primary**
Special Issues
Mets to liver are fed primarily by **hepatic artery* (which would be
route of intra-arterial chemotherapy or embolization).
*Intra-op U/S – <u>most sensitive method</u> of picking up liver mets
(detects 3–5 mm)
****Resectable liver mets pre-op*
Resect if completely resectable and leaves adequate liver
function (need 1 cm margin) - number of tumors, size,
and location are not factors if you can get complete
resection (even bi-lobar lesions)
****Wedge** vs. **formal liver resection** depends on location,
number and liver reserve *(eg **mets to segments 1 and*
*2** → left hepatic lobectomy + caudate resection if*
sufficient liver reserve)
5-YS after resection of isolated liver mets – 35%
Poor prognostic indicators for liver mets:
Disease free interval < 12 months
> 3 tumors
CEA > 200 (ug/L)
Size > 5 cm
Positive nodes
Synchronous primary and liver met
****Colorectal CA invasion of adjacent organs** (T4) **should be*
resected <u>en bloc</u> (eg partial bladder resection, pancreas, liver,
****duodenum*, any other organ) → this is stage II if pt has
negative nodes and no mets; **should <u>not</u> cut across tumor w/*
resection (even if you have to perform a Whipple)
Colon perforation from obstruction
MC in **cecum** (Law of LaPlace tension = pressure x diameter)
*Suspected colo-vesicle fistula – cystoscopy (best test)

*False-positive fecal occult blood test – beef, Vit C, iron, antacids, cimetidine

****Radiation Proctitis** (radiation colitis)
1) **Acute radiation proctitis** (1st few weeks) - diarrhea and tenesmus
Tx: conservative Tx (steroid enemas) unless perforation (rare)
2) **Late radiation Proctitis** (months to years)
Sx's: **bleeding** (MC Cx), **obstruction**, **fistula** or **ulcer** (get Bx)

**Dx: CT scan, proctoscopy
   a) ****Bleeding from rectum – <u>Formalin fixation</u> of rectum** *(best Tx)*; argon beam, cautery, epi injection, rectal resection (last resort)
   b) **Obstruction** from **strictures – Tx:** Low residue diet, possible steroids; stricture **dilatation**, local trans-anal **excision** if refractory (6-8 weeks); **divert** w/ ostomy (last resort)
   c) **Fistulas** (usually conservative Tx)
   <u>Avoid</u> APR for radiation proctitis

3) **Late radiation <u>Colitis</u>** (eg XRT for previous ovarian CA) - If you need surgery (eg obstruction), bowel resection only when safe, o/w bypass

Lower GI Bleeding
    Melena or hematochezia (both can occur w/ UGI bleed)
        Stool guaiac can stay positive up to 3 weeks after bleed
    Hematemesis – bleeding from pharynx to ligament of Treitz
    Melena – tarry stools (need as little as 50 cc of blood)
    *Azotemia after GI bleed – bacterial **urea production** from intra-luminal blood (↑ BUN)
    *Hemoglobin absorption from GI tract can result in *jaundice*
    *Note – a small bowel source for LGIB is rare
    Tx: **NGT** (make sure you get back bile) or **EGD** to R/O UGI source
        Proctoscopy to look for hemorrhoids
        *Vasopressin and **octreotide** to slow bleeding if hypotensive
        Stages of LGIB (guidelines):
            1) In **persistent shock** (SBP 60 despite blood transfusions)
                → **OR for total abdominal colectomy** (R/O **UGIB** w/ NGT + proctoscopy to R/O hemorrhoids 1st)
            2) **Massive LGIB** (SBP 90 despite multiple blood transfusions)
                → **Angio** (find which side) then **OR** or select embolization
            3) **Moderate LGIB** (BP 120) → **colonoscopy** (can Tx w/ clips)
            4) **Mild LGIB** (or moderate LGIB and can't find source) →
                Upper and **lower endoscopy**
                Angiography – bleeding must be > 0.5 cc/min
                *Tagged RBC scan – bleeding must be ≥ 0.1 cc/min
                    (**most sensitive test); good for hard to find bleeds
                Video capsule study
                Meckel scan (technetium-99 pertechnate scintography)
                Push endoscopy – upper endoscopy using a rigid over-tube to prevent coiling in stomach → gets further down small bowel
Diverticulosis bleeding
    MCC of lower GI bleed
    MC on **left side**
    Arterial bleeding from disrupted **vasa rectum**
    Usually causes **significant bleeding** (75% stop spontaneously; 25% recur)
    Tx: **Endoscopic Tx** (epi, careful cautery, clip), surgery if that fails
        Recurrent bleeding → resection
Angiodysplasia bleeding
    MC on **right side**
    Venous bleeding
    Bleeds usually less severe than diverticular (rarely massive) but higher recurrence (75%)
    *Soft signs of angiodysplasia on angiogram – tufts, slow emptying
    20% of pts w/ angiodysplasia have **aortic stenosis**
    Tx: **Endoscopic Tx** (epi, cautery, clip), surgery if that fails
        Aminocaproic acid for diffuse disease (eg small + large bowel)
        Recurrent bleeding → resection (unless diffuse disease)
Small bowel bleeding (rare) – angiodysplasia, tumor, Meckel's, Crohn's
*Meckel's Diverticulum is the MCC of painless lower GI bleeding in children and teenagers.

**Polyps
  Hyperplastic polyps – MC polyp; no CA risk
  Tubular adenoma – MC intestinal neoplastic polyp (75%)
      Usually pedunculated
  Villous adenoma – most likely to be symptomatic
      Usually **sessile** and larger than tubular adenomas
      50% of villous adenomas have **cancer**
  Increased CA risk – > 2 cm, sessile, and villous lesions
  Most **pedunculated polyps** are removed endoscopically
  Sessile polyps may need segmental resection (stain area w/ methylene
      blue so you can find it at time of resection)
  If not able to get all of the polyp, need segmental resection (MC w/ sessile)
  High-grade dysplasia – basement membrane is intact (carcinoma in situ)
  Intra-mucosal cancer – into muscularis mucosa (carcinoma in situ → still
      not through basement membrane)
  Invasive cancer – into submucosa (T1)

  *Polypectomy shows T1 lesion – polypectomy adequate if:
      Margins clear (2-3 mm)
      Well differentiated
      No vascular / lymphatic / neuro invasion
      → O/W need a formal colon resection
  **Extensive low rectal villous adenomas with atypia
      Trans-anal excision as much of polyp as possible
      ***No APR unless CA is present (if T1 CA is present, trans-anal
          excision may still be adequate, see below)*
  ***Pathology shows T1 lesion after **trans-anal excision** of low villous
      adenoma → trans-anal excision adequate if:*
      Clear margins (2-3 mm)
      Is **well differentiated**
      No vascular / lymphatic / neuro invasion
      → O/W need formal rectum resection
  Pathology shows T2 lesion or greater after trans-anal excision of **rectal
      polyp** → pt needs APR or LAR (pre-op chemo-XRT if T3 or T4)

**Peutz-Jeghers syndrome *(AD)*
  Sx's: melanotic **mucocutaneous** (oral) + **skin pigmentation** (patches);
      freckles
  Path
      GI hamartomatous polyps (entire GI tract) – can cause obstruction
          → 1st presentation often **intussusception**
      ***Have increased risk of **extra-intestinal malignancies** (eg
          pancreas, liver, lungs, breast, ovaries, uterus, and testicles)*
      MC cancer w/ Peutz-Jeghers – **breast CA
      ***No significant increased risk of colon CA → NO prophylactic
          colectomy*
      Some increased risk of **intestinal malignancies**, but not significant
          enough to warrant prophylactic resection (related to
          adenomatous changes in hamartomatous polyp)
      Mean survival – 57 years of age
  Screening
      GI - EGD and **colonoscopy** every 1-2 yrs; remove polyps if **> 5 cm,**
          if **hemorrhagic,** or that look **malignant**
      Also need screening for uterus, ovary, cervix, breast, and testicles

**_Familial adenomatous polyposis_ (FAP)
All have cancer by age 40 (**100% lifetime risk**); autosomal dominant
Mutation in **APC tumor suppressor**
Polyps <u>not</u> present at birth
Polyps are present in **puberty** (**1000's**, carpet the colon)
Do <u>not</u> need colonoscopy for surveillance with suspected FAP → just need
    flexible sigmoidoscopy to check for polyps (teens)
  **_Need_ total colectomy_ prophylactically at age 20
Also get **duodenal peri-ampullary polyps** and **adenocarcinoma** → need
    to check duodenum for polyps and CA w/ EGD every 1-2 years
    (remove polyps if found)
  **Newly discovered FAP (hundreds of polyps on sigmoidoscopy)
    1)   Perform **complete colonoscopy** and metastatic w/u
        CT scan - look for associated ***desmoid tumors** (eg Gardner's)
    2)   Need **EGD** to look for duodenal polyps or CA
    3)   Offer genetic counseling to rest of the family
  **Surgery
    **_Total proctocolectomy, rectal mucosectomy, and ileo-anal pouch_
    Lifetime **proctoscopy** surveillance of **residual rectal area** and EGD
      (every 2 years) to look for **polyps / tumors**
    Total proctocolectomy w/ end ileostomy also an option
    **_Following colectomy, MCC of death w/ FAP is peri-ampullary CA_
      of duodenum (would need Whipple)
  **Gardner's syndrome (FAP variant, APC gene)
    1) **Colon CA**
    2) **Osteomas** (odd **bumps on forehead** or other bony
      protuberances, benign – leave alone)
    3) ****Desmoid tumors** - benign but <u>locally invasive</u>
      High recurrence rate (70%)
      Tx: often <u>not</u> able to perform WLE due to local invasion
        **_If involving significant small bowel or mesentery,_
          excision not indicated due to high recurrence,
          morbidity, bleeding risk, fistula rate and risk of short
          bowel syndrome
      If not resectable - **Sulindac + Tamoxifen**; poss. chemo
  Turcot's syndrome (FAP variant) – **colon CA and **brain tumors**

**Lynch syndromes (hereditary non-polyposis colon cancer, HNPCC)
  Autosomal dominant, fewer polyps than APC (< 100)
  **_Defects in DNA mismatch repair genes_ (hMSH2, hMLH1, hPMS1, etc)
  Predilection for right-sided (eg cecal CA) and **multiple colon CA's
  80% lifetime risk of developing colorectal CA
  Lynch I – just colon CA risk
  Lynch II – also risk of ovarian, endometrial, bladder, stomach, pancreas
  **Amsterdam criteria ("3, 2, 1")
    3 relatives (1 first degree relative to the other 2)
    over **2** generations
    1 relative w/ cancer before age 50
  Amsterdam II criteria same as I except includes any combination of CA
    (endometrial, gastric, small bowel, ovarian, renal, brain, ect.)
  Need **surveillance colonoscopy**:
    1) Starting at age 21 or 10 years before primary relative got CA
    2) Every 2 years until age 40, then every year
  **Total colectomy should be performed with the 1st colon CA operation
  Need surveillance program for the other types of tumors also

MCC stoma stenosis – ischemia, Tx: dilatation
MCC fistula near stoma – Crohn's Disease
MC stomal infection – Candida
**Dark stoma after APR – re-operate and revise (indicates vascular
  compromise, can end up w/ necrosis or stricture)

Rectum and Anus

497. **Eight days after internal hemorrhoid resection your pt is alarmed by a small amount of blood smear on toilet paper. Which of the following is true
   a. This is likely a bleeding diverticulum
   b. This is likely ischemic colitis
   c. This is likely a peptic ulcer
   d. The patient would likely benefit from fiber supplements

   Answer d. ***This pt has **sloughing of eschar** from his **hemorrhoidectomy**. **Fiber supplements** and **improved hydration** help avoid local trauma. Significant bleeding needs an exam under anesthesia.*

498. *A 32 yo man undergoes discectomy for a ruptured lumbar disc. He has required heavy narcotic use and post op day 5 he is noted to have blood in his stools. Which of the following is true:
   a. The patient likely has a aorto-enteric fistula
   b. The patient is likely bleeding from a sigmoidal artery
   c. The patient likely has a colon cancer
   d. The patient likely needs stool softeners

   Answer d. This pt most likely has an **anal fissure** related to constipation and straining from large hard stools. Surgery (especially back surgery) can cause this problem which is compounded by heavy narcotic use.

499. *A 50 man presents with pain on defecation and some red streaking after bowel movements. You perform anoscopy which feels tight and notice some piled up anoderm in the posterior midline along the anal margin. There is a small tear there as well. The initial treatment for this patient is:
   a. Sitz baths, lidocaine jelly, stool softeners, nitrate paste
   b. Abdominoperineal resection
   c. Low anterior resection
   d. Lateral subcutaneous internal sphincterotomy

   Answer a. The initial Tx of **anal fissure** (piled up anoderm is the **sentinel pile** associated with these) is medical with Sitz baths, lidocaine jelly, stool softeners, increasing fluid intake and nitrate paste. Topical calcium channel blockers have marginal success. Botox has high recurrence. ***The Tx of choice for **anal fissures** refractory to medical Tx is ****lateral subcutaneous internal sphincterotomy**. This considered the most effective therapy for anal fissures.*

500. *All of the following are true of procidentia except
   a. Initially treated w/ laxatives
   b. Initially treated w/ high fiber diet and stool softeners
   c. Secondary to pudendal neuropathy
   d. The Altemeier procedure is good for frail patients

   Answer a. Laxatives are *contraindicated* in pts w/ **rectal prolapse** (procidentia). Conservative medical Tx is indicated for rectal prolapse that reduces spontaneously. Pts that have to manually reduce or who cannot reduce the prolapse (incarcerated rectal prolapse) require surgery.

501. *An 82 yo multiparous woman from a nursing home has severe dementia, COPD, and requires oxygen. She presents with fecal incontinence and on exam her rectum slides below her anus. You are able to reduce it manually. The most appropriate surgical strategy in this patient would be:
   a. Perineal rectosigmoidectomy
   b. Open low anterior resection (LAR) and pexy
   c. Laparoscopic low anterior resection and rectopexy
   d. Anterior mesh rectopexy

Answer a. This patient has **rectal prolapse** (procidentia). For young and fit pts, **LAR (recto-sigmoid resection** w/ pexy, laparoscopic or open) offers the best chance of long-term success (< 10% recurrence).

For the elderly and frail patient, however, the *Altemeier procedure (perineal rectosigmoidectomy)* avoids a laparotomy. The redundant rectum and sigmoid are manually prolapsed through the anus, are resected with primary anastomosis and then returned to the abdomen.

502. *A 32 yo woman continues to suffer from severe fecal incontinence 3 months after delivery. All of the following are true except:
    a. Initial treatment is w/ a high fiber diet and bulk
    b. Sphincteroplasty is good for *neurogenic* anal incontinence
    c. Vaginal delivery is the MC traumatic cause of fecal incontinence
    d. The external sphincter is tightened w/ anterior sphincteroplasty

    Answer b. There is no good Tx for **neurogenic anal incontinence** (eg spinal cord injury) except possible colostomy.

    Anal incontinence due to abdomino-perineal descent that is refractory to medical Tx is best treated w/ **anterior sphincteroplasty** (anterior portion of external anal sphincter is tightened).

503. **A 50 yo man presents with a 4 cm anal mass above the dentate line. Your biopsy comes back as cloacogenic cancer. The most appropriate next step is:
    a. Abdominoperineal resection
    b. Laser fulgration
    c. Chemo-XRT (5-FU and mitomycin, plus XRT)
    d. Low anterior resection

    Answer c. **The most appropriate Tx of *anal canal squamous cell CA (cloacogenic CA is a variant of squamous cell CA)* is the **Nigro protocol**, which consists of *5-FU* and **mitomycin**, plus **XRT**. This cures 80%. **Surgery is NOT the initial Tx of choice.*

Anus arterial supply – inferior rectal artery
Venous drainage
    Above dentate – internal hemorrhoid plexus
    Below dentate – external hemorrhoid plexus
Nodal Drainage
    Superior and **middle rectum** – IMA nodes
    Lower rectum – IMA nodes (primarily), also to internal iliac nodes
    Anal canal (above dentate) – internal iliac nodes (pelvic nodes), inguinal
    Anal margin (below dentate) – inguinal nodes
Dentate line – transition from columnar to stratified squamous epithelium
*Anal canal** – area proximal to dentate
*Anal margin** – area between the dentate line and anal verge
*Anal verge** is the opening of the anus to the skin surface of the body
External anal sphincter is the continuation of the **puborectalis muscle**
Internal anal sphincter is the continuation of the **muscularis propria**
Central tendon separates vagina and external sphincter

Hemorrhoids

Left lateral, right anterior, and right posterior hemorrhoidal plexuses

External hemorrhoids can cause pain when they thrombose

Are distal to dentate line

Covered by sensate squamous epithelium - pain, swelling, itching

Do not band external hemorrhoids (painful)

Internal hemorrhoids cause bleeding or prolapse

Primary – slides below dentate w/ strain

Secondary – prolapse reduces spontaneously

Tertiary – prolapse must be manually reduced

Quaternary – can't reduce

Tx:

High fiber diet, stool softeners, sitz baths, lidocaine jelly

Surgical indications: thrombosed external hemorrhoid (Tx: **< 72 hrs** – *elliptical excision*, **> 72 hrs** – *lance open* to relieve pain), recurrent bleeding, large external component, moderate to severe pain

1) **Band** (in office) primary and secondary internal hemorrhoids

2) **Hemorrhoidectomy** for tertiary + quaternary internal hemorrhoids

Resect down to *internal sphincter* in all 3 areas (take mucosa and submucosa)

Post-op – stool softeners, bulk fiber, sitz baths, lidocaine jelly

Cx's

Urinary retention (MC Cx following hemorrhoidectomy, 20%)

Pelvic musculature spasm after local anesthesia wears off

Tx: place urinary catheter

***Eschar can slough** post-op causing **light bleeding late** (5-10 days) Tx: **stool softeners** and **hydration** to avoid local trauma; avoid ASA and NSAIDs; **Significant bleeding** needs exam under anesthesia*

Anal fissure

Caused by a **split in the anoderm** from large, hard stools

90% in **posterior midline**

Sx's:

Straining bowel movements (eg constipation due to heavy narcotic use after back surgery, perineal surgery, etc)

Pain and **bleeding** after defecation

Chronic ones usually have a **sentinel pile**

Anoscopy + rectal exam to confirm Dx (**pain** reproduced **exam**)

Medical Tx (90% heal) - sitz baths, bulk and water hydration, lidocaine jelly, stool softeners (Colace), NTG cream (for chronic ones)

Avoid suppositories (cause irritation, pain)

***Surgical Tx - lateral subcutaneous internal sphincterotomy**

Do NOT go past the dentate line

Do NOT go through the mucosa

Do NOT cut external sphincter

***Do not perform sphincterotomy w/ Crohn's disease*

Feel for groove between internal and external sphincter

Use 11 blade to make a transverse cut

Fecal incontinence is the most serious Cx of surgery

Lateral or recurrent fissures → Worry about Crohn's, STD's, or anal CA

*Rectal prolapse

Secondary to **pudendal neuropathy** and **laxity of anal sphincter + pelvic floor**

RFs – laxative abuse, multiparous, straining, females, long standing diarrhea, age, COPD (coughing)

Prolapse starts 6–7 cm from anal verge

Types

Full-thickness rectal prolapse – entire rectum protruding through anus
Mucosal prolapse – just rectal mucosa (not entire wall)
Internal intussusception – rectum collapses but does not exit anus
Tx:
High fiber diet and **stool softeners** (prevent straining)
For **full thickness prolapse** (all layers of bowel wall) <u>and</u> have to manually reduce or **can't manually reduce** →
1) *Old frail lady* → *Altemeier* procedure (*perineal rectosigmoidectomy; pull rectum / sigmoid out anus, resect w/ primary anastomosis*)
2) *Good condition pt – low anterior resection* and **pexy** of residual colon

*Anal incontinence

Neurogenic (gaping hole w/ laxity of levators, eg spinal cord injury)
No good treatment (possible colostomy)
Abdominoperineal descent
Trauma to levator ani, puborectalis, and external anal sphincter muscles; **anus** falls below **levators**
MCC – vaginal childbirth
Medical Tx; high fiber diet, bulk (limit to 1 BM/d)
Surgery - ****Anterior Sphincteroplasty** (*tightens* **external sphincter**)
**Pudendal nerves in lateral walls – avoid dissection there
Stenosis post-op (MC Cx)
Tx: sitz baths, bulk, lidocaine jelly, stool softeners
Anal dilatation under anesthesia over several weeks

**Anal cancer

Association with **HPV** and previous **XRT**
The **dentate line** is an important landmark for how SCCA is treated

1) ****Anal Canal** Lesions (<u>above</u> dentate line)
**Squamous Cell CA (SCCA; eg *Cloacogenic*, Epidermoid CA, Mucoepidermoid, Basaloid)
RFs – HIV, HPV, and immunosuppression
Sx's: pruritis, bleeding, palpable mass
Tx: ****Chemo-XRT 1st line** (<u>NOT</u> surgery)
**Nigro protocol (*5-FU + mitomycin*) + *XRT* (*cures 80%*).
Adenocarcinoma – Tx same as low rectal CA, APR usual, possible WLE for T1 tumors (see rectal CA for criteria)

2) **Anal Margin** Lesions (<u>below</u> dentate line)
Better prognosis than anal canal CA
Squamous cell and **Basal cell** CA treated similar to other skin CA
Squamous cell CA
Sx's: ulcerating, slow growing; MC Met's – inguinal nodes
Tx:

Lesions < 5 cm (T1 and T2) and negative nodes →
WLE w/ 1-2 cm margin (*No APR → follow below*)
Lesions > 5 cm (T3), **involving sphincter** (T4; fixed lesion), **positive nodes**, *or* **recurrence** →
Chemo-XRT (5-FU + cisplatin)
Sphincter preservation in 80%; **APR** if above fails
5-YS w/ positive nodes – 80%

*Perianal Fistulas (fistula-in-ano)

    Sx's - usually Hx of abscess, now with soiling and drainage

    Inter-sphincteric (70%), arise from a **peri-anal abscess**
        These do <u>not</u> involve the external anal sphincter
        Located between the internal and external anal sphincters
        Tx: **Fistulotomy** (open tract and curettage out, healing by
            secondary intention)

    Trans-sphincteric (20%), arising from as **ischio-rectal abscess**
        Goes through external anal sphincter
        Tx: **Lower 1/3** of external anal sphincter – fistulotomy (as above)
            Upper 2/3 of external anal sphincter - **draining seton stitch**
                (allows drainage and promotes fibrosis of tract) or **rectal*
                advancement flap (*No fistulotomy - risk of <u>incontinence</u>)

    Supra-sphincteric (5%), arising from a **supra-levator abscess**
        Tx: **draining seton stitch** or **rectal advancement flap** as above

    Extra-sphincteric (5%) - usually the result of trauma, Crohn's, colon CA,
        XRT, diverticulitis; Tx: varies, rectal advancement flap often used

    Draining setons should be strongly considered in pts w/: recurrent or
        multiple fistulas, anterior fistulas in women, ***Crohn's***, previous
        sphincter injury or impaired incontinence
    Should avoid fistulotomy in pts w/ Crohn's
    Avoid <u>cutting</u> setons in general

    *Tx for asymptomatic fistula-in-ano w/ Crohn's - observation
    The most serious Cx that can occur from fistula surgery is **<u>incontinence</u>*
        *as a result of damage to the **external anal sphincter***
    Pts w/ **inflammatory bowel disease (ie Crohn's or UC) suffering from*
        active proctitis or inflamed peri-anal disease should <u>not</u> undergo
        rectal advancement flap due to poor healing.

    Goodsall's Rule
        Posterior fistulas (90% of fistulas) connect to anus at posterior
            midline
        Anterior fistulas connect to anus in a straight line
        Fistulas that are <u>not</u> posterior and in midline → need to R/O
            inflammatory bowel DZ, CA

<u>**Abscesses**</u> (peri-rectal and peri-anal)

    Superior to **levator ani muscles** → drain through the **rectum**
    Inferior to **levator ani muscles** → drain through the **skin**
    Abx's for cellulitis, DM, pt's w/ hardware (eg prosthetic valve)
    WTD dressings and try to heal from the bottom up
    A Horseshoe abscess does <u>not</u> need an extensive incision, will drain
        through the opening you make

**Anorecto-vaginal fistulas

    Etiologies: Obstetrical trauma (MCC), others - infection, IBD, XRT, CA
    Simple (low to mid vagina), usually from obstetrical **trauma or **infection**
        Tx: Many obstetrical ones heal spontaneously (give it 6-8 wks)
              Inflammatory bowel DZ - try 6-8 wks of aggressive Tx
              **Rectal advancement flap (trans-anal approach) if medical Tx
                fails (flap of rectal mucosa and internal sphincter is
                advanced and used to cover fistula hole)
    **Complex: (high in vagina)
        Tx: Abdominal or combined perineal approach usual
              **Resection *and re-anastomosis of rectum, close vagina*
                primarily, interpose omentum between rectum and
                vagina, ileostomy

Hernias and Abdominal Wall

504. *All of the following are true except
    a. The shelving edge is formed by the internal abdominal oblique fascia
    b. The MC organ found in women w/ sliding hernias is ovary
    c. The MC organ found in men w/ sliding hernia is cecum
    d. The MC Cx following hernia repair is urinary retention

    Answer a. ***External abdominal oblique*** *fascia forms the* ***shelving edge***

505. *All of the following are true of inguinal hernia repair except:
    a. The vas deferens runs medial to the cord structures
    b. Patients with severe COPD can undergo local inguinal hernia repair with injection of the ilioinguinal nerve
    c. Testicular atrophy following inguinal hernia is most commonly due to thrombosis of the spermatic artery
    d. The most commonly injured nerve with laparoscopic inguinal hernia repair is the genitofemoral nerve

    Answer c. *Testicular atrophy* following inguinal hernia is most commonly due to **thrombosis of the spermatic veins**. This injury most commonly occurs during dissection of a large distal hernia sac.

506. *A 55 yo man returns to clinic following Lichtenstein (mesh) hernia repair with persistent right groin pain. You perform a physical exam and obtain a CT scan, both of which show no signs of hernia recurrence or infection. The pain seems to be reproduced with tapping just medial to the anterior superior iliac spine. This most likely represents injury to the:
    a. Ileo-inguinal nerve
    b. Genitofemoral nerve
    c. Sciatic nerve
    d. Lumbosacral plexus nerves

    Answer a. The MC injured nerve (or entrapped nerve) with inguinal hernia repair is the **ilioinguinal nerve**. Tx is with ilioinguinal nerve blocks, which can be therapeutic and diagnostic. If the pain recurs after nerve blocks (local anesthetics and steroids) and NSAIDs, **neurectomy** is indicated.

507. *At reoperation for a recurrence of an inguinal hernia following laparoscopic repair, the most common location for the recurrent hernia is:
    a. Lateral
    b. Medial
    c. Anterior
    d. Posterior

    Answer b. Laparoscopic mesh hernia repair has a 5% recurrence. The MCC is **separation of mesh from fascia medially**. Need at least a 3 cm overlap of the fascia and mesh with adequate fascia fixation (*avoid* making the mesh too small and make sure attached medially; need it tension free)

508. **A 65 yo woman presents with a tender mass just <u>below</u> the inguinal ligament. This most likely represents:
    a. An inguinal hernia
    b. An obturator hernia
    c. A ventral hernia
    d. A femoral hernia

    Answer d. A mass below the inguinal ligament is c/w a **femoral hernia**. **Femoral canal boundaries: Superior** – inguinal ligament, **Inferior** – pectineal ligament, **Medial** – lacunar ligament (attaches to pubis; connect the inguinal and pectineal ligaments), **Lateral** – femoral vein

283

509. **During repair of a femoral hernia through an inguinal approach, you try to reduce the bowel but are unsuccessful. The most appropriate next step is:
      a.   Pull on the bowel until it gives
      b.   Resect the bowel through a femoral exploration
      c.   Divide the rectus muscle
      d.   Divide the inguinal ligament

Answer d. **If you are unable to reduce the bowel for a **femoral hernia** through an inguinal approach, **divide the inguinal ligament**, reduce the bowel (making sure its viable 1st), and then repair the inguinal ligament.*

510. *A 65 yo woman presents with a tender medial thigh mass. The pain increases with internal rotation of the thigh. This most likely represents:
      a.   A Spigelian Hernia
      b.   An obturator hernia
      c.   A lumbar Hernia
      d.   A Richter's Hernia

Answer b. This scenario is c/w **obturator hernia**. The Howship-Romberg sign is pain w/ internal rotation of thigh, classic for obturator hernia.

Inguinal Anatomy
External abdominal oblique fascia
> Forms the **inguinal ligament** (inferior portion of inguinal canal → *shelving edge*)
> Forms roof (anterior portion) of inguinal canal
> You cut through this to get to the inguinal canal

Internal abdominal oblique fascia
> Muscle portion forms **cremasteric muscles**
> Fascia combines w/ transversalis fascia to form the **conjoined tendon,** which serves as the floor of the inguinal canal

Transversalis fascia
> Along w/ **conjoined tendon** forms inguinal canal floor
> Beneath this are the femoral vessels

Conjoined tendon
> Composed of the aponeurosis of the internal abdominal oblique and transversus abdominis muscles (transversalis)
> Along w/ the transversalis muscle, forms the inguinal canal floor

Inguinal ligament (Poupart's ligament)
> Arises from **external abdominal oblique fascia**
> Runs from anterior superior iliac spine to the pubis
> This is anterior to where the femoral vessels exit the pelvis
> Forms inferior portion of inguinal canal

Lacunar ligament – where inguinal ligament splays and insert into pubis
> Connects the inguinal and pectineal ligaments (forms an arc)
> Femoral vessels and nerve go through the arc (between inguinal and pectineal ligaments

Pectineal ligament (Cooper's ligament)
> Posterior to the femoral vessels (lies right against the bone)

Internal ring – entrance to canal from peritoneum
External ring – exit from canal into scrotum

Hesselbach's triangle - rectus muscle, inferior inguinal ligament, inferior epigastric vessels
> **Direct hernias** – inferior and medial to epigastric vessels
>> From weakness in abdominal wall; rare in females
>> Higher **recurrence** than indirect
> **Indirect hernias** - superior and lateral to epigastric vessels
>> **MC type**
>> From persistently *patent processus vaginalis*
>> Higher risk of **incarceration** than direct

Pantaloon hernia – direct and indirect components
Incarcerated hernia – can lead to bowel strangulation; should be
repaired emergently if it can't be reduced
Sliding hernias
Visceral peritoneum and retroperitoneal organ make up part
of the sac
Males (MC gender for sliding hernia) – <u>cecum or sigmoid</u> usual
Females – <u>ovaries</u> (MC) or fallopian tubes usual
Bladder can also be found
Females w/ ovary in canal
Ligate round ligament (lets ovary fall back into pelvis)
Return ovary to peritoneum; biopsy of ovary if looks abnormal
Vas deferens – runs medial to cord structures
RFs for adult inguinal hernias – age, obesity, lifting, COPD (coughing),
constipation, straining (BPH), ascites, pregnancy, peritoneal dialysis

Inguinal Hernia Repair

Bassini – conjoined tendon + transversalis fascia (superior) approximated
to *shelving edge* (inferior); reconstructs floor of the inguinal canal
Cooper's ligament repair – conjoined tendon + transversalis fascia
(superior) approximated to *pectineal ligament* (inferior, posterior)
Need relaxing incision in external abdominal oblique fascia
Can use for *femoral hernias*
Lichtenstein – mesh reforms inguinal canal floor; sewn between conjoined
tendon and inguinal ligament; recurrence decreased (↓ed tension)
Hernias in infants and children (up to 18 yrs)
Just perform high ligation (nearly always indirect)
Open sac prior to ligation to make sure nothing important is in there
Severe COPD w/ incarcerated inguinal hernia
Can repair under local w/ anesthetic injection into ilioinguinal nerve
(medial to anterior superior iliac spine) and direct groin injection
Trouble reducing incarcerated inguinal hernia at time of repair →
divide inguinal ligament at internal ring (best option; repair it later)
You find a femoral hernia when exploring inguinal hernia and can't
reduce contents → Tx **cut through inguinal ligament** and floor of
inguinal canal to free bowel; end up w/ **Cooper's Ligament Repair**
Cx's: *Urinary retention* – MC early Cx following hernia repair
Tx: foley, leg bag if persistent
Recurrence rate – 1%, lower w/ mesh
Testicular atrophy (from ischemic orchitis, <1%) - MC from
dissection of <u>distal part</u> of hernia sac (beyond pubic tubercle) w/
vessel disruption and *thrombosis of spermatic cord veins*
RFs – redo hernias, large hernias
Pain after hernia – MC compression of *ilioinguinal nerve*
Tx: local infiltration can be diagnostic and therapeutic
If that doesn't work go in and resect nerve (neurectomy)
Cord lipomas – remove
Ilioinguinal nerve injury
MC nerve injury after inguinal hernia repair
Loss of cremasteric reflex; numbness on ipsilateral penis,
scrotum and inner thigh
Nerve usually injured at external ring
Nerve is anterior to cord structures
Genitofemoral nerve injury
MC nerve injury w/ laparoscopic hernia repair
Genital branch - branches to cremaster (motor) +
scrotum (sensory); runs posterior / inferior to cord
Femoral branch - branches to upper lateral thigh (sensory)
Runs lateral to iliac vessels

Laparoscopic inguinal hernia repair

Inferiorly, make sure to staple mesh to **inguinal ligament** – avoid area
where the spermatic cord and epigastric vessels enter inguinal canal
(although due need staples medial to this to avoid recurrence)
MCC of recurrence after laparoscopic hernia repair →
Medial separation of mesh from fascia at inguinal ligament
MCC - mesh is *too small*
Laparoscopic inguinal hernia repair compared to open repair has:
Reduced immediate post-op pain
Earlier return to work
Greater intra-op Cx's, especially **life threatening** (anesthetic related
and injury to blood vessels)

Femoral hernia

Sx's: mass just below inguinal ligament
Femoral canal boundaries:
Superior – inguinal ligament
Inferior – pectineal ligament
Medial – lacunar ligament (attaches to pubis; connect the inguinal
and pectineal ligaments)
Lateral – femoral vein
Femoral canal structures - NAVEL (lateral to medial) – femoral nerve,
femoral artery, femoral vein, empty space, lymphatics
High risk of incarceration → may need to **divide inguinal ligament** to
reduce bowel
Hernia passes under the inguinal ligament
Have characteristic **bulge** on anterior-medial thigh **below ligament**
Usually repaired w/ **Cooper's Ligament** repair

Ventral hernias

Can be major operations; presents as a **large abd mass** after operation
CT scan to confirm ventral hernia
RFs – obesity, smoking, COPD, previous hernia repair
Laparoscopic repair w/ mesh (best option; majority repaired this way)
No mesh w/ bowel compromise – just repair enterotomy and close
(abx's, back in 6 weeks)
0.1% risk of placing veress needle or trocar into bowel / blood vessel
Recurrence rate for laparoscopic mesh repairs – 5%.
RFs for recurrence – larger hernias, longer OR time, previous
repair, obesity (BMI > 40)
MCC for recurrence - separation of mesh from posterior fascia
MC Cx after ventral hernia repair – seroma (bulge), leave unless very
symptomatic (Tx: aspiration)
Skin graft placed over bowel after necrotizing fasciitis and now has
ventral hernia → leave it alone
Most studies show a lower wound infection rate, reduction in ileus, shorter
length of stay, and longer OR time w/ laparoscopic mesh ventral
hernia repair compared to open repair.

Obturator hernia (anterior pelvis)

Herniation through **obturator canal**
Elderly women, multiparous, bowel gas below pubic ramus
Howship-Romberg sign - inner thigh pain w/ internal rotation *(classic)*
Dx usually made at time of surgery for small bowel obstruction
Tx: Operative reduction, may need mesh; check other side for defect

Incisional hernia – MC type to recur; inadequate closure is MCC
Umbilical hernia: RFs – African-Americans; males; obesity or ascites in adults
Tend to **close spontaneously in children** (esp if < 2.5 cm)
Delay repair until **age 5**
Risk of incarceration is in adults, not children

Urology

511. **All of the following are true except:
   a. The seminal vesicles are connected to the urethra
   b. Ejaculation failure after proctocolectomy is due to disruption of pelvic sympathetic nerves
   c. Tx for transitional cell CA of the renal pelvis is radical nephroureterectomy
   d. Seizures following TURP are most likely due to hyponatremia

   Answer a. *The **seminal vesicles** are connected to the **vas deferens**.
   Ejaculation failure after proctocolectomy is due to disruption of **pelvic sympathetic nerves.**

512. *All of the following are true of kidney stones except:
   a. Calcium oxalate stones are MC
   b. Uric acid stones are radiolucent and are likely to appear in pts w/ gout, ileostomies, or myeloproliferative disorders
   c. Initial Tx of choice for intractable nephrolithiasis is extra-corporeal shock wave lithotripsy (ESWL)
   d. Magnesium ammonium phosphate stones are associated staph aureus

   Answer d. Magnesium ammonium phosphate stones (struvite) are associated **proteus infections** (produce urease)

513. **A 32 yo man presents with a painless testicular mass that has been present for about 3 months. All of the following are true except:
   a. This is unlikely to be testicular torsion
   b. The patient should have an orchiectomy via trans-scrotal approach
   c. Seminoma is the most likely malignant tumor
   d. The patient should have an orchiectomy via trans-inguinal approach

   Answer b. This most likely represents a testicular tumor. An important concept is that you do not want to disrupt the lymphatic plane in these pts, which means you do not want any scrotal incisions (or biopsies).

   Tx of choice of this mass is **orchiectomy via trans-inguinal approach (the testicle and attached mass are your biopsy specimen).

514. *All of the following are true except:
   a. 90% of seminomas have Beta-HCG elevation
   b. Seminoma is the MC testicular tumor
   c. Seminoma is extremely sensitive to XRT
   d. Seminoma is NOT associated w/ AFP elevation

   Answer a. Only 10% of seminomas have beta-HCG elevation

515. *All of the following are true of prostate cancer except:
   a. Stage IA disease in an 80 yo man requires no additional treatment
   b. A normal PSA is < 4
   c. PSA should go to zero 24 hours after prostatectomy
   d. Seizure after TURP is most likely related to hyponatremia

   Answer c. PSA should go to zero 3 weeks after prostatectomy (half-life is 3 days). Normal PSA is < 4.

   Stage IA disease after TURP (examination of specimen from TURP) is managed by observation in the elderly. Younger pts (> 10 year expected life span) should consider other options.

516. **A 50 yo man comes to your clinic w/ aching scrotal pain. You examine the pt and get an U/S which shows a left sided varicocele. Which of the following tumors is most likely give the presentation:
    a. Testicular seminoma
    b. Lung CA
    c. Pancreatic CA
    d. Renal cell CA

    Answer d. **A **new varicocele** on the left side may be a sign of **left sided renal cell CA**. The left gonadal vein drains into the left renal vein and the right gonadal vein drains into the IVC. A new left varicocele is worrisome for RCCA compressing the left gonadal vein. A new right sided varicocele is worrisome for an abdominal or pelvic mass causing pressure.
    ****Varicoceles** cause **reduced fertility**
    **Hydrocoeles and Spermatoceles do not affect fertility

517. *All of the following are true of renal cell carcinoma except:
    a. They can synthesize erythropoietin
    b. Partial nephrectomy is indicated for tumors < 4cm if creatnine is > 2.5
    c. When growing into the IVC, IVC reconstruction is usually needed
    d. The classic presentation is pain, abdominal mass, and hematuria

    Answer c. Although these tumors have a predilection for IVC invasion, they usually do not attach to the walls and can be plucked out of the IVC at the time of nephrectomy. ***Partial nephrectomy** is indicated for tumors < 4 cm if creatnine is > 2.5.

518. *All of the following are true of bladder cancer except:
    a. The MC is transitional cell carcinoma
    b. Schistosomiasis infection is associated w/ bladder squamous cell CA
    c. Transitional cell carcinoma limited to the submucosa can be treated with intra-vesicle BCG or trans-urethral resection
    d. Transitional cell carcinoma with invasion of the muscle (T2) is best treated with wedge resection

    Answer d. ***Transitional cell CA** with muscle invasion requires total cystectomy and formation of an ileal conduit.

519. **All of the following are true except:
    a. Oncocytomas and angiomyolipomas are benign renal tumors
    b. Spermatoceles do not affect fertility
    c. Preoperative phimosis should be treated w/ a dorsal slit to open
    d. Tx for vesicoureteral reflux is ileal conduit

    Answer d. Tx for vesicoureteral reflux is re-implantation of ureter into the bladder ****Preoperative phimosis** is treated w/ a **dorsal slit** to open

Gerota's fascia – fascia that encloses the kidney
****Anterior to posterior structures** (VAP) – renal vein, renal artery, renal pelvis
    ****Right renal artery** crosses posterior to the IVC
    ****Left renal vein** crosses anterior to the aorta (MC)
Ureters cross **over iliac vessels**
Left renal vein – can be ligated from IVC
    Has collaterals (left adrenal vein, left gonadal vein, left ascending lumbar vein)
    Right renal vein does not have these collaterals and cannot be safely ligated
Epididymis – connects to vas deferens
***Seminal vesicles** – are connected to the vas deferens
MCC renal insufficiency following surgery – hypotension intra-op
****Erection** – parasympathetic; ****ejaculation** – sympathetic
    Ejaculation failure after proctocolectomy is due to disruption of the **pelvic sympathetic ganglia

Kidney Stones

Sx's: severe colicky pain, restlessness

Dx: **UA** – blood or stones; **Abd CT** – stones, hydronephrosis; 90% opaque

Types of stones

1) **Calcium oxalate stones** (radio-opaque)

MC kidney stone (75%)

↑ed after **terminal ileum resection** due to **oxalate reabsorption** in colon

2) **Magnesium ammonium phosphate stones** (radio-opaque)

Struvite stones

Associated w/ **kidney infections** and **urea splitting organisms** such as *Proteus mirabilis (urease)*

Can cause **staghorn calculi** that fill the renal pelvis

3) **Uric acid stones** (radio-lucent)

RFs – gout, ileostomies, short gut

W/ ileostomy, loss of alkaline fluid from ileostomy lowers urinary pH and volume, leading to uric acid stone formation

4) **Cysteine stones** (radio-dense to radiolucent)

Associated w/ **congenital disorders** of cysteine metabolism

Prevention –Tiopronin (↓s rate of cysteine solidification)

ESWL indications - intractable pain or infection, progressive obstruction, progressive renal damage, solitary kidney, > 6 mm (not likely to pass); Tx: **ESWL** *(best Tx; extracorporeal shock wave lithotripsy)*

**Testicular cancer

MCC cancer death in men 25-35

Vast majority of solid tumors of testicles are malignant

90% of tumors are **germ cell** – seminoma or non-seminoma

Undescended testicles (cryptorchidism) – ↑s risk of testicular CA

MC get seminoma

Sx's: painless hard mass *(classic)* ± gynecomastia

Dx: Cardinal finding is *mass in substance of testis*

U/S *(1ˢᵗ test)* – make sure not a hydrocoele (will transluminate if so)

Labs *(get before orchiectomy so you have levels)* – **AFP, B-HCG,** and **LDH** (correlates w/ tumor bulk)

Orchiectomy - through an **inguinal incision** (*not* trans-scrotal → do not want to disrupt lymphatics); **The testicle and attached mass are the biopsy specimen**

Do not stick a needle through scrotum to get Dx

Overall 5-YS survival – 90%; seminoma better than non-seminomatous

Seminoma

MC testicular tumor

10% have beta-HCG elevation

No AFP elevation (if elevated, Tx like non-seminomatous)

Spreads to retroperitoneum

Seminoma is extremely sensitive to XRT

Tx: **All stages get – Orchiectomy + Retroperitoneal XRT** *(para-aortic and ipsilateral pelvic)*

Chemo (cisplatin, bleomycin, etoposide) reserved for either systemic mets or bulky retroperitoneal nodes

Non-seminomatous testicular CA

Types – teratoma, choriocarcinoma, yolk sac, embryonal

AFP and **beta-HCG** – elevated in 90%

Spreads hematogenously to **lungs**; spreads to **retroperitoneum**

XRT never used as primary Tx for non-seminomatous

Tx: **All stages get – Orchiectomy + Retroperitoneal Node Dissection** (is prophylactic if stage I)

Stage II or greater (beyond testicle): add **Chemo** (cisplatin, bleomycin, etoposide)

MC location for primary extra-gonadal germ cell tumor – mediastinum (see Thoracic Chp)

Prostate Cancer

MC CA in US for men; 2nd MCC CA death in men (#1 - lung CA)

Sx's: asymptomatic (MC), obstructive, irritative (eg frequency, dysuria) hematuria, erectile dysfunction

Screening - mortality benefit from screening <u>not</u> established (DRE or PSA)
- PSA - not very specific or sensitive; can be ↑ed w/ prostatitis, BPH, chronic catheterization

Dx: TRUS w/ Bx (6-12 Bx's) – histology correlates w/ prognosis

Path:
- MC site – posterior lobe
- MC mets – bone (osteoblastic - x-ray shows hyperdense area)
- Many pts impotent after resection; can get incontinence

Tx:
- Stage I (Tia is non-palpable, not on imaging, *TURP specimen*) +
  - Stage II (T1 or T2 - both confined to capsule of prostate) *either:*
    1) Watchful waiting (esp age >75 or limited life expectancy) <u>or</u>:
    2) XRT <u>or</u>;
    3) Radical prostatectomy w/ pelvic LN dissection (if lifespan >10 yrs)
  - Stage III (extends thru capsule) or Stage IV (invades adjacent structures or mets) → XRT + androgen ablation

Androgen deprivation options:
1) Bilateral orchiectomy *(best therapy)*
2) GnRH analogues (leuprolide, goserelin) – cause ↓ FSH and ↓LH
3) Anti-androgens (flutamide, bicalutamide) – block androgen receptor

XRT can help w/ bone pain or local recurrence

W/ prostatectomy, PSA should go to 0 after 3 weeks (1/2 life 3 days) → if not, get bone scan to check for mets

Prognosis - High PSA, high Gleason grade and ↑ed age are predictors of mets

Renal cell carcinoma (RCCA; **hypernephroma**)

MC primary tumor of kidney
- MC kidney tumor – mets from breast CA

RF – smoking

Sx's: abd pain, mass and hematuria *(classic triad)*

Dx: CT chest/abd/pelvis - tumor disrupts renal contour
- *Can often be fairly certain about RCCA based on CT scan but can <u>not</u> exclude RCCA w/ CT scan
- *Biopsy <u>not</u> useful* – hard to DDx from oncocytoma; also high risk of bleed (unfavorable risk-benefit ratio)
- Essentially all renal masses need some sort of resection (<u>cysts</u> are observed unless complex)

Path
- Solid tumor – 90-95% solid renal masses are RCCA
  - ± necrosis, ± calcification
  - MC subtype – clear cell (75%)
- MC mets – lung (30% have mets at time of Dx)
- Paraneoplastic syndromes:
  - Erythrocytosis from erythropoietin secreting tumors
  - HTN from renin secreting tumors
  - Stauffer syndrome – ↑ed LFTs; improves after successful resection
- Wide range of 5-year survival – related to size + degree of spread:
  - Stage I (< 4 cm)   > 95%
  - Stage IV (eg mets to lungs)   5%
- Oncocytoma - benign tumor
- Angiomyolipoma - benign hamartoma; occur w/ tuberous sclerosis

Tx:
  Radical nephrectomy – Tx of choice for majority; takes kidney,
      adrenal gland, fat, Gerota's Fascia, and regional nodes
    Consider partial nephrectomy if:
      1) RCCA on **limited area of kidney** (eg < 4 cm) *and;*
      2) If total nephrectomy would result in **dialysis** (eg pt creatnine
          2.5)
  Bilateral small tumors – partial nephrectomies (avoid dialysis)
  Chemo-XRT (doxorubicin based), interferon, IL-2 (all marginal)
  Sunitinib (for mets or unresectable RCCA)
      Multi-targeted receptor tyrosine kinase (MRTK) inhibitor
  Special situations
    Isolated lung mets – resection
    RCCA has predilection for growth into IVC (even right atrium)
        Pull tumor thrombus out of IVC (± cardiopulmonary bypass)
    Transitional cell CA of renal pelvis – Tx: radical nephroureterectomy

Bladder cancer
  Males (4:1); prognosis based on stage and grade
  RFs – smoking, aniline dyes, cyclophosphamide, occupational exposure
  MC type – transitional cell CA (90%)
  Sx's: **painless hematuria** (*classic*)
  Dx: **UA cytology, cystoscopy**
  Tx:
    T1 (**muscle *not* involved**)
        Intravesical BCG (or valrubicin) or **transurethral resection**
    T2 or greater (**muscle involved**):
      1) **Cystectomy** (w/ ileal conduit) + bilateral pelvic node
          dissection *and;*
      2) **Chemo-XRT** (MVAC: methotrexate, vinblastine, Adriamycin
          cisplatin)
      Men – include **prostatectomy** in resection
      Women – include **TAH + BSO** and **anterior vaginal wall**
    Mets – chemo-XRT only
  Overall 5-YS after cystectomy – 60% (5-YS for T1 tumors – 95%)
  Squamous cell CA of bladder – schistosomiasis

Testicular torsion
  Peaks in 15 yo population
  Involved testis often not viable at exploration
  Torsion MC is towards midline
  Dx: **U/S** – can be used to aid in Dx (shows no blood flow to testis)
      If suspicion high → **skip U/S and immediate detorsion**
  Tx: **Trans-scrotal incision**, then **de-torse testis**
      Bilateral orchiopexy if testicle viable
      If not, resection and orchiopexy of contra-lateral testis
      100% viable if within 6 hours

Benign prostatic hyperplasia (BPH)
  Usually arises in **transitional zone**
  Sx's: nocturia, frequency, dysuria, weak stream, urinary retention
  Dx: DRE – enlarged prostate; TRUS
  Initial Tx
    Alpha blocker – terazosin (Hytrin), relax smooth muscle
    5-alpha-reductase inhibitors – finasteride (Proscar), inhibits
        conversion of testosterone to dihydrotestosterone (inhibits
        prostate hypertrophy)

Surgery (TURP – trans-urethral resection of prostate)
>**Indications** – recurrent UTI's, gross hematuria, stones, renal insufficiency, failure of medical Tx
>>*Post-TURP syndrome* (ie **seizures**) - *hyponatremia* secondary to irrigation w/ water (as opposed to normal saline); can precipitate **seizures** from cerebral edema; Tx: careful correction of Na with diuresis (see Fluid / Electrolytes Chp)
>
>Most pts w/ TURP have **retrograde ejaculation**

*Neurogenic bladder (spastic bladder)
>MC secondary to spinal injury
>Accidental voiding, often of large amounts of urine
>Injury above T-12
>Tx: *surgery to increase bladder resistance*

*Neurogenic obstructive uropathy (flaccid bladder)
>Incomplete emptying of the bladder, can have frequency
>Injury below T-12; can occur with APR
>Tx: *intermittent catheterization*

Urinary Incontinence
>*Stress incontinence* (often w/ cough, sneeze)
>>**MC type of incontinence; MC in women**
>>Due to **pelvic floor weakness** leading to hypermobile urethra or **loss of sphincter mechanism**
>>RFs – multiparous women, age, obesity, prostatectomy
>>Tx: **Kegel exercises** to strengthen pelvic floor
>>**Alpha-adrenergic agents**
>>Surgery for **urethral suspension or pubovaginal sling** (best)
>
>*Overflow incontinence*
>>Incomplete emptying and enlarged bladder (MC type in males)
>>**Obstruction** (eg BPH) leads to distention and leakage
>>Tx: medical Tx of BPH, possible TURP

Other urologic diseases
>****Varicocele** – abnormal enlargement of veins draining testis (MC on left)
>>**New onset left sided varicocele** – worrisome for **renal cell CA** (left gonadal vein inserts into left renal vein, obstruction by renal tumor causes varicocele)
>>Can also be from other **intra-abdominal, pelvic, or retroperitoneal malignancy** placing pressure on **gonadal veins**
>>Is found in scrotum on **posterior portion** of testicle (different from testicular tumor)
>>****Reduced fertility** due to thrombosis/compression/warmth
>>>→ **improved fertility w/ high spermatic vein ligation**
>
>****Spermatocele**
>>**MC cystic structure of scrotum**
>>Fluid filled cystic structure superior and separate to testis along epididymus
>>Tx: surgical removal if symptomatic; ****These do not impair fertility**
>
>**Ureteropelvic obstruction** – Tx: pyeloplasty (relieves obstruction)
>***Vesicoureteral reflux** – Tx: re-implantation into bladder w/ long bladder muscle portion (prevents reflux)
>***Ureteral duplication**
>>**MC urinary tract abnormality**
>>Tx: re-implantation in bladder if obstructed
>>*Not a contra-indication to kidney donation for TXP*

Ureterocele
> MC at junction of ureter and bladder; MC in females
> MC associated w/ **ureteral duplication**
> Sx's: UTI's, retention
> Tx: resect and re-implant ureter in bladder if sx's

Hypospadias – ventral urethral opening
> Tx: repair at 6 months with penile skin

Epispadias – dorsal urethral opening Tx: surgery

Horseshoe kidney – usually joined at lower poles
> Cx's: UTI, urolithiasis, hydronephrosis
> Tx: may need pyeloplasty for obstruction

Persistent urachus – connection between umbilicus and bladder
> 10% have bladder outlet obstruction (eg **wet umbilicus**)
> Dx: **voiding cystourethrogram** (will also show any obstruction)
> Tx: resection of sinus and cyst w/ closure of bladder; relieve any
> > obstruction

Epididymitis – inflammation or infection of epididymis
> **MCC sudden scrotal pain**
> **U/S** – increased blood flow to epididymis
> **MC infection** – Chlamydia; others – gonorrhea, E coli (Tx: abx's)

Pneumaturia
> **MCC** – diverticulitis and subsequent formation of colo-vesical fistula

WBC casts – seen w/ pyelonephritis and glomerulonephritis

RBC casts – just w/ glomerulonephritis

Priapism
> Tx: aspiration of corpus cavernosum w/ dilute epinephrine
> May need to create a communication through glans w/ scalpel to
> > relieve
> RFs – sickle cell anemia, hypercoaguable states, trauma,
> > intracorporeal injections for impotence, sildenafil

SCCA of penis – standard care is penectomy w/ 2-cm margin

IV Indigo carmine or methylene blue – used to check for urine leak

Phimosis found at time of laparotomy – *Tx: need dorsal slit*

Erythropoietin – ↓ production in pts w/ chronic renal failure **(low Hct)**

Peyronie's Disease – thick plaques in tunica albuginea cause penile
> curvature;
> Tx: **conservative Tx** for up to 1 year (colchicines, Vit E)
> If that fails to relieve sx's, need **Nesbit operation** (tissue on opposite
> > side of plaque is shortened to straighten curve – *plaque is not
> > excised*)

Gynecology

520. *A 28 yo old woman presents to the ED w/ severe abd pain, abd distension, a systolic BP of 60 despite 2 liters of lactated ringers, and a heart rate of 120. The hematocrit comes back at 18. The most appropriate next step is:
   a. Go to OR
   b. FFP and go to the ICU
   c. Send a beta-HCG
   d. Abdominal CT scan

   Answer a. Sometimes you can't wait for a Dx. The most appropriate step here is to go to the OR and figure it out in there. This is highly suspicious for a ruptured ectopic pregnancy.

521. **A 23 yo woman with previous pelvic inflammatory disease presents to the ER w/ acute abd pain. All of the following are true in this pts work-up except:
   a. Unruptured ectopic pregnancy should undergo salpingectomy
   b. A 7 cm tubo-ovarian abscess from pelvic inflammatory disease should undergo percutaneous drainage
   c. Ruptured graafian cysts should be followed
   d. Ovarian torsion requires detorsion and assessment of viability

   Answer a. Unruptured **ectopic pregnancy** should undergo salpingotomy (removal of the ectopic pregnancy), not salpingectomy (which is removal of the fallopian tube). Another option is to abort the pregnancy w/ MTX.
   Ovarian torsion (adnexal torsion) requires detorsion and assessment of viability
   A 7 cm tubo-ovarian abscess should undergo percutaneous drainage

522. **All of the following are true except:
   a. The fallopian tube (ampullary portion) is MC site of ectopic pregnancy
   b. The round ligament maintains anteversion of the cervix
   c. First trimester bleeding with a closed os and no heartbeat on U/S is consistent w/ missed abortion
   d. Seizures are usually the first system of magnesium toxicity

   Answer d. Respiratory depression is associated w/ **magnesium toxicity**
   The fallopian tube (ampullary portion) is MC site of **ectopic pregnancy**
   The round ligament maintains anteversion of the cervix
   First trimester bleeding with a closed os and no heartbeat on U/S is consistent w/ missed abortion

523. *A 21 yo sexually active woman presents with abd pain and discharge. On pelvic exam and she has cervical motion tenderness and discharge. Her Beta-HCG is negative The Tx should be:
   a. Ceftriaxone and doxycycline
   b. Bactrim
   c. Vancomycin
   d. Levofloxacin

   Answer a. This pt most likely has **pelvic inflammatory disease** related to Chlamydia or Gonorrhea. Tx is with ceftriaxone and doxycycline.

524. *A 25 yo woman complains of cyclical rectal bleeding, You perform anoscopy and find a blue mass at 5 cm above the dentate line (3 cm above the levators) Given the likely diagnosis, all of the following are true except:
   a. Sx's of this condition are dysmenorrhea, infertility and dyspareunia
   b. Ovaries are the MC site
   c. This lesion requires low anterior resection
   d. This lesion can be treated with hormonal manipulation

Answer c. This pt has **endometriosis**, which is usually controlled with OCP's. A blue rectal mass in a young female pt who presents with rectal bleeding should alert you to endometriosis.

525. **All of the following are true of ovarian cancer except:
   a. Ovarian CA w/ peritoneal mets is usually treated primarily w/ total abdominal hysterectomy, bilateral oophrectomy, resection of peritoneal metastases, and omentectomy
   b. Debulking therapy can be effective
   c. Mucin ovarian tumors are associated w/ pseudomyxoma peritonei
   d. Risk factors for ovarian cancer include oral contraceptive pills (OCPs)

   Answer d. Use of OCPs lowers the risk of ovarian CA.

   ***Ovarian CA w/ peritoneal mets* is usually treated primarily w/ total abdominal hysterectomy, bilateral oophrectomy, resection of peritoneal metastases, and omentectomy.** You should try to remove all the carcinomatosis and leave residual tumor deposits < 1 cm. Intra-peritoneal chemotherapy is effective for ovarian CA w/ peritoneal mets

526. **A 55 yo post-menopausal woman has a newly discovered ovarian tumor on the right side. All of the following are true except:
   a. CA confined to bilateral ovaries is stage I disease
   b. An ovarian mass associated with ascites and right hydrothorax is best treated w/ a peritoneal drain and pleurodesis
   c. Serous tumors are the MC ovarian tumor overall
   d. The clear cell type of ovarian CA has the worst prognosis

   Answer b. *Meige's syndrome* consists of a pelvic ovarian tumor (classically fibroma) that causes **ascites** and **hydrothorax. Tumor excision** cures syndrome and relieves the ascites and hydrothorax

   CA confined to *bilateral ovaries* is *stage I disease*

527. *All of the following are true of ovarian CA except:
   a. Intra-peritoneal chemotherapy can be effective for ovarian CA
   b. Omentectomy is indicated with surgery for ovarian CA
   c. The MC site of initial spread of ovarian CA is the contra-lateral ovary
   d. Ovarian CA is usually diagnosed at an early stage

   Answer d. Ovarian CA is usually diagnosed late.

528. **All of the following are true except:
   a. A suspicious incidental ovarian cyst discovered at the time of laparoscopic cholecystectomy should be managed w/ 4 quadrant wash (send for cytology) plus biopsy of any associated mass, the omentum and any suspicious areas
   b. High grade cervical intra-epithelial neoplasia following conization biopsy requires hysterectomy
   c. The MC vaginal CA in young girls is sarcoma botryoides
   d. Stage II vulvar CA requires bilateral labial resection.

   Answer b. **High grade cervical intra-epithelial neoplasia following conization biopsy requires no further therapy.**

   A suspicious incidental ovarian cyst discovered at time of laparoscopic cholecystectomy should be managed w/ 4 quadrant wash (send for cytology) plus biopsy of any associated mass, the omentum and any suspicious areas. **Oophrectomy should not be performed at this time**

Stage II vulvar CA *requires* **_modified radical_ **vulvectomy** *(entire vulva removed including* **bilateral labia majora / minora** *and clitoris) +* _bilateral inguinal/femoral LN_ *dissection*

Normal Anatomy
Fallopian tubes carry ovum from ovaries to uterus
    Ampullary portion of fallopian tube -*MC site of **ectopic pregnancy**
*Ligaments
    *Round ligament – maintains **anteversion** of uterus
        Starts at uterus, goes through inguinal canal, eventually attaches to labia majora
    Infundibular ligament - has **ovarian vessels** (artery, vein) + nerve
        Fold of peritoneum that extends out from ovary to pelvic wall
    Broad ligament – contains **uterine vessels** (artery, vein)
        Connects the sides of the uterus to the floor and walls of pelvis
    Cardinal ligament – holds cervix and vagina in place at base of broad ligament; Contains **uterine artery and vein**
U/S – often study of choice for Dx of disorders of female genital tract
*Mittelschmerz
    Rupture of **graafian follicle** or follicular swelling
    *Pain can be confused w/ appendicitis
    Occurs 14 days after 1st day of menses
    Negative pelvic exam and negative U/S
    Tx: nothing; if already in OR for RLQ pain and you find this, perform appendectomy and close

*Abortions
*Missed
    Dx: 1st trimester bleeding, closed os, U/S – positive sac, no heartbeat Embryo or fetus has died but no miscarriage yet
Threatened – 1st trimester bleeding, positive heartbeat
    Possibly due to **sub-chorionic hematoma** – Tx: bed-rest
Incomplete – abortion tissue protrudes through os
Ectopic (see below for management)
    Acute abd pain, positive beta-HCG, and negative U/S for sac
    Other sx's – missed period, vaginal bleeding, hypotension
    RFs – previous tubal manipulation, PID, previous ectopic, smoking
    MC location – ampullary portion of fallopian tubes
    Life-threatening – hemorrhage and shock can occur

Ectopic Pregnancy
1) **Abdominal/pelvic pain**
2) **Positive B-HCG**
3) **U/S cannot find conception**
4) **Hypotension**
The above = **ruptured ectopic pregnancy** → go to the OR
May be able to see ectopic pregnancy on U/S
Laparoscopy as a 1st step usual
Un-ruptured ectopic pregnancy: Tx - salpingotomy, evacuate hematoma, hemostasis, repair tube; can also try medical Tx (eg methotrexate) to try and terminate pregnancy
Ruptured ectopic pregnancy – salpingectomy if unstable; o/w salpingotomy as above

Best time for surgery in pregnancy is 2nd trimester
Too early risk **spontaneous abortion** (1st trimester, 10-15%)
Too late risk **preterm labor** (3rd trimester, 10-15%)
1% risk of fetal demise in 2nd trimester w/ surgery *(best time)*

*Pregnancy w/ acute cholecystitis
    Initial Tx - → abx's and NPO *(**95% treated without intervention)*

*Pregnancy w/ appendicitis
    MC problem requiring surgery with pregnancy
    May have **RUQ pain** in 3rd trimester - appendix moves **towards RUQ** w/
        pregnancy; pain may be exacerbated w/ pt lying on **right side**
    Dx **Get an U/S 1st** (diameter > 7, thickness > 2)
    Laparoscopic appendectomy if 1st or 2nd trimester; open usual for 3rd
    If open appendectomy, **mark site of incision over the site of maximal**
        pain before you put pt to sleep - ___appendix is displaced superiorly___
        ___by uterus___
    High appendix **rupture, premature labor** (10-15%) and **fetal loss** (5-10%)
        w/ appendicitis in pregnancy

Pelvic inflammatory disease
    Increased risk of **infertility** and **ectopic pregnancy**
    Sx's: lower abd pain, N/V, fever, vaginal discharge
    MC in **first 1/2 of menstrual cycle**
    RFs – multiple sexual partners
    Dx: cervical motion tenderness *(best),* adnexal tenderness, GS + cultures
        (Gonococcus, Chlamydia)
    Tx: ceftriaxone + doxycycline (admit if severe)

**Tubo-ovarian abscess
    Sx's: fevers and chills; RFs - previous PID, IUD use
    Dx: **Cervical motion tenderness** and **adnexal mass** on pelvic exam
        Get **B-HCG** to R/O ectopic pregnancy
        U/S for diagnosis (≥ 6 cm usually require drainage)
    Tx: ****percutaneous drain** *(esp. if > 6 cm)* **+ abx's** (doxycycline,
        ceftriaxone); If you have to operate (can't get drain in or ruptured
        abscess) → laparotomy, evacuate abscess, washout, place drains

**Ovarian torsion (adnexal torsion)
    Sx's – sudden lateralized lower quadrant pain, N/V; Dx: U/S
    **Tx: relieve torsion, check for viability; resection if vascular necrosis

**Incidental ovarian tumor or cyst when performing another procedure
    4 quadrant wash and send for cytology; biopsy mass, omentum and any
        suspicious areas
    If original procedure elective (eg laparoscopic gastric bypass) – may
        abort procedure depending on findings (eg peritoneal studding)
    If non-elective – finish procedure
    **Do _NOT_ perform oophrectomy at initial procedure

*Endometriosis
    Sx's: **dysmenorrhea, dyspareunia** and **infertility** *(classic)*
        Rectal involvement can cause bleeding during menses → rectal
            endoscopy shows **blue mass*
        Catamenial PTX – endometriosis in lung (causes recurrent PTX)
    MC site – ovaries
    Many women w/ **infertility have endometriosis**
    Tx: progesterone, OCP's, Danazol, NSAID's

**Ovarian cancer
    MCC of gynecologic CA death (non-breast CA)
    2nd MC gynecologic CA (#1 - endometrial CA)
    ↓ed risk – OCPs, bilateral tubal ligation, multiparous
    ↑ed risk – nulliparity, late menopause, early menarche, unopposed post-
        menopausal estrogen replacement; BRCA, HNPCC, Ashkenazi Jews
    Often a **delay in Dx** (60% stage III or IV at Dx); 80% **post-menopausal**
    Sx's: pelvic or abd pain, bloating, feeling full, painful sex, urinary sx's
    Dx: **U/S** and **CA-125**; diagnostic laparoscopy
    *MC type – serous tumors
    *Worst prognosis ovarian CA – clear cell type
    *Best prognosis ovarian CA – malignant germ cell tumors
    MC mets to ovary (ie Krukenberg tumor) – GI CA (**colon CA** MC; if from
        stomach CA, path will show **signet ring cells**)
    *Meige's syndrome – pelvic ovarian tumor (classically fibroma) that
        causes <u>ascites + hydrothorax</u> (MC on right); **tumor excision cures*
        syndrome
    **Stage

I	Confined to ****one or <u>both</u> ovaries**
II	Disease **confined to pelvis**
III	Spread **throughout abdominal cavity** or **positive nodes**
IV	Distant **mets**

        Bilateral ovary involvement still **stage I
        *MC initial regional spread – contra-lateral ovary
    *Tx - all stages get:
        1) **Total abd hysterectomy + bilateral salpingo-oophrectomy**
        2) **Pelvic** and **para-aortic LN dissection**
        3) **Omentectomy**
        4) **4 quadrant washes + Bx's** (under right diaphragm, peri-colic
           recess, pelvic sidewall)
        **Debulking tumor (cyto-reduction of carcinomatosis) – is effective
           and improves prognosis for advanced CA (helps chemo-XRT);
           tumor nodules left behind should be **< 1 cm**
        *Chemo - cisplatin + paclitaxel for residual disease
           *can give intra-peritoneal chemo
        XRT – of some benefit (for residual disease after surgery)
    Overall 5-YS – 35% (late stage at Dx)

Endometrial cancer
    MC gynecologic CA in US (non-breast CA)
    Sx's: vaginal bleeding; *vaginal bleeding in postpartum pt is endometrial*
        CA until proved otherwise (need endometrial Bx)
    RFs: nulliparity, obesity, unopposed estrogen, Tamoxifen
    MC type – endometrioid CA
    Worst prognosis – clear cell
    Dx: endometrial curettage or brush Bx; D&C (**routine screening** w/ RF)
    Tx:
        Stage I (limited to endometrium only) – TAH + BSO
           Abdominal approach, <u>not</u> vaginal
        Stage II, III, and **IV** or **high grade tumors** →
           1) TAH + BSO + para-aortic / pelvic LN dissection
           2) post-op XRT
    Overall 5-YS – 75% (early stage at Dx)

**Cervical cancer

Sx's: vaginal bleeding, painful sex, discharge

PAP smear has greatly decreased incidence of cervical CA

<u>All</u> associated w/ **HPV** (MC HPV 16 and 18)

MC type – squamous cell CA; goes to **obturator nodes 1st**

Dx: **PAP smear** – looks for cervical intraepithelial neoplasia (CIN) or
dysplasia; if present, need a Bx (called colposcopy Bx)

Colposcopy Bx – if high grade CIN (microscopic disease w/o
basement membrane invasion) or if more invasive lesion found
(eg CIS), need conization Bx

Conization Bx – inner lining of cervix is removed

If no basement membrane (BM) invasion (eg carcinoma is situ
or high grade CIN) → **that is all that is necessary*

Stage

CIS full-thickness epithelium; no stromal or BM invasion

I   cervix only

II   upper 2/3 of vagina

III pelvic sidewall, lower 1/3 vagina, hydronephrosis, positive nodes

IV   bladder or rectal invasion (IVA), mets (IVB)

Tx:

***Microscopic Disease** (<u>no</u> basement membrane invasion, eg CIS or
CIN) - **Conization Bx only*

Stages I and II

Total abdominal hysterectomy (TAH) + **pelvic LN dissection**

Stages III to IV - **chemo-XRT *only*** (cisplatin based); if that fails need
<u>pelvic exenteration</u> (TAH+BSO, vagina, rectum, bladder)

Can **leave ovaries** w/ cervical CA (unless pelvic exenteration)

Overall 5-YS – 75% (early stage at Dx due to Pap smear)

Vaginal cancer

MC type – squamous cell CA

Sarcoma Botryoides – rhabdomyosarcoma that occurs in young girls

Tx: resection usual

MC vaginal tumor – invasion from surrounding or distant structure

**Vulvar cancer

MC type – SCCA; goes to <u>inguinal nodes</u> 1st, need **2 cm margins**

Tx: **Paget's, VIN III or higher** (vulvar intra-epithelial neoplasia), or
carcinoma in situ – all premalignant (Tx: WLE)

Stage I (< 2 cm) →

WLE + <u>ipsilateral</u> inguinal and femoral node dissection

Stage II (> 2 cm) or **Stage III** (spread beyond vulva or positive nodes)

***modified radical* vulvectomy** (entire vulva removed
including **bilateral labia majora / minora** and clitoris)
+ <u>bilateral</u> inguinal/femoral LN dissection

Overall 5-YS – 75%

Other GYN Disorders

Post-menopausal vaginal bleeding: Dx – endometrial Bx (suspicious for
endometrial CA)

Uterine Prolapse (procidentia) – uterus protrudes through vagina

RFs – multiparity; Tx: weight loss. D/C smoking (↓ cough), pessary,
vaginal hysterectomy

Polycystic Ovarian Disease

Sx's – amenorrhea, infertility, hirsutism; Tx: **clomiphene** citrate

Uterine leiomyomas (eg fibroids)

Sx's: under hormonal influence; bleeding (MC Sx), recurrent
abortions, infertility; Tx: GnRH analogues (eg **leuprolide**)

Ovarian cysts - <u>septated</u>, <u>solid</u> components, <u>papillary projections</u> or
<u>increased vascular flow</u> on Duplex U/S are all worrisome for CA

529. *All of the following are true except
    a. The middle cerebral artery is connected to the posterior cerebral artery by the posterior communicating artery
    b. Injury w/ neuropraxia usually recovers
    c. Epidural hematomas are MC caused by torn bridging veins
    d. Hemi-transection of the spinal cord is most likely to result in ipsilateral motor and contra-lateral pain and temperature loss

Answer c. *Epidural hematomas** are most commonly caused by bleeding from the **middle meningeal artery** (see Trauma section).

*Circle of Willis
Circle of arterial circulation in the brain such that if one artery is occluded, the communicating arteries will still allow blood flow
Vertebral arteries – coalesce to form a single **basilar artery**
    Basilar artery branches into two **posterior cerebral arteries**
Posterior communicating arteries - these connect **middle cerebral arteries** to **posterior cerebral arteries**
Anterior cerebral arteries – branches of **middle cerebral arteries**
    Connected to each other through one **anterior communicating artery**
The **internal carotid artery** becomes the **middle cerebral artery**

Broca's area – speech motor, posterior part of anterior lobe
Wernicke's area – speech comprehension, temporal lobe
Pituitary adenoma, undergoing XRT, pt now in shock
    Dx: pituitary apoplexy Tx: **steroids**
Diaphragm innervation – **phrenic nerve** (cervical nerve roots 3–5)
Microglial cells – brain macrophages

*Nerve injury
Neuropraxia – mildest form of injury (MC injury)
    No axon or myelin sheath injury but interruption of **conduction impulse**
    Temporary loss of function (motor >> sensory)
    Generally all recover
    Mildest form – foot falls asleep (pressure on sciatic nerve)
    Severe – blunt trauma (make take 6-8 weeks to recover)
*Axonotmesis
    ***Disruption of axon** w/ preservation of myelin sheath
    Paralysis and loss of sensation
    MC w/ crush injury
    Wallerian degeneration of nerve occurs (antegrade degeneration towards end plate)
    Nerve has to regenerate for recover (1 mm/day) – can take weeks
Neurotmesis
    Worst form of injury - severe contusion, stretch, complete laceration
    ***Disruption of axon and myelin sheath**
    May not recover or may need surgery for recovery
*Regeneration of **peripheral nerves** occurs at rate of **1 mm/day***
    Central nerves do not regenerate
Nodes of Ranvier – bare sections between myelin sheath cells; allow salutatory propagation of action potentials
Sensory – 1st to recover after nerve damage

Subarachnoid hemorrhage (SAH, non-traumatic causes listed below)
  Sx's: severe HA (thunderclap), vomiting, confusion, LOC, seizures
  Etiology – cerebral aneurysms (85%, branch points) and AVMs (10%)
  Tx: Prevent **re-bleeding** (open clips or endovascular coils) and
      Prevent **vasospasm** (calcium channel blocker, volume, phenylephrine)

Spinal cord injury
  Complete cord transaction – areflexia, flaccidity, anesthesia
      Autonomic paralysis below level of transection
  Spinal shock (neurogenic shock) – **hypotension, normal or slow heart
  rate,** and **warm extremities** (vasodilated)
      Occurs w/ spinal cord **injuries above T5** (loss of sympathetic tone)
      Tx: fluids initially, may need phenylephrine drip (alpha agonist)
  Brown-Sequard syndrome (incomplete cord transection; hemi-section of
      cord) **MCC** – penetrating injury
      Loss of (occurs below level of injury):
          Ipsilateral motor
          Contra-lateral pain and temperature
      About 90% recover to ambulation
  Cauda equina syndrome – pain and weakness in lower extremities
      Loss of bowel or bladder function
      Due to compression of lumbar nerve roots

  Doral nerve roots (posterior) – generally afferent; carry *sensory* neurons
      Spinothalamic tract – pain and temp
  Ventral nerve roots (anterior) – generally efferent; carry *motor neurons*
      Corticospinal tract – motor
      Rubrospinal tract – motor

Brain tumors
  Sx's: HA, seizures, progressive neuro deficit, persistent vomiting
  Adults – 2/3 supra-tentorial
  Children – 2/3 infra-tentorial
  MC primary brain tumor – gliomas
      MC subtype – glioblastoma multiforme (uniformly fatal)
  MC mets to brain – lung
  MC brain tumor in children – medulloblastoma
  MC mets to brain in children – neuroblastoma

Spine tumors
  MC benign; MC overall – neurofibroma
  Intra-dural tumors more likely benign
  Extra-dural tumors are more likely malignant
  Paraganglioma – can secrete norepinephrine

Myelomeningocele
  Neural cord defect – herniation of spinal cord and nerve roots through
      defect in vertebra; looks like big sac off vertebral column
  If sac ruptured – surgery needed to prevent infection of spinal cord
  MC in lumbar region

GABA (Gamma-Amino-Butyric Acid) – chief neuro-inhibitory neurotransmitter in
    brain; GABA analogues have anti-convulsing, anti-anxiety, relaxing effects

Orthopaedics

530. *A man suffers a minor dog bite and presents 4 days later with pain in a semi-flexed left 2nd digit, tendon sheath tenderness, pain w/ passive motion and swelling in the finger. The most appropriate next step is:
    a. Amputation
    b. Continued antibiotics
    c. FNA
    d. Mid-axial longitudinal incision and drainage

    Answer d. *Supporative Flexor Tenosynovitis is one of the few orthopedic emergencies. It is caused by an infection in the flexor tendon sheath of the hand. Infection here can rapidly destroy the finger's flexing ability. Tx: ****mid-axial longitudinal incision and drainage** (avoid lateral incision along finger – the nerves are there).

531. **All the following are true of supra-condylar humeral fractures in children except
    a. Type III will need percutaneous wire fixation
    b. Type II fractures will likely need wire fixation
    c. Type I fractures can just be placed in a sling
    d. Type I fractures need wire fixation

    Answer d.
    **Type III fractures will need wire fixation
    **Type II will also most likely need wire fixation
    **Type I can just be treated w/ a sling

532. *A 20 yo man falls on an outstretched hand and now complains of tenderness in the "snuff box" of his right hand. You get an XR but it is negative. The most appropriate next step is:
    a. Spica cast up to the elbow, repeat films in 2 weeks
    b. Exploration
    c. Nothing
    d. Tape fingers together

    Answer a. Snuff box tenderness is worrisome for a scaphoid bone Fx. These Fx's are hard to see on X-ray. They are at high risk for avascular necrosis. Tx for a pt w/ snuff box tenderness and a negative X-Ray is a cast up to the elbow w/ F/U XR in 2 wks.

533. **A 59 yo woman undergoes an abdomino-perineal resection which takes 12 hours. Post-operatively, you note she has a foot drop on the right. All of the following are true except:
    a. Proper patient positioning could have likely prevented this problem
    b. This patient should have a fasciotomy
    c. This problem is related to the common peroneal nerve
    d. A foot brace may benefit this patient

    Answer b. ****This patient likely suffered a common peroneal nerve** injury where the peroneal nerve wraps around the leg at the level of the fibula. This occurred from compression of this area while in the lithotomy position.

    The common peroneal nerve bifurcates into the **deep peroneal nerve (dorsiflexion, sensation in 1st toe web-space) and **superficial peroneal nerve** (foot eversion).

534. **A 24 yo man suffers a supracondylar humeral Fx. Six hours after the event, the pt has his arm reduced and placed in a sling. Shortly afterwards, the patient develops severe forearm swelling and pain. The arm is tense. You have trouble finding distal pulses. The most appropriate next step in management is:

a. Emergent open reduction and internal fixation
b. Emergency repair of the brachial artery
c. Angiogram and stent placement
d. Forearm fasciotomies (S-shaped for volar compartment, longitudinal for dorsal compartment)

Answer d. Compartment syndrome (****Volkmann's contracture** in this case) can occur after the interruption of blood flow, a delay (4-6 hours), and then restoration of blood flow. This pt needs forearm fasciotomies to the volar and dorsal compartments.

**Forearm fasciotomy
> Volar incision – **curvilinear (lazy S shape) so that all of the major nerves and arteries are decompressed
> Dorsal incision - **Longitudinal incision (linear)
The vessel involved in **Volkmann's contracture is the **anterior interosseous artery.**

535. **Anterior dislocation of the shoulder is most likely to injure the:
    a. Subclavian vein
    b. Subclavian artery
    c. Axillary nerve
    d. Thoracic duct

Answer c. **Anterior shoulder dislocation is most likely to injure the **axillary nerve.**

536. **Posterior dislocation of the hip is most likely to injure the:
    a. Femoral artery
    b. Femoral vein
    c. Sciatic nerve
    d. Femoral nerve

Answer c. **Posterior hip dislocation is most likely to injure the **sciatic nerve**

537. *All of the following are true except:
    a. Tx for an isolated anterior ring Fx (eg pubic rami) w/ minimal ischial displacement is weight-bearing as tolerated (WBAT)
    b. Salter-Harris III Fx's (crosses the epiphyseal plate) should undergo closed reduction
    c. Humeral spiral Fx's (mid-shaft) are at risk for radial nerve injury
    d. Femur Fx associated w/ tachypnea is most likely from fat embolus

Answer b. Salter-Harris III Fx's (crosses the epiphyseal plate) should undergo open reduction and internal fixation (ORIF)

Humeral spiral Fx's (mid-shaft) are at risk for **radial nerve injury (weak wrist and finger extension)

538. **All of the following are true except
    a. Acute pain w/ ankle ecchymosis and a lump behind the knee in a tennis player is most likely a plantaris muscle tendon rupture
    b. Calcaneus Fx is associated w/ lumbar Fx's in 10% and radius Fx's in 5%
    c. The MC injured nerve w/ lower extremity fasciotomy is the superficial peroneal nerve
    d. Petechiae, hypoxia and mental status changes after setting a long bone Fx suggests ETOH intoxication

Answer d. ****Petechiae, hypoxia and mental status changes** *after setting a long bone Fx suggests* **fat embolism**

The MC injured nerve w/ **lower extremity fasciotomy *is the* **superficial peroneal nerve** *(lateral compartment; affects foot eversion)*

Brachial Plexus
Ulnar nerve
Motor - wrist flexion and intrinsic musculature of hand;
Finger abduction (spread fingers);
Sensory - 5th and ½ 4th fingers, back of hand
Injury – claw hand; involved in **cubital tunnel syndrome** at elbow
Median nerve
Motor - thumb apposition (anterior interosseous, the OK sign), thumb abduction, finger flexors
Sensory - most of palm; 1st 3½ fingers on palmar side
Nerve involved in **carpal tunnel syndrome** at wrist
Injury – decreased thumb movement, fingers will be extended
Radial nerve
Motor - Wrist extension, finger extension, thumb extension, triceps
**No intrinsic hand muscles
Sensory – 1st 3½ fingers on dorsal side
Musculocutaneous nerve – motor to biceps, brachialis, coracobrachialis
Axillary nerve – motor and sensory to deltoid (abduction)

Lower extremity nerves
Obturator nerve	hip adduction
Superior gluteal nerve	hip abduction
Inferior gluteal nerve	hip extension
Femoral nerve	knee extension

Bone Sections
Diaphysis – midsection, shaft
Metaphysis - epiphyseal growth plate (between diaphysis and epiphysis)
Epiphysis – rounded end of long bone

Herniated Lumbar Disc
Sx's **Back pain** aggravated by activity, can **radiate down leg**
Herniated disc is **nucleus pulposus**
Certain movements ↑ inter-vertebral pressure at disc (eg attempting to rise out of a chair and bending over at waist)
Often have a history of chronic back pain.
L1 to L3 nerves - weak hip flexion
*L4 nerve (MC type L4–5 disc) - weak knee extension (quadriceps), weak patellar reflex
*L5 nerve (L5–S1 disc) - weak dorsiflexion (foot drop), ↓ sensation in big toe web space
S1 nerve (S1–S2 disc) - weak plantarflexion, weak Achilles reflex, ↓ sensation in lateral foot
Dx: **MRI** *(best test)*
Tx: 90% treated w/ **NSAID's and pain meds**
With time, disc shrinks on its own, decompressing spine
Failure of conservative Tx (6 weeks) - consider surgery
Surgical decompression removes of part of disc (**discectomy**)
Consider emergent decompression for severe cord compression (ie cauda equina syndrome) - loss of bowel or bladder function, saddle anesthesia, loss of movement, progressive muscle weakness, increasing pain, disc fragments in the cord; Tx: **dexamethasone**, surgical **decompression**

Fractures

Salter Harris Fracture Types in children
>> **Type I and I** – closed reduction
>> **Type III, IV, and V** – crosses epiphyseal plate
>>> Can affect growth plate of bone;
>>> Need open reduction and internal fixation (ORIF)

> Fx's assoc. w/ **avascular necrosis** – scaphoid, femoral neck, talus (ankle)
> Fx's assoc. w/ **non-union** – clavicle, 5th metatarsal (Jones' Fx)
> Fx's assoc. w/ **compartment syndrome** – supracondylar humerus, tibia
> *RF for non-union* – smoking (#1)
> **Spine Fx's** (see Trauma Chp)

Upper Extremity

> **Prolonged hand ischemia** (eg laceration of radial and ulnar arteries) -
>> Motor function can remain in digits after prolonged ischemia because
>> motor groups are in proximal forearm.

> *Shoulder dislocation*
>> **Anterior** (MC, 90%) Tx: closed reduction
>>> Risk of **axillary nerve injury**
>> **Posterior** (seizures, electrocution). Tx: closed reduction
>>> Risk of **axillary artery injury**
>> Surgery for either of above if **displaced humeral Fx** also present

> **Scapula Fx**: Tx: sling unless **glenoid fossa** involved, then need ORIF

> *Proximal humeral Fx*
>> **Non-displaced** Tx: sling; **Displaced or comminuted** Tx: ORIF
>> Risk of **axillary nerve damage**

> **Mid-shaft humeral Fx** – Tx: sling (almost all)
>> Surgery only for failed reduction or neurovascular events
>>> *Risk of **radial nerve damage***

> **Supracondylar humerus Fx**
>> **Adults** → ORIF
>> **Children**
>>> **Type I** (non-displaced) – closed reduction
>>> **Type II and III** (partially and totally displaced) – closed
>>>> reduction and internal fixation w/ Kirschner wire
>>> *Risk of **brachial artery damage***
>> Risk of **Volkmann's Contracture** (ie compartment syndrome, below)

> **Colles' Fx** – fall on outstretched hand, distal radius Fx ± distal ulnar
>> dislocation; *MC Fx in children*
>> Tx: **closed reduction** for vast majority (adults + children)

> *Combined radial and ulnar Fx*
>> **Adults** – ORIF
>> **Children** – **closed reduction** preferred
>> Risk of **ulnar and radial nerve damage** w/ forearm Fx's

> **Scaphoid Fx** (eg wrist Fx; perilunate wrist Fx)
>> **MC carpal bone Fx** – <u>scaphoid</u> (MC Fx in wrist)
>> Snuffbox tenderness *(classic);* can have **negative x-ray**
>> Tx:
>>> **Negative X-ray** – *all pts get spica cast to elbow*, follow-up X
>>>> –rays in 2 weeks to look for Fx healing (occult Fx)
>>> **Non-displaced Fx** (scaphoid or lunate) - spica cast to elbow, 6-
>>>> 8 wks
>>> **Displaced Fx** (<u>scaphoid or lunate</u>) – ORIF
>>> Risk of **avascular necrosis** w/ scaphoid (Tx: hip bone graft)

> **Volkmann's contracture**
>> Supracondylar humerus Fx → occludes *anterior interosseous
>> artery* → closed reduction of Fx → artery opens → reperfusion
>> injury, edema, and *forearm compartment syndrome* (<u>flexor</u>
>> compartment most affected; volar)

Sx's: **pain in forearm w/ passive extension**; weakness; tense
forearm, hypoesthesia; loss of pulse is late finding
Tx: **fasciotomy** (both volar and dorsal compartments)
**Forearm fasciotomy
Volar incision – **curvilinear (lazy S shape) so that all of the major
nerves and arteries are decompressed
Dorsal incision - **Longitudinal incision (linear); Need to open both
the mobile extensor wad and extensor digitorum communis
muscle group compartments
Carpal tunnel syndrome
Median nerve compression by **transverse carpal ligament**
Tx: splint, NSAIDs, steroid injections; transverse carpal ligament
release if refractory
Trigger finger
Tenosynovitis of flexor tendon that catches at MCP joint when trying
to extend finger
Tx: splint, tendon sheath steroid injections (not tendon itself – risk
necrosis); If refractory → **release pulley system at MCP joint**
**Suppurative tenosynovitis
Infection that spreads along flexor tendon sheath (can **destroy
tendon**); can occur after minor trauma (eg cat or dog bite)
Sx's (4 classic signs)
1) **tendon sheath tenderness**
2) **pain w/ passive motion**
3) **swelling along sheath**
4) **semi-flexed posture of involved digit**
**Tx: → mid-axial longitudinal incision and drainage, abx's
*Paronychia – bacterial infection where nail and skin meet on digit; painful
Infection can proceed underneath nail-bed (**erythema, swollen**)
Tx: abx's; warm soaks; ***remove nail** if purulent underneath

Lower extremity
**Pelvic fractures
MC associated injury – closed head injury
Need to Tx **life threatening hemorrhage** from pelvic Fx 1st
Need to assess whether or not the **pelvic ring is stable**
**Isolated pubic rami Fx's do not require ORIF (Tx WBAT)
Bilateral rami Fx's w/ minor displacement do not require ORIF
Generally need **≥ 2 significant Fx's or dislocations** for ring to be
unstable requiring **ORIF**
*Hip dislocation (risk of **avascular necrosis**, avoid delayed reduction)
Posterior (MC 90%) – internal rotation, adduction, shortened leg
Tx: closed reduction; risk of ***sciatic nerve injury**
Anterior – external rotation, abduction, shortened leg
Tx: closed reduction; risk of injury to ***femoral artery or nerve**
Hip Fx (ie femoral head and acetabulum)**;** almost all treated **surgically**
High mortality in **pts aged > 65** (20% mortality in 6 months)
Femoral neck Fx – external rotation, abduction, shortened
ORIF or partial arthroplasty (hemiarthroplasty)
Risk of **avascular necrosis** if open reduction delayed
Femoral shaft Fx – ORIF w/ intramedullary rod (adults + children > age 6)
Children aged < 6 - spica cast
*Lateral knee trauma – can injure the following:
Anterior cruciate ligament
Posterior cruciate ligament
Medial meniscus
Medial collateral ligament
**Posterior knee dislocation – closed reduction
All pts need angiogram to R/O popliteal artery injury
Patellar Fx - Tx: **long leg cast** for most; **ORIF** if comminuted

Tibial plateau, tibial shaft, and **tibia-fibula Fx's**
> Tx: **ORIF** unless open Fx, then need **external fixator**
> Risk of **compartment syndrome** w/ tibial plateau Fx

*__*Plantaris muscle rupture__* – pain and mass below popliteal fossa
> (contracted plantaris) and ankle ecchymosis. Unnecessary for normal
> function so not repaired (eg *__*tennis players__*, still be able to walk on it
> unlike Achilles' tear)

*__*Achilles tendon tear__* – re-attachment in OR usual

*__*Calcaneus Fx__* (heel)
> Tx: **cast immobilization** if non-displaced
> **ORIF** for <u>any</u> displacement
> Risk of **compartment syndrome** of foot
> > *__*10% have lumbar spine Fx's, 5% distal forearm Fx's__* (from fall)

__MC injured nerve w/ lower extremity fasciotomy__** – superficial peroneal
> nerve (foot eversion)

__Foot-drop after:__**
> **Lithotomy position** (compression of side of leg while in stirrups) or;
> **Fibula head Fx** or;
> **Crossing legs for long period** (temporary dysfunction)
> → **__**common peroneal nerve for all__** (Tx: foot brace for foot drop)
> Common peroneal nerve wraps around the neck of the fibula and
> > divides into the deep and superficial peroneal nerves

Swollen erythematous knee, sexually active – aspirate to R/O infection
> (gonorrhea)

__Fat embolism__**
> Sx's: **__**petechiae, hypoxia,__** and **mental status changes** (confusion) –
> > *classic triad*; other sx's similar to PE (following long bone Fx)
> **Sudan red stain** – fat in sputum and urine
> **MCC** – lower extremity (hip and femur) Fx's or ortho procedures
> **Tx:** supportive; may need to intubate

Lower leg compartments
> **Anterior** (Arteries/Nerves) – anterior tibial artery, deep peroneal nerve
> **Lateral** (Nerves) – superficial peroneal nerve
> **Deep posterior** (Arteries/Nerves) – posterior tibial artery, peroneal artery,
> > tibial nerve
> **Superficial posterior** (Nerves) – sural nerve

__Compartment syndrome__**
> **__**MC in anterior compartment of leg__** (get foot-drop) after **restoration of
> vascular compromise**
> **High risk Fx's** – supracondylar fracture (Volkmann's contracture), tibial
> > plateau Fx, calcaneus Fx, elbow dislocations
> > Any injury resulting in **interruption** and then **restoration** of blood
> > > flow; **__**can also occur from large crush injuries__**
> Is a **reperfusion injury** mediated by **PMNs**
> Can occur in any muscle compartment (*pressure in compartment exceeds
> > capillary filling pressure* – get **rhabdomyolysis**):
> Sx: **Classic scenario** – Fx w/ loss of blood flow → repair (> 4-6 hours later)
> > → **pain** and **swelling** soon post-op
> > 1st **finding** – <u>pain</u> w/ passive motion
> > > Others – swelling; paresthesias → anesthesia → paralysis →
> > > > poikiothermia → pulseless (late finding)
> > > **Distal pulses** can be <u>present</u> w/ compartment syndrome → last
> > > > thing to go
> Dx:
> > **Based on clinical suspicion** (if suspected → fasciotomy)
> > Pressure **> 20 mmHg** abnormal

Tx:

**Fasciotomy (for leg - medial incison for superficial + deep posterior
and lateral incision for anterior + lateral compartments)
With fasciotomy, you are through the fascia when the **muscle bulges**
Incise the **total length of compartment** (eg the length of the leg)
Remove all dead tissue (myoglobinuria if you don't resect)
Alkalinize urine for myoglobinuria; watch for hyperkalemia
**MC injured nerve w/ lower extremity fasciotomy - *superficial
peroneal*

Bone tumors

MC bone tumor – mets (**MC - breast**, #2 prostate)
Tx: ORIF w/ impending Fx (> 50% cortical involvement); then XRT
Colon CA rarely goes to bone
XRT for painful bony mets
Pathologic fractures – Tx: ORIF
MC primary malignant bone tumor – multiple myeloma
Tx: chemo for systemic disease
*MC bony tumor overall – osteochondroma
*MC bony malignant tumor – osteosarcoma
Presence of **pain** w/ any bone lesion (other than a Fx) is highly suggestive
of malignancy
Most impt prognostic indicator for sarcomas – tumor grade
Malignant Bony tumors
Osteosarcoma (osteogenic sarcoma)
MC primary malignant bony tumor (35%)
MC at **knee (50%)**; **Young pts** (80% aged < 20 years)
Tx: **limb-sparing resection in 90%**; consider **pre-op chemo-
XRT** (doxorubicin-based; see Skin and Soft Tissue Chp)
Overall 5-YS – 65%
Chondrosarcoma - Can arise from **osteochondroma**
Ewing's Sarcoma
MC in adolescents; **painful swelling**
MC location proximal **diaphysis of femur** (long bones)
Tx: *Chemo-XRT is mainstay of Tx*
Chemo – Doxorubicin based (ifosfamide, etoposide)
**all pts get chemo due to high rate of micro-metastases
Then XRT ± resection (can usually spare limb)

Torus fracture – buckling of metaphyseal cortex in children (eg distal radius)
Tx - cast (3 weeks)
Open fractures – washout, abx's, external fixation, soft tissue coverage

Infectious Arthritis

Arthrocentesis – > 50,000 WBCs highly suspicious for infectious arthritis
Tx: **Abx's** (Vancomycin usual unless worried about gonorrhea)
Surgical drainage indicated in most cases, esp w/ larger joints

Pediatric Surgery

539. **All of the following are true except:
    a. Elevated alkaline phosphatase in a child is due to bone growth
    b. Surfactant is effective for respiratory distress syndrome
    c. The gallbladder is considered part of the midgut
    d. Newborns are at increased risk for cutaneous infection due to impaired PMN chemotaxis

    Answer c. The gallbladder is part of the foregut (proximal to Ampulla).

540. *The maintenance fluid for a 25 kg girl would be:
    a. 45 cc/hr
    b. 65 cc/hr
    c. 85 cc/hr
    d. 105 cc/hr

    Answer b. 65 cc/hr (40 cc/hr for 1st 10 kg, 20 cc/hr for 2nd 10 kg, 1 cc/hr for each kg after that).

541. A neonate has a large hemangioma on his face. All of the following are appropriate in this patient's management except:
    a. These lesions can usually be observed initially
    b. These lesions usually regress
    c. A hemangioma filling the ear canal should be observed
    d. Persistent large hemangiomas after age 8 will likely need treatment

    Answer c. Hemangiomas causing a functional deficit (eg eyelid, ear canal) should be removed.

542. A 3 yo child has a 0.5 cm hemangioma on her lateral nare that has been present since she was 2 years old. The most appropriate Tx is:
    a. Multiple pulse dye laser treatments
    b. Excision and flap closure
    c. Steroid injection
    d. Observation

    Answer d. Observation is generally indicated for most congenital **hemangiomas** until age 5-6.

543. All of the following are true except:
    a. Congenital lobar emphysema is due to failure of bronchial cartilage to develop, resulting in air-trapping
    b. Bronchogenic cysts are abnormal lung tissue outside lung (MC in mediastinum)
    c. CCAM are due to overgrowth of bronchial tissue and are usually connected to the airway
    d. The systemic arterial supply should be addressed last when resecting pulmonary sequestrations

    Answer d. The **systemic arterial supply** should be resected 1st when resecting **pulmonary sequestrations.**

544. *A 2 yo boy in the ED has a new inguinal mass. All the following are true except:
    a. Sedation will help reduce inguinal hernias
    b. Inguinal hernias should be fixed 2-3 weeks after reduction
    c. To reduce an inguinal hernia manually, the child should be placed in trendelenburg position w/ knees bent
    d. Extension into the internal ring differentiates an inguinal hernia from a hydrocoele

Answer b. Inguinal hernias in children should be fixed 24-48 hours after a reduction. Incarcerated hernias (unable to reduce) should be repaired the same day as discovery to avoid infarction (emergency procedure).

545. *A 2 yo is brought in for an umbilical hernia. All of the following are true except:
    a. This pt should have surgery at about age 5 if the hernia fails to close
    b. This patient is at high risk for incarceration
    c. These hernias are increased in African-American patients
    d. These hernias are increased in premature patients

    Answer b. Children with umbilical hernias are at low risk for incarceration.

546. *All of the following are true of cryptorchidism (undescended testicle) except:
    a. Complications include infertility, torsion and testicular CA
    b. The MC location is the inguinal canal
    c. CA risk is reduced if the testicle(s) are brought into the scrotum
    d. Division of the spermatic vessels is indicated at re-operation for orchiopexy if inadequate length is still an issue

    Answer c. Risk of testicular CA remains the same even if the testicle is brought into scrotum (lifetime surveillance). The blood supply to the **vas deferens** collateralizes to the testicles if the spermatic vessels are ligated.

547. *A 15 yo boy develops sudden, severe scrotal pain and a high-riding right testicle. The next appropriate step is:
    a. Bilateral exploration of testicles through inguinal incision
    b. Unilateral exploration of testicle through inguinal incision
    c. Bilateral exploration of testicles through scrotal incision
    d. Unilateral exploration of testicle through scrotal incision

    Answer c. Tx of choice for testicular torsion is to pexy the involved testicle if still viable (otherwise resection) and to pexy the contra-lateral testicle (through a *scrotal incision*, unlike inguinal incision for testicular mass)

548. *All of the following are true of neuroblastoma except:
    a. N-myc and diploid tumors confers a worse prognosis
    b. The MC location is the adrenal gland
    c. Catecholamine secretion is common
    d. Primary neuroblastomas that cross midline are considered stage II

    Answer d. Primary tumors that cross the midline are considered stage III

549. *All of the following are true of Wilms' Tumor except::
    a. Most important prognostic indicator is tumor grade (anaplastic worse)
    b. Is the MC kidney tumor in children
    c. Lung mets are initially treated w/ resection
    d. Rupture of tumor during resection can *up-stage* the tumor

    Answer c. Tx for lung mets from Wilms' Tumors initially is whole lung XRT

550. *A 2 yo girl presents w/ painless rectal bleeding. You perform an exam, including DRE, which is normal. Given the most likely cause, which of the following tests will be best to make the diagnosis:
    a. Abdominal CT
    b. MRI
    c. 99m-Tc-pertechnate scan
    d. EGD

    Answer c. Meckel's diverticulum is the MCC of painless LGIB in children. It is best diagnosed w/ a Meckel scan (99m-Tc-pertechnate scan)

551. A newborn has a gross defect in his abd wall. All of the following are true except:
   a.   Gastroschisis is due to rupture of an umbilical vein
   b.   Omphalocele is a failure of embryonal development
   c.   Retention sutures are indicated if having trouble returning the bowel to the abdomen at primary closure
   d.   The most serious complication is sepsis

   Answer c. If having trouble returning the bowel to the abdomen for either **gastroschisis** or **omphalocele**, a silastic silo should be placed (contains the abdominal contents outside the abdomen) which is gradually tightened over time (stretches abdominal wall and makes room for intestines).

552. *A 2 yo boy in the ED has abd distension, pain, vomiting and currant jelly stools. The maximum barium column height and maximum air pressure when trying to reduce an intussusception with an air-contrast enema are:
   a.   Column height 1 meter, air pressure 120 mmHg
   b.   Column height 2 meters, air pressure 240 mmHg
   c.   Column height 2 meters, air pressure 240 mmHg
   d.   Column height 2 meters, air pressure 240 mmHg

   Answer a. The max column height of barium when trying to reduce an **intussusception** is **1 meter**. The max air pressure if you are using an air contrast enema is **120 mmHg**. If the intussusception does not reduce with those maximums (can keep it there for about an hour), take pt to OR and do it manually. You risk perforation if you go higher than these values. If the intussusception is not completely relieved despite pneumatic attempt, you need laparotomy for manual reduction.

553. *A newborn infant fails to pass meconium in the 1st 24 hours of life and subsequently gets progressive abd distension. Plain films which show distended loops of small bowel, but no air-fluid levels. The colon is totally decompressed. The transition point is in the RLQ. On exam, the child has an anus located in the proper position. The most appropriate next test is:
   a.   Upper GI series
   b.   Barium enema
   c.   Enteroclysis
   d.   Rectal biopsy

   Answer b. The scenario is most consistent w/ **meconium ileus**. The obstruction occurs in the terminal ileum. No air-fluid levels form because the bowel contents stick to the bowel wall instead of pooling (thick meconium). Barium enema can make the Dx as well as relieve the obstruction. **N-acetylcysteine enemas** usually work better than barium.

554. *A 3 week old infant who is otherwise healthy is brought to the ED for vomiting of greenish fluid. The most appropriate next test is:
   a.   Upper GI series
   b.   Barium enema
   c.   Enteroclysis
   d.   Rectal biopsy

   Answer a. Bilious vomiting in any child in the first 2 years of life requires an upper GI series to rule out **malrotation**. This is done _**emergently**_. Characteristic finding on UGI - **duodenum does _not_ cross midline

555. *A newborn infant fails to pass meconium in the 1st 24 hours of life and subsequently gets progressive abd distension. Your order plain films which show a distended colon. On exam, the child has an anus located in the proper position and on rectal exam there is explosive release of watery stool. The most appropriate next test is:

a. Upper GI series
b. Barium enema
c. Enteroclysis
d. Rectal biopsy

Answer d. The scenario is most consistent with **Hirschsprung's disease**. Dx of Hirschsprung's Disease is made w/ rectal biopsy, which shows absence of ganglion cells in the myenteric plexus.

556. *A 3 week old male infant is brought to the ED for repeated forceful vomiting such that it hits the wall opposite the child. On exam, you notice a small protuberance in his RUQ. The vomiting is non-bilious. The most appropriate next test is:
    a. Upper GI series
    b. Ultrasound
    c. Enteroclysis
    d. Abdominal CT scan

Answer b. Projectile vomiting and "olive" in the RUQ is most consistent w/ **pyloric stenosis**. Dx is best w/ U/S. *These pts get hypochloremic, hypokalemic metabolic alkalosis.*

557. *A newborn has severe respiratory distress immediately following birth. CXR shows loops of bowel filling the left chest. All of the following are true except:
    a. Patients with this problem have about a 50% survival overall
    b. The incidence is increased on the left side compared to right
    c. Both lungs are dysfunctional
    d. Repair immediately after birth is indicated

Answer d. The above scenario is most consistent w/ **congenital diaphragmatic hernia.** This lesion is associated w/ a 50% overall survival. These pts should be stabilized <u>before</u> repair (high frequency ventilation, inhaled NO, ECMO)

558. *A newborn suffers from severe aspiration and choking w/ feeds. You try to place an NG tube and cannot get it down. CXR shows the NG tube stops in the mid-esophagus and a distended stomach. The following are true of the most likely Dx except:
    a. The MC type is Type C
    b. Tx generally requires right thoracotomy and end to end anastomosis
    c. The MC post-op Cx is leak
    d. Delayed repair is indicated for low birth weight or sepsis

Answer c. *The MC post-op Cx from repair of TEF is GERD:*
*Type C TEF is MC and involves a proximal esophageal pouch and a distal TEF. You cannot pass an NGT because it gets held up in the pouch. Tx of TEF generally involves **right thoracotomy** w/ end to end **anastomosis** of the esophagus and closure of the trachea.*

559. **Treatment for a type I choledochal cyst is:
    a. Careful follow-up
    b. Cystogastrostomy
    c. Cystoduodenostomy
    d. Cyst resection and hepatic-jejunostomy

Answer d. **Choledochal cysts** need to be resected because of the risk of forming cancer in the cyst and the risk of cholangitis and pancreatitis. A hepatico-jejunostomy should be performed for Type I cysts. These form from abnormal reflux of pancreatic enzymes.

Embryology and Development

Foregut – includes lungs, esophagus, stomach, pancreas, liver, gallbladder, bile duct, duodenum proximal to and including ampulla

Midgut – includes duodenum distal to ampulla, small bowel, large bowel to distal ⅓ of transverse colon

Hindgut – includes distal ⅓ of transverse colon to anal canal

Midgut rotates 270 degrees counterclockwise during normal development

Umbilical vessels – **2 umbilical arteries** (from iliac arteries) and **1 umbilical vein** (drains to portal system and IVC)

↑ed **alkaline phosphatase** in children vs. adults from **bone growth**

Respiratory Distress Syndrome (RDS; eg hyaline membrane disease): Tx – surfactant

Immunity at birth

IgA – from mothers milk

IgG – only immunoglobulin to crosses placenta

****PMNs** have **impaired chemotaxis** (children at risk for **cutaneous** infections)

Maintenance intravenous fluid rate

4 cc/kg/hr for 1st 10 kg
2 cc/kg/hr for 2nd 10 kg
1 cc/kg/hr after above

Maintenance Fluid Type

Neonates – D10 1/4 normal saline (no potassium)

Infants – D10 1/4 normal saline (no potassium until making urine)

Toddlers and school age – D5 1/2 normal saline w/ 20 mEq K

Effective fluid resuscitation

Neonates and infants – urine output of 2-3 cc/kg/hr

Toddlers and school age – urine output of 1 cc/kg/hr

Children (<6 months) have only **25% the GFR capacity of adults** – poor concentrating ability, careful w/ potassium containing fluids

MCC childhood death – trauma

Trauma bolus – 20 cc/kg x 2, then blood 10 cc/kg

Tachycardia – best indicator of shock in children

Neonate	>150
Age 0-1 year	>120
Rest	>100

Initial fluid resuscitation w/ dehydration (eg **pyloric stenosis) – normal saline 20 cc/kg

Most commons (in childhood unless o/w stated)

MC malignancy – leukemia (ALL)

MC tumor – hemangioma

MC tumor in newborn – sacrococcygeal teratoma

MC solid tumor class – CNS tumors

MC intra-abdominal tumor – neuroblastoma

MC in child <2 years – neuroblastoma

MC in child >2 years – Wilms tumor

MC kidney tumor – Wilms' Tumor

MC liver tumor – hepatoblastoma (70% liver tumors in children malignant)

MC lung tumor – carcinoid

MCC duodenal obstruction – malrotation

MC in newborns (<1 week) – duodenal atresia

MC after newborn period (>1 week) – malrotation

MCC colon obstruction – Hirschsprung's disease

MCC painful lower GI bleeding – benign anorectal lesions (fissures, etc)

MCC painless lower GI bleeding – Meckel's diverticulum

MCC Upper GI bleeding in years 0–1 – gastritis, esophagitis
MCC Upper GI bleeding 1 year to adult - esophageal varices, esophagitis
Double bubble sign (gastric + duodenal dilatation on AXR) – malrotation,
duodenal atresia, or annular pancreas

****Hemangioma**

MC tumor of childhood and infancy

Appears at birth or shortly after

Usually rapid growth w/ first 12 months of life but then involutes

MC sites - head and neck

Tx: ****Observation** – most resolve by **age 5-6** (85%)

Treatment indications:

1) Has **uncontrollable growth** *or:*

2) **Impairs function** (airway, eyelid or ear canal) *or:*

3) **Persistent after age 8**

4) **Ulceration** and **recurrent bleeding**

Tx if indicated:

**Oral steroids (*best Tx*; possible lesion injection as adjunct)

Pulsed dye laser (better for more superficial lesions without
significant volume, eg port-wine stains)

Consider resection if steroids not successful

Rare cx's of hemangioendothelioma (infants; usually liver hemangiomas)

Kasabach-Merritt syndrome – consumptive **coagulopathy** (high
PT, PTT) and **thrombocytopenia**; newborns

Tx: **embolization** and **steroids** *(best Tx)*; surgery rare

CHF (A-V shunting) – Tx: **embolization** and **steroids;** surgery rare

Congenital capillary malformation (port wine stain) Tx– pulsed dye laser

Congenital Vascular Malformations (AVMs)

Arterio-venous (**MC type to cause sx's** and **MC requiring Tx**)

Surgical indications: hemorrhage, ischemia to affected limb, CHF,
functional impairment, limb-length discrepancy (AVM limb longer)

Tx: **embolization** (may be sufficient) and/or **resection** if sx's

Congenital anomalies of the lung

Congenital lobar emphysema (hyperinflation)

Sx's: resp distress or hypotension (same mechanism as tension PTX)

Bronchus cartilage fails to develop – get air trapping w/ expiration

MC location – LUL

Dx: **CXR** - hyperinflation of lobe; compression of other structures

Tx: **lobectomy**

*Bronchogenic Cysts

Sx's: can compress airways w/ **resp distress** or become **infected;**
Newborns can become very ill

Are **extra-pulmonary** cysts formed by **abnormal lung tissue**
(parenchyma, cartilage) **Are not connected to airway*

MC cyst of mediastinum

MC location – right side near carina

Often contain milky liquid; malignant degeneration reported

Tx: **cyst resection**

Congenital cystic adenomatoid malformations (CCAM)

Sx's: newborns - resp distress, older children - infection

Rapid decompensation can occur w/ ventilator – need
emergent decompression by removing cyst

From **overgrowth of bronchiole tissue** (no cartilage; columnar
epithelium); **MC** in lower lobes

Usually **intra-pulmonary**; can get air-trapping

Connected to airway bronchus

Malignant degeneration reported

Tx: lobectomy

Pulmonary sequestration
>Sx's: FTT, resp distress (tachypnea), infection, CHF, hemorrhage
>>Has **continuous murmur** (DDx- AVM, sequestration, PDA)
>Dx: **CT angio** - lung mass w/ anomalous blood supply
>Path
>>**Lung tissue** but <u>not</u> connected to airway and has *******systemic arterial blood supply*** (lung tissue can be intra-lobar or extra-lobar)
>>**MC location** - LLL, ***but <u>no</u> connection to airway*
>>*Anomalous arterial supply*
>>>*MC off thoracic aorta*
>>>Can also come off **abdominal aorta** (celiac) through **inferior pulmonary ligament**
>>**Intra-lobar sequestration** – pulmonary venous connection
>>**Extra-lobar sequestration** – systemic venous drainage usual (MC - **azygos vein**)
>>May have malignant change
>*Tx: *need to ligate systemic arterial supply 1st; lobectomy (or resection of mass if extra-lobar)*

*<u>Pulmonary arterio-venous malformation</u> (AVM) – continuous murmur
>Tx: embolization 1st line now

<u>Hydrocoele in children</u>
>Formed from persistent **tunica vaginalis**
>Can have connection to peritoneum (**processus vaginalis**, communicating hydrocoele) or not (non-communicating)
>Most disappear by 1 year
>Can be in **inguinal canal** or **scrotum**
>U/S - hydrocoele will <u>transluminate</u> if in scrotum (bowel from hernia will not)
>**Surgical indications:**
>>1) At **age 1 year** if not resolved *or;*
>>2) **Communicating** (persistent processus vaginalis; size waxes/wanes)
>Tx: **resect hydrocoele + ligate processus vaginalis** (inguinal approach)

<u>Inguinal hernia in children</u>
>Due to persistent **processus vaginalis; MC in males,** MC on **right**
>Can cause **SBO** or bowel strangulation w/ incarceration
>**RFs** – prematurity
>Varying degrees – can go all the way to the scrotum or stop short
>*Lump in inguinal canal (eg intestine, cecum) at <u>internal ring</u> differentiates hernia from hydrocoele*
>Tx:
>>**Incarcerated Hernia** (high risk age **< 1 year**) – tender, firm swelling
>>>**Manual Reduction** (firm steady pressure) w/ **sedation**
>>>>**Trendelenburg** position (head down) w/ **knees bent**
>>>**Emergent operation** if not able to reduce incarceration
>>>**If reduced → admit, repair within next 24-48 hours**
>>**Non-incarcerated** - elective repair within 1 week
>>Repair – ****<u>high ligation</u>** (to age 16 or so) ; make sure testicle in scrotum at end of procedure
>>Explore **contra-lateral side** if **left sided, female,** or child **< 1 year**

<u>Umbilical hernia</u>
>Failure of closure of linea alba
>Most will close by age 3
>↑ed in African Americans, prematurity, males
>Rarely cause incarceration
>Tx: surgery if not closed by **age 5**, if **incarceration,** or if pt has a **VP shunt**

**Undescended testicles (cryptorchidism)
- Path
  - **MC location** – 90% in inguinal canal
    - Can be anywhere in retroperitoneum, ectopic or vanished
    - 30% bilateral; **inguinal hernias** common
  - **Risks** of undescended testicle:
    - **Testicular CA** (5 x if unilateral, 10 x if bilateral, get **seminoma**)
      - ****CA risk stays the same even if testicles brought into scrotum**
    - **Infertility, Torsion**
  - Tx: **Medical Tx:** hCG injections (variable success); **wait 4-6 mos** after birth before surgery
- **Surgery**
  - **Orchiopexy** through **inguinal incision** (if testicle in canal); attach testis to **scrotum**; **high ligation** of inguinal canal
  - If not able to get testicles down (from inadequate length of cord structures)→ close, wait 6 months and try again
    - ****If won't come down again, perform **division of spermatic vessels** (away from testis) to get length, then attach to scrotum (blood supply to **vas deferens** keeps testicles alive)
  - ***Adult cryptorchidism** - resect testicle, almost all non functional

**Neuroblastoma
- **MC extra-cranial solid malignancy in children**
- **MC malignancy in infancy period**
- **MC age ≤ 2** (50%)
- Sx's
  - **MC presentation** – asymptomatic mass
  - Other sx's – diarrhea, **raccoon eyes** (orbital mets), **HTN, unsteady gait** (opsomyoclonus syndrome)
- Path
  - From **neural crest cells** - small round blue cells in **rosette pattern**
  - **MC location** – adrenal gland; also occurs along sympathetic chain
  - 90% secrete **catecholamines** (check UA-VMA, HVA, metanephrines)
  - 50% have **metastases** at Dx (lung and bone)
  - Disease spectrum: ganglioneuroma (benign)→ ganglioneuroblastoma (malignant)→ neuroblastoma (most malignant)
  - ****Worse prognosis** (categorized into low, moderate, and high risk)
    - **Age > 18 months**
    - **Tumor grade** (poor histology, high mitosis index, diploid tumor)
    - **Mets**
      - ****N-myc oncogene** amplification (regulates microRNAs)
- Dx: **CT chest/abd/pelvis** - ± calcifications; **compresses** renal parenchyma rather than invades (DDx vs. Wilms' tumor)
  - **MIBG** – can locate tumors
- ****Stage IV-S**   1) **Age < 1** and;
  - 2) **Localized** tumor (stage I or II) and;
  - 3) **Distant mets** (liver, skin, bone)
- Tx: **Low Risk** - resection only
  - **Moderate or High Risk**
    - 1) **Neoadjuvant chemo** (DECC) - doxorubicin, etoposide, cisplatin + cyclophosphamide (then **retinoic acid** if high risk) – neoadjuvant Tx can downstage tumors
    - 2) **Resection**
    - 3) **XRT** for residual DZ (if high risk, XRT to primary area)
- **Overall 5-YS** – 40%

*Wilms' tumor (nephroblastoma, is a <u>kidney</u> tumor)
> **MC kidney tumor in children**
> **MC age > 2** (mean 3 years)
> Sx's **MC presentation** – asymptomatic mass
>> Other- <u>hemi-hypertrophy</u> (high association w/ Wilms) hematuria, HTN
> Path: 10% bilateral
>> ***Most impt prognostic indicator** – tumor grade (<u>anaplastic</u> worst)
> Dx: **Abd CT** – **replacement** of renal parenchyma - <u>not</u> displacement and <u>no</u> calcifications (DDx vs. neuroblastoma)
> Tx: **resection** and chemo <u>+</u> XRT
> ***Lung mets** – *Tx whole lung XRT (resection if that fails)*
> Chemo (VAD) – vincristine, actinomycin, doxorubicin
> **IVC extension** - occurs through **renal vein**, **can <u>extract</u> from IVC*
> **Avoid rupture** of tumor w/ resection - can ↑ stage
> **Overall 5-YS** – 90%

<u>Hepatoblastoma</u> - MC malignant liver tumor in children (80%)

*Meckel's diverticulum
> **MCC of painless lower GI bleeding in children aged ≤ 2 years**
> **MC presentation in adults** – obstruction
>> Obstruction from **intussusception** or **volvulus**
>> Can also get diverticulitis
> **2's**
>> 2 feet from ileo-cecal valve
>> 2 inches in length
>> 2% of population
>> Usually present in 1st 2 years of life with **bleeding**
>> 2% symptomatic
>> 2 **tissue types** (pancreatic and gastric)
>>> MC – **pancreatic**
>>> Most likely to be symptomatic – **gastric** (causes bleeding)
> Is a **true diverticula** (involves all layers of bowel wall)
> Persistent vestigial remnant of **omphalomesenteric duct** (ie **persistent vitelline duct)**
> Found on anti-mesenteric border of small bowel
> Dx: **Meckel scan** (99-Tc-pertechnate) if trouble locating (mucosa lights up)
> Tx:
>> **Incidental** → usually not removed unless **gastric mucosa** suspected (diverticulum feels **thick**) or has a very **narrow neck**
>> **Diverticulectomy** – for uncomplicated diverticulitis (base <u>not</u> involved)
>> **Segmental resection** for diverticulitis and:
>>> 1) **Complicated** (eg perforation)
>>> 2) **Neck of diverticulum is > 1/3 diameter of bowel lumen** (don't want to narrow lumen)
>>> 3) **Base** involved

*Gastroschisis
> Congenital **abdominal wall defect**
> Etiology – **intrauterine rupture of **umbilical vein** (most likely)*
> RFs – high risk pregnancies, low birth weight
> Path
>> Almost always **right of midline** near umbilicus
>> **No peritoneal sac**
>> **Stiff bowel** from exposure to amniotic fluid
>> 10% have **congenital anomalies** *(less than omphalocele)*
> Tx:
>> **Saline soaked gauzes** (prevent <u>fluid loss</u> from exposed bowel)
>> Fluid resuscitation, prophylactic abx's, repair when stable
>> **At operation:**

Place bowel back in abdomen and close primarily (as long as it
is not tight and the bowel is not compromised)
Often can't get primary repair and have to attach a *silastic
silo* to abdominal wall:
Contains abdominal contents outside body
Progressively tightened over days-weeks to stretch abd
cavity wall and make room for intestines
Primary closure at a later date
*Check for other abnormalities (MC - *intestinal atresia)*
MC serious complication – sepsis
Mortality – 10%

Omphalocele
Congenital **abdominal wall defect**
Etiology – **failure of embryonal development**
Path
Midline defect
Has **peritoneal sac w/ umbilical cord attached**
50% have associated **congenital anomalies** (eg Down's, cardiac, GI
and neuro; causes *worse prognosis then gastroschisis*)
Can contain bowel, liver, spleen, etc
Tx:
Saline soaked gauzes (prevent fluid loss from exposed bowel)
Fluid resuscitation, prophylactic abx's, repair when stable
At operation:
Place bowel back in abd and close primarily (as long as bowel
is not compromised)
Often can't get primary repair and have to attach a *silastic
silo* to abdominal wall: (same method as gastroschisis)
Check for other abnormalities (eg **malrotation**)
MC serious complication – sepsis
Mortality – 20% (mainly increased due to assoc. congenital anomalies)

Patent Urachus – connection between umbilicus and bladder
Patent Omphalomesenteric Duct (Vitelline duct)
Connects ileum and umbilicus; can **drain sucus out umbilicus**
Tx: resection of the persistent duct
Persistent Omphalomesenteric Vessels (Vitelline vessels)
Artery passes from umbilicus to aorta; **Vein** from umbilicus to portal vein
MC presents w/ torsion of bowel w/ possible strangulation, necrosis
Tx: de-torse bowel w/ resection if necrotic, ligation of persistent vasculature
Omphalitis
Infection of **umbilical stump** after birth
Can lead to portal vein thrombosis (↑LFTs, possible variceal bleeding)
Tx: anticoagulation for acute portal vein thrombosis; abx's for infection

Necrotizing enterocolitis (NEC)
Sx's: **Bloody stools** after **1st feeding in premature neonate** (*classic*)
Others – feeding intolerance, distension, lethargy, vomiting
RFs: prematurity, hypoxia, hypotension, anemia, polycythemia, sepsis
Dx:**Serial AXR's** (Q 6 hours) - check for free air, **pneumotosis**
(pathognomonic), portal vein air
Lateral decubitus best to look for free air
Initial Tx: NPO, IV fluids, prophylactic Abx's, NGT, TPN (medical Tx
usually for 2 weeks); serial exams and AXR's (Q 6 hours)
Indications for OR: free air, peritonitis or clinical deterioration
→ resect dead bowel and bring up ostomies
Extremely ill and can't tolerate laparotomy – **place drain** in NICU
Pneumotosis and/or portal venous air by themselves are not
indications for drain or laparotomy
Mortality 10%

Can get late **stenosis** at previous NEC areas
Need **barium contrast enema** and **upper GI w/ SBFT** before taking down
   ostomies to R/O distal obstruction from stenosis
At risk for **short bowel syndrome** later in life

**Intussusception
   MC age – 3 months to 3 years
   Sx's: **RUQ pain, 'sausage mass'** and **abd distention**
      Currant jelly stools (from vascular congestion, <u>not</u> an indication for
         resection)
   Path: Invagination of one loop of intestine into another (**MC – ileocolic**)
      Lead points in children:
         MC – *enlarged Peyer's Patches*
         Others – Meckel's diverticulum, lymphoma
      Recurrence after reduction – 15%
         Surgery if occurs <u>after 2nd time of reduction</u>
   Tx: ***Reduce w/ air-contrast enema**
      90% successful (<u>no</u> surgery required if reduced)
         **Max pressure with air-contrast enema – 120 mmHg
         **Max column height with barium enema – 1 meter (3 feet)
         ↑**perforation risk beyond these values** → need laparotomy
            w/ manual reduction if you have reached these values
         Incompletely relieved intussusception despite above –
            laparotomy for manual reduction
      Need to go to OR with **peritonitis, free air,** if **unable to reduce,** or
         occurs a **3rd time** - usually don't require resection unless
         associated with lead point (eg Meckel's) or perforation
   Adult w/ intussusception – *most likely has **malignant lead point (eg
      colon CA, metastatic melanoma)* → *OR for **resection** (<u>no</u> reduction)*

*Hirschsprung's disease
   MCC colonic obstruction in infants; <u>Males</u> (4:1)
   Sx's: **Infants fail to pass meconium in 1st 24 hours** (MC Sx)
      Others sx's - distention, constipation, vomiting
      Can get **explosive release of watery stool** w/ anorectal exam
   Dx:***Rectal biopsy (best test)** – *diagnostic (suction cup biopsy)*
      *Absence of ganglion cells in myenteric plexus
   Path: **Failure of neural crest cells to migrate in caudal direction**
      Disease starts in rectum, moves proximal; in 5% entire colon affected
   Tx: ***Resect rectum and distal colon to a point proximal to where
      ganglion cells appear** (margins to path to confirm ganglion cells)
      May need **colostomy initially** (eg Hirschsprung's colitis)
      Pull-through procedure (connect good residual colon to anus, eg
         Soave or Duhamel procedure)

*Meconium ileus
   Thick meconium (ie **1st stool**) causes **distal ileal obstruction**
   Sx's: abd distention, bilious vomiting; high association w/ **Cystic Fibrosis**
   Dx:
      AXR – dilated small bowel loops <u>without</u> air-fluid levels (meconium
         is too thick to separate from bowel wall); ground glass or 'soap
         suds' appearance; colon is decompressed
      N-acetylcysteine or **gastrografin enema** (see below)
      Sweat chloride test or **PCR for Cl channel defect** (cystic fibrosis
         transmembrane conductance regulator, CFTR)
   Path
      Can cause **ischemia** or perforation w/ **meconium pseudocyst** or
         free **perforation**
      Can cause **late strictures** (from ischemia)
   Tx: **Fluid resuscitation important** (osmotic load w/ gastrografin enema
      will draw fluid, can cause hypotension)

Empiric abx's and NGT
**Gastrografin or N-acetylcysteine enema *(best test and best Tx)*
Effective in 80%, done under fluoroscopy
Can make Dx and potentially Tx
Surgical indications:
Failure of enema to relieve obstruction
Peritonitis (eg perforation or necrosis)
Clinical deterioration
If surgery required, manual decompress (milk meconium out) and
place tube enterostomy for <u>N-acetylcysteine antegrade enemas</u>

*Imperforate anus
Associated w/ **VACTERL** (see TE Fistula above)
High (fistulizes <u>above</u> levators)
Meconium in **urine or vagina** (fistula to bladder, vagina or prostatic
urethra)
Tx: colostomy, later anal reconstruction w/ **posterior sagittal
anoplasty*
Low (fistulizes <u>below</u> levators, perineal skin)
Tx: **posterior sagittal anoplasty* (pull anus down into sphincter
mechanism), **no colostomy needed**
Need post-op **anal dilatation** to avoid **stricture**

*Malrotation
MCC duodenal obstruction in children (90% occur at age ≤ 1 year)
Sx's: sudden onset of **bilious vomiting** *(hallmark)*
**Bilious vomiting in any child in first 2 years of life requires upper
GI series to R/O malrotation; needs to be done *emergently*
Path
Failure of normal counter clockwise rotation (270°)
Ladd's bands cause **duodenal obstruction**, coming out from right
retroperitoneum
Volvulus is associated w/ compromise of SMA, leading to **infarction
of entire small bowel**
Dx: **UGI** *(best test)* – duodenal-jejunal junction displaced to the right (may
not cross midline); corkscrew duodenum; ± obstruction
Tx:* Ladd's procedure
Resuscitation
Resect Ladd's bands
Counterclockwise rotation of bowel (assess viability)
Place and fix **cecum in LLQ** (cecopexy)
Place and fix **duodenum in RUQ**
Appendectomy
*Duodenal webs may be present w/ malrotation and can cause
persistent bowel obstruction after Ladd's procedure

**Pyloric stenosis
Usually presents at **3–12 weeks;** first born white **males;** often Family Hx
Sx's: **projectile vomiting** *(classic, non-bilious)*; feel '**olive mass'** in
stomach (the pylorus), dehydration
U/S – pylorus ≥ **4 mm thick,** ≥ **14 mm long**
**Get hypochloremic, hypokalemic metabolic alkalosis
Tx:
**Fluid Resuscitate <u>before</u> OR
Normal saline bolus (20 cc/kg)
D5 1/2 normal saline at 1.5 x maintenance then used
Potassium replaced as needed <u>after</u> UOP is established
**Pyloromyotomy – RUQ incision; divide vein of Mayo, proximal
extent of myotomy should be circular muscles of stomach

**Duodenal atresia
>MCC duodenal obstruction in newborns (< 1 week)
>MC intestinal atresia
>MC type – distal to ampulla of Vater
>Etiology – failure of recanalization of duodenum (not vascular accident)
>Sx's: causes **bilious vomiting**, feeding intolerance, scaphoid abdomen
>>80% distal to ampulla – bilious vomiting
>>20% proximal to ampulla – non-bilious vomiting
>**Associated anomalies**
>>**Duodenal webs** (look for these intra-op)
>>**Down's syndrome** (20% have Down's)
>>Cardiac, renal, and GI anomalies (eg malrotation)
>RFs - **polyhydramnios** on pre-natal U/S
>Dx: **AXR** – shows *double-bubble sign* (classic, duodenum and stomach)
>Tx: Resuscitation
>>****Duodeno-duodenostomy** or duodeno-jejunostomy
>>****Duodenal webs** can cause persistent obstruction after repair (Tx: resection of web via longitudinal duodenostomy)

Intestinal atresia (jejunal and ileal)
>*Etiology – result of *intrauterine vascular accident* (→ ischemia and atresia)
>**Pre-natal U/S** – polyhydramnios
>Sx's: bilious emesis, distention; most do not pass meconium
>Dx: AXR – bowel distension w/ distal decompression
>Tx: resection w/ **primary anastomosis** or bring up **ostomies** if too damaged (look for **multiple lesions**)

Cystic duplication
>MC in **ileum**; MC on **mesenteric border**; Tx: **resect cyst**

*Diaphragmatic hernias
>MC on **left side** (80%); **overall survival 50%**
>Usually have severe **pulmonary hypertension** and **pulmonary hypoplasia**
>80% have **associated anomalies**: cardiac, neuro, malrotation
>*Both lungs are dysfunctional (one from compression by bowel and contra-lateral lung dysfunction from pulm HTN)*
>Sx's: respiratory distress; risk of barotrauma
>Dx: **Prenatal** – U/S; **CXR** - bowel in chest (may see NGT in chest)
>Tx:
>>**High frequency ventilation**
>>**Inhaled NO**, possible **ECMO** (extracorporeal membrane oxygenation)
>>*Stabilize before operating*
>>Surgery through **abdominal approach**:
>>>Need to reduce bowel and repair diaphragmatic defect ± mesh
>>>Look for malrotation
>>*Bochdalek's hernia (MC) – located posterior-lateral*
>>**Morgagni's hernia** (rare) – located anterior-medial (retrosternal);
>>>MC in **adults** (pressure creates hernia)- majority asymptomatic, leave alone unless symptomatic
>>**Eventration** – failure of diaphragm to fuse

**Tracheoesophageal fistulas
>Sx's: Newborn **spits up feeds**, excessive **drooling**
>>Respiratory sx's w/ feeding (aspiration, choking)
>>**Can't place NG tube in stomach** (classic)
>RFs – males, diabetic mothers, polyhydramnios, < 2500 g
>Dx   **CXR/AXR** (almost always give Dx) – contrast studies rarely needed
>>**Distal atresia** – gasless abdomen
>>**Proximal atresia** – distended stomach

ECHO, renal U/S, spinal and limb X-rays to R/O VACTERL
Type C (MC type -85%)
> **Proximal esophageal atresia** (blind pouch) and **distal TEF**
> **AXR** – distended stomach

Type A (2nd MC type -10%)
> Esophageal atresia and <u>no</u> fistula
> AXR – gasless abdomen

**VACTERL anomalies = Vertebral, Anorectal (MC - imperforate anus), Cardiac anomalies, TE fistula, Renal Disorders, and Limb anomalies

Initial Tx
> Replogle tube (just goes into proximal segment)
> Semi-upright position *(never prone)*
> If intubation required, place gastrostomy tube (G-tube)

**Surgery - **Right thoracotomy w/ resection of atretic segment and primary anastomosis of esophagus; close hole in trachea

Infants that are **premature, < 2500 gm, or sick** → Replogle tube, treat respiratory sx's, delayed repair

**MC Cx of repair – <u>GERD</u>

Survival related to **birth weight** and **associated anomalies**

****Choledochal cysts**
> **Young females** of **Asian descent** usual
> Sx's: episodic **abd pain, jaundice,** and **RUQ mass** (*classic,* triad in 50%)
>> Other sx's – **pancreatitis, cholangitis**
>
> **Path** - from abnormal **reflux of pancreatic enzymes** during uterine development; 90% extra-hepatic
>> 5-10% **CA risk** (cholangiocarcinoma)
>
> **Types**
>> **Type I:* (MC – 85%) saccular or **fusiform dilatation** of common bile duct (CBD) w/ normal intrahepatic duct.
>> **Type II:** isolated **diverticulum** off CBD
>> **Type III or Choledochocele:** arise from dilatation of **duodenal portion of CBD** or where pancreatic duct joins
>> **Type IV:** dilation of both **intra-hepatic / extra-hepatic** biliary system
>> **Type V or Caroli's disease:** dilatation of **intra hepatic** ducts *only*
>
> ****Tx:**
>> **Type I* – cyst excision, **hepatico-jejunostomy** (roux-en-Y) and **cholecystectomy**
>> **Type II* – cyst **excised completely** and choledochotomy closed **primarily**
>> **Type III** – trans-duodenal approach w/ **marsupialization or cyst excision**; careful identification of ampulla → may need sphincterotomy for adequate drainage
>> **Type IV** (partially intrahepatic) and **type V** (Caroli's disease, totally intrahepatic) → individualized; will need **partial liver resection, hepatico-jejunostomy,** or **liver TXP**

Biliary atresia
> MCC **neonatal jaundice requiring surgery**
> MC indication for **Liver TXP in children**
> **Jaundice > 2 weeks** after birth suggests atresia (**refractory to phototherapy**)
> Path - ↑ed **conjugated bilirubin,** ↑ LFTs
> Dx   **Liver Bx** *(best test)* – peri-portal fibrosis, bile plugging, late cirrhosis
> Tx: **Extra-hepatic ducts** *only*→ **Kasai procedure** (hepaticoporto-jejunostomy) - 1/3 get better, 1/3 go on to liver Txp, 1/3 die
>> If **intra-hepatic ducts involved** → liver TXP

Teratoma (dermoid cyst)
Are likely congenital but can present later in life
Can be **germ cell** or **embryonal tumor:**
>>**Germ cell** – occur is testes and ovaries
>>**Embryonal** – MC along midline (eg sacrococcygeal)
MC location – sacrococcygeal teratoma
MC type in newborns – sacrococcygeal teratoma
MC type in adolescents – ovarian
At risk for **malignancy** - **↑ *AFP or beta-HCG* indicates *CA***
Can be cystic, solid, or mixed
Tx: excision

*Sacrococcygeal teratomas
MC in **females;** presents as a **pre-sacral mass**
90% benign at birth (almost all have exophytic component)
Great potential for malignancy (**adenocarcinoma**)
AFP – good marker to follow for recurrence if malignant
2-month mark is a huge transition
>>< 2 months old → 10% malignant
>>> 2 months old → 60% malignant
CT scan to assess abdominal and pelvic extent
Tx: *Coccygectomy*

*Lymphadenopathy
Usually acute suppurative adenitis associated w/ URI or pharyngitis
>>**If fluctuant** → FNA, culture and sensitivity, abx's
>>May need incision and drainage if it fails to resolve
Chronic causes – cat scratch fever, atypical mycoplasma
Asymptomatic: Abx's for 10 days → excisional biopsy if no improvement
>>**This is lymphoma until proved otherwise**

Other Disorders
Pectus excavatum (sinks in)
>>Sternal osteotomy, strut placed (Nuss procedure places strut w/o osteotomy)
>>Repair if causing respiratory symptoms or emotional stress
>>Possible improvement of pulmonary dynamics
Pectus carinatum (sticks out, pigeon chest) - strut not necessary; repair for emotional stress (not shown to improve pulmonary dynamics)
***Congenital tracheomalacia**
>>Elliptical fragmented rings (rather than C shaped)
>>Usually w/ associated **TEF or esophageal atresia**
>>Sx's: expiratory wheeze; can have dying spells w/ feeding
>>>gets better in **1-2 yrs** but surgery need surgery if dying spell
>>Dx: **CXR** – narrowing on lateral
>>>**Awake bronch –** A-P dimension collapses (last test to be performed)
>>**Indications for surgery** (rarely need surgery):
>>>*Dying spell* (MC indication for surgery)
>>>**Respiratory sx's** (eg recurrent infections)
>>>**Unable to wean from vent**
>>Tx: *Aortopexy* (*best*, aorta sutured to back of sternum, opens up trachea)
Choanal atresia - obstruction of choanal opening in nose by bone or mucus membrane, usually unilateral; Sx's: intermittent **respiratory distress**, poor suckling: Tx: **surgical excision** of obstruction

Skin and soft tissue

560. **All of the following are true except:
    a. Melanin is formed in keratinocytes
    b. Stretch marks are due to dermal collagen damage and associated neovascularization
    c. Krause's end-bulbs are involved in cold sensation
    d. Cushing's Syndrome striae are due to loss of both collagen and tensile strength

    Answer a. Melanin is formed by **melanocytes** in epidermis basal layer.
    ***Stretch marks** are due to **dermal collagen damage** and associated neovascularization*
    ***Cushing's Syndrome striae** are due to **loss of collagen** and tensile strength*

561. **A 45 yo woman presents to your office with a lump in her right axilla that she has noticed for 3 months. She denies any sx's and has had no recent infections. Mammogram is normal. A complete exam reveals no other suspicious lesions. The mass is about 2 cm in diameter, feels hard, and is not painful. There is no surrounding erythema. The most appropriate next step is:
    a. Antibiotics
    b. Core needle biopsy
    c. Close follow-up
    d. Sentinel lymph node biopsy

    Answer b. This mass needs to be biopsied. Abx's are not indicated because there has been no antecedent illness and the mass is not inflammatory. Also it would be unusual for an inflammatory mass to last 3 months. Sentinel lymph node biopsy is not indicated. You could resect the mass (excisional biopsy) if the core needle biopsy was indeterminate.

562. **Core needle Bx in the above pt comes back as melanoma. You cannot find any skin lesions on the patient's body. The most appropriate next step is:
    a. Formal axillary lymph node dissection
    b. nothing
    c. Mastectomy
    d. Chemo-XRT only

    Answer a. There are a couple of possibilities with this scenario. First is that there is a melanoma primary somewhere and you cannot find it (some melanomas are non-pigmented). Second is that the primary melanoma has regressed spontaneously and the lymph nodes are all that is left of the disease (best scenario). **Error on the side that gives the best chance of survival, which is a **formal axillary lymph node dissection**.

    Note that the dissection for melanoma is different than for breast cancer. For melanoma, you are trying to remove all the disease which means you need to take **level I, II, and III lymph nodes.

    With breast CA, you only need to sample level I and II nodes. You are not trying to remove all the disease w/ breast CA, but merely staging the pt.

563. *A 65 yo man has a 1 cm diameter dark colored lesion on his arm that looks different according to the patient. You perform a physical exam and find no other lesions. The next appropriate step is:
    a. Resection with 1 cm margin
    b. Punch biopsy
    c. IL-2 therapy
    d. Scrape top layer off and send to cytology

Answer b. Because you do not know if this is melanoma or not, resection with a margin is not indicated (also, margins are based on depth of lesion, not width). Scraping off the top layer would be inappropriate because you would not be getting the depth of the lesion. The best answer is punch biopsy (although you could also just resect the lesion without margins, and then go back for a re-resection if it turns out to be cancer). The **punch Bx** should be at the most abnormal looking spot or thickest area

564. **The punch biopsy in the above pt comes back as melanoma that invades 2 mm deep. You perform a physical exam (axillary region) and find no clinically positive nodes. Mets work-up is negative. The most appropriate next step is:
    a.   SLNBx and resection of the primary with 2 cm margin
    b.   Axillary lymph node dissection + resection of primary w/ 2 cm margin
    c.   SLNBx and resection of the primary with 1 cm margin
    d.   Axillary lymph node dissection + resection of primary w/ 1 cm margin

    Answer a. Sentinel lymph node biopsy is indicated for lesions > 1 mm deep w/ clinically negative nodes. A melanoma 2 mm (1-4 mm) deep requires a 2 cm margin with resection.

    Primary excision (or re-excision) for **melanoma:
    Melanoma in situ (Hutchinson Freckle if on face)- 0.5 cm margin OK
    Thin melanoma (< 1 mm)   1 cm margin
    Intermediate melanoma (1-4 mm)   2 cm margin
    Thick melanoma (> 4 mm)   2-3 cm margin

565. *All of the following are true of melanoma except:
    a.   Blue is the most ominous color
    b.   Melanoma is the MC metastasis to small bowel
    c.   Ulceration indicates a better prognosis
    d.   Melanoma on the anterior scalp is most likely to metastasize to the parotid gland and anterior cervical chain

    Answer c. Ulceration indicates a worse prognosis.

    Parotid Basin Melanoma (ear, temple, forehead, anterior scalp) has a 20% metastasis rate to **parotid gland (need superficial parotidectomy)
    < 1 mm deep - superficial parotidectomy
    > 1 mm deep - SLNBx and superficial parotidectomy
    clinically positive nodes - superficial parotidectomy and MRND

566. *All of the following are true except:
    a.   An appropriate margin for a forearm 2 cm basal cell CA is 0.5 cm
    b.   Morpheaform is the *least* aggressive basal cell CA due to collagenase production
    c.   A 2 cm margin is indicated for Marjolin's Ulcers
    d.   A 2 cm anterior scalp squamous cell CA w/ clinically negative nodes should undergo primary resection and superficial parotidectomy

    Answer b. **Morpheaform** is the most aggressive **basal cell CA**

567. **A pt has a 5 cm mass in his anterior thigh. All of the following are true except
    a.   MRI is indicated before any biopsy
    b.   Core needle biopsy is preferred in most cases
    c.   The most important prognostic factor for sarcoma is node status
    d.   If open Bx is indicated, the incision should be along the long axis of the extremity

    Answer c. ****Tumor grade** is the most important prognostic factor for sarcoma. **Sarcomas *rarely* have nodal involvement.

568. **All of the following are true of sarcomas except:
    a. The MC soft tissue sarcoma is malignant fibrous histiosarcoma
    b. The MC mets location is lung
    c. Most extremity soft tissue sarcomas require amputation
    d. Complete resection of a retroperitoneal sarcoma allows the best chance for survival

Answer c. 90% of extremity sarcomas can be treated without amputation. ****Complete resection** *(w/ negative margins) of a retroperitoneal sarcoma allows the best chance for survival (take what you have to, eg kidney)*

569. All the following are good prognostic indicators of metastatic sarcoma except:
    a. Disease-free interval < 12 months
    b. < 4 lesions
    c. Primary lesion control
    d. Doubling time > 20 days

Answer a. A disease-free interval > 12 months has a better prognosis.

570. *All of the following are true except:
    a. Resection is the procedure of choice for Kaposi's Sarcoma (KS)
    b. Alveolar subtype is the worst prognosis rhabdomyosarcoma
    c. The MC location for osteosarcoma is the knee
    d. A painful lesion comprised of blood vessels and nerves near the terminal aspect of the digit is consistent w/ glomus tumor

Answer a. Surgery is not the Tx of choice for KS. These lesions should be palliated (HAART AIDS Tx, systemic interferon alpha, XRT, ect).

**Alveolar subtype is the worst prognosis rhabdomyosarcoma
A painful lesion comprised of **blood vessels and nerves** near the **terminal aspect of the digit** is consistent w/ **glomus tumor

571. **All of the following are true of Merkel Cell carcinoma except:
    a. It is a locally aggressive neuroendocrine skin CA
    b. Has common mets to bone and LN's
    c. Keratin antibodies show peri-nuclear pattern
    d. Nodes do not need to be assessed

Answer d. ***These red to purple skin tumors are **very aggressive** w/ local invasion and metastases to lymph nodes and distant sites (bone MC).*

572. *All of the following are true except:
    a. Refractory hyperhydrosis requires ligation of T1-T4 sympathetic ganglia
    b. Ganglion cysts typically occur over joints and require removal of check valve
    c. Verruca vulgaris (wart) is usually best treated with salicylic acid
    d. Intra-lesional steroid injection after excision if generally the best Tx for keloids

Answer a. Refractory hyperhydrosis requires ligation of T2-T4 sympathetic ganglia; ligation of the T1 ganglia would result in Horner's syndrome.

**Intra-lesional steroids after excision if generally the best Tx for keloids

573. *All of the following are true of sacral decubitus ulcers except
    a. Flaps should not be performed in patients w/ active infection
    b. Stage II decubitus ulcers will likely require a flap
    c. Bone involvement after flap placement requires long term antibiotics
    d. Stage III ulcers are full thickness down to the subcutaneous fat

Answer b. Stage II decubitus ulcers do not require a flap

574. *All of the following are true except
   a.   Tx of choice for refractory retroperitoneal fibrosis is freeing of the ureters w/ omental wrapping
   b.   The MC retroperitoneal tumor is lymphoma
   c.   Hypertrophic scar tissue frequently goes beyond the original injury
   d.   Peritoneal blood following trauma is absorbed through fenestrated lymphatic channels

Answer c. Hypertrophic scar tissue does not go beyond the original injury. **Keloids** do go beyond the original injury.

Skin Components
Epidermis (top layer) – consists of stratified squamous epithelium
Dermis – collagen, elastic fibers, scaffold for epidermis
Mechano-receptors
   Pacinian corpuscles – deep pressure
   Ruffini's corpuscles – warmth, skin stretch (slippage of objects)
   ***Krause's end-bulbs** – cold
   Meissner's corpuscles – light pressure and tactile sense
Eccrine sweat glands – aqueous sweat (thermal regulation, is hypotonic)
Apocrine sweat glands – milky type sweat
   Highest concentration in palms and soles
   Most sweat released is a result of the sympathetic nervous system via acetylcholine
Lipid-soluble drugs – have increased skin absorption
Dermis is composed primarily of **Type I collagen** (tensile strength)
Tension – the resistance to stretching (collagen)
Elasticity – the ability to regain shape (branching proteins can stretch out to twice normal length)
***Cushing's Syndrome Striae – **decreased collagen* results *in loss of tensile strength* and elasticity
***Stretch Marks – damage to **dermal collagen w/* blood vessel *dilatation* and *neovascularization*
Tissue expanders work by local recruitment, thinning of dermis and epidermis, and mitosis (more cells)
***MCC of pedicled or anastomosed free flap necrosis* – venous thrombosis
***Blood supply to skin for myocutaneous flap* – underlying muscle perforators
Trans-rectus abdominal myoplasty (TRAM Flap)
   ***Blood supply* – superior epigastric vessels* (can't use if previous CABG w/ IMA use)
   Cx's – necrosis, ventral hernia, bleeding, infection
   ***Most important determinant of TRAM flap viability* – peri-umbilical muscle perforators to skin

UV radiation
Damages DNA (oxygen free radical formation breaks up DNA)
UVB – *most damaging type*
Melanin - single best factor for protecting skin from UV radiation
   Absorbs UV radiation and dissipates energy as heat

Skin Lesion Dx
   1) **Punch biopsy** (need to get down to subcutaneous fat)
      No shave biopsy, need to get depth
      Face, hands or feet (cosmetic regions or hard to close areas) – always want punch Bx
      Consider punch Bx for lesions in any location (easy office procedure)

Biopsy at **thickest spot** or **most abnormal looking**
2) **Excisional Bx** w/ 1 mm margin for other areas (as long as it is small)
    Make sure you are into **subcutaneous fat** (need full thickness)
Fix in **Formalin**, paraffin embedded permanent section, H + E stain, (**not** frozen section)

Melanoma
Lung MC met location
Melanoma MC metastasis to small bowel
RFs – fair complexion, easy sun-burning, previous skin CA or XRT
MC site for melanoma – **back** (men), **legs** (women)
Blue worst color in terms of malignant potential
Worse survival - ↑ number of nodes; location on back or posterior arms/ neck/scalp (BANS), ocular, mucosal, ulcerated, men, ↑ mitotic rate
Originates from **melanocytes** (neural crest cells) in epidermis basal layer
Axillary lymph node melanoma w/ no primary → Tx: complete ALND
Markers: **S-100** protein and **HMB-45**
No MOHS surgery for melanoma
Signs of melanoma transformation (ABCD rule)
    Asymmetrical
    Border irregularity (angulations, notching, ulceration, bleeding)
    Color change (blue most ominous, red, darkening)
    Diameter (> 6 mm or enlargement)
Types of Melanoma
    Lentigo maligna (eg Hutchinson's freckle) – **melanoma in situ;** least aggressive, radial growth 1st; usually an elevated nodule
    Superficial spreading melanoma (MC type) intermediate malignancy
    Nodular – most aggressive; increased mets and deep growth at Dx: Blue-black w/ smooth borders; occurs anywhere
    Acral lentigo – very aggressive; usually ***palms, soles* or *subungal*** African-Americans
Mets w/u:
    All intermediate (> 1 mm) and **thick** (1-4 mm) require -
        Chest/Abd/Pelvic CT, LFT's and LDH (marker for metastasis)
Nodal DZ w/u -
    All intermediate (> 1 mm) and **thick** (1-4 mm) get **SLNBx;**
        Exception - **clinically positive nodes**, then perform formal lymphadenectomy
    Thin melanoma (< 1 mm) that need **SLNBx**
        Ulceration
        Regression on path (was deeper at one point but regressed)
        If into **reticular dermis**
        Has **high mitotic rate**
    Nodal DZ but can't find primary → formal lymphadenectomy; either had regression of primary or is non-pigmented melanoma
Tx:
    Primary excision (or re-excision) **for melanoma:**
        Melanoma in situ (only in epidermis;

Hutchinson Freckle if on face)	0.5 cm margin OK
Thin melanoma *(< 1 mm)*	1 cm margin
Intermediate melanoma *(1-4 mm)*	2 cm margin
Thick melanoma *(> 4 mm)*	2-3 cm margin

        Need to get down to underlying **muscle fascia** (not through it; elliptical incision w/ 3:1 ratio length to width)
        If going across a **joint,** make an **S-shaped incision**
        In-transit mets - resection
    Formal lymphadenectomy of nodal drainage areas
        Indicated for **positive SLNBx** or **clinically positive nodes**
        You are trying to clear tumor from these areas (not sample)

4 general nodal basins - inguinal, axillary, cervical, parotid
**Scalp and face anterior to pinna *(including ear)* and superior to lip
→20% have mets to **parotid gland** – *all need* **superficial parotidectomy**; *if clinically positive nodes or positive SLNBx* need **superficial parotidectomy + MRND**
*Subungal melanoma
*Remove the nail and get a punch Bx
Thumb melanoma → amputate at the DIP joint
Any other finger melanoma → amputate at the PIP
Toe melanoma→ amputate at the MTP joint
Systemic Tx
Dacarbazine *(1ˢᵗ line)* for positive nodes (stage IIIb) or mets (IV)
IL-2, and **tumor vaccines** can be used for **nodes** or **mets** (marginal)
**Axillary lymph node shows melanoma but no primary – *Tx: axillary lymph node dissection (Take level I, II and III nodes – trying to clear all the nodes here)*

Basal cell

*MC malignancy in US (4x MC than squamous)
From epidermis – basal epithelial cells
Pearly, rolled appearance, slow growth, ulcerative deep invasion
*Rare mets or nodal spread
MC type – nodular form
Morpheaform most aggressive which has **collagenase** production
Tx: Need **0.3 - 0.5 cm margins**

**Squamous cell CA

Erythema, papulonodular with crust, ulceration, red-brown color
Mets - Melanoma > Squamous cell CA > Basal cell CA
RFs - post-XRT, old burn scars (Marjolin's ulcer), actinic keratosis
RFs for mets – poorly differentiated, ↑ depth, immunosuppressed
Tx: ****Need *1 cm margins* for most**
Cosmetic location or high risk - Mohs surgery (margin mapping w/ conservative slices; <u>NOT</u> used w/ melanoma); minimizes resection area (eg on face)
Need **2 cm margins for:* **Marjolin's ulcer**, **Penile CA** (penectomy, possibly partial if distal lesion) and **Vulvar CA**
**Nodes
Indications for prophylactic nodal dissection:
1) **> 2 cm** in circumference *or:*
2) **> 4 mm** deep *or:*
3) ****All Parotid Basin Lesions** (****ear**, temple, forehead, anterior scalp) – 20% risk of parotid nodal involvement (****all need prophylactic superficial parotidectomy**)
Clinically positive nodes → regional lymph node dissection
Parotid basin lesion w/ clinically positive nodes → superficial parotidectomy + MRND
Chemo-XRT - if neuro, nodal, or vessel invasion or positive margins

**Soft tissue sarcoma

*MC sarcoma – malignant fibrous histiosarcoma (#2 liposarcoma)
MC site – extremities (50%); 50% in **children**
RFs – **Asbestos** (mesothelioma), **PVC and arsenic** (angiosarcoma), **Chronic lymphedema** (lymphangiosarcoma); **XRT**
*Desmin – marker for rhabdomyosarcoma
Hematogenous spread, <u>not</u> to lymphatics (nodal mets rare)
Do <u>not</u> need lymph node dissection
*MC mets – lung
**Most impt prognostic indicator – *tumor grade* (undifferentiated worse) part of staging sarcomas

MRI of primary area for <u>all</u> potential sarcomas <u>before Bx</u> to r/o neuro, bone, or vascular invasion

Biopsy:
  1) **Core needle biopsy** (*best Dx method*, along long axis plane of future incision for en bloc resection; 95% accurate)
  2) If core needle <u>not</u> feasible or insufficient tissue:
     Longitudinal Excisional biopsy if < 4 cm → then go back for margins if sarcoma
     Longitudinal Incisional biopsy if > 4 cm (resect biopsy skin site if biopsy shows sarcoma)
     Both of above along *long axis plane of future incision* for en bloc resection (ie incision along **long axis** of extremity)

Tx:
  Need elliptical incision and margins around previous Bx site
  Want 2-3 cm margin for tumor
  90% do <u>not</u> need amputation → try for perform limb-sparing rsxn
  Complete resection best chance for survival
  *Pre-op XRT (50 Gy) ± chemo (**doxorubicin** based) - may allow limb sparing surgery*
  Post-op chemo-XRT indications (doxorubicin based) - **high-grade, close margins, or tumors > 5 cm**
  XRT decreases local recurrence; no real effect on survival
  Chemo has not improved survival
  5-YS w/ complete resection – 40%

Special Issues:
  Isolated mets w/o evidence of systemic DZ (eg lung or liver) → resect as long as you leave enough of the organ to live
  Local recurrence→ re-stage (same as above) resection if resectable
  Distant recurrence (eg lung) → re-stage, resection if resectable
  Best prognosis mets:
     Disease free interval > 12 months
     < 4 mets
     Doubling time > 20 days
     Complete resection
     Primary control
  Head and neck sarcomas
     MC in **pediatric population** (**MC type** - rhabdomyosarcoma)
     Difficulty w/ margins due to proximity to vital structures (eg carotid, spinal cord)
  Retroperitoneal sarcoma
     MC retroperitoneal sarcoma – *liposarcoma*
     R/O lymphoma (lymphoma is MC retroperitoneal tumor - night sweats, fever or chills, adenopathy)
     Want en bloc resection - Take everything you have to (eg kidney, spleen, colon, portion of liver); <25% resectable w/ negative margins due to proximity to vital organs
     Best chance for survival is a negative margin resection
     Midline incision for pelvic and retroperitoneal sarcomas
     Poor prognosis for retroperitoneal sarcomas due to:
        Delay in <u>Dx</u>
        Difficulty w/ <u>total resection</u> and getting negative margins
        Difficulty getting <u>XRT</u> retroperitoneal (bowel in the way)
     Local recurrence 40%
     Often have pseudocapsule but don't shell out → leaves residual tumor
  Visceral sarcomas: MC type – leiomyosarcomas

Kaposi's sarcoma (KS; highly vascular sarcoma)
ALL are caused by **human herpes virus 8** (HHV 8)
From **lymphatic endothelium** that forms vascular channels
MC neoplasm in AIDS pt
MC sites - oral and **pharyngeal** mucosa (odynophagia,
dysphagia; bleeding); others skin, respiratory or GI
Slow growing - rarely causes death w/ AIDS
Tx:
Surgery not Tx of choice– primary goal is **palliation**
Exceptions - intestinal hemorrhage
HAART Tx (see Infection Chp) shrinks AIDS related KS
Systemic Tx: interferon-alpha
Local Tx: XRT, intra-lesional vinblastine
**Childhood rhabdomyosarcoma
MC soft tissue sarcoma in children – rhabdomyosarcoma
Can manifest in head, ear, neck, vagina, extremities and trunk
(poorest prognosis)
MC subtype – embryonal
**Worst prognosis subtype – alveolar*
Botryoides tumor – vaginal rhabdomyosarcoma (sx's –
bleeding)
MC malignant aural tumor of childhood
Neurofibromatosis (von Recklinghausen's DZ; autosomal dominant)
Affects **neural crest cells** (schwann cells, endoneurial
fibroblasts)
Disordered **skin pigmentation** (café au lait spots, axillary
freckling)
< 10% actually get CA
1) **Type I NF** (**neurofibromin** mutation)
a) **CNS** (acoustic neuroma)
b) **Peripheral nerve sheath** (neurofibroma, neurolemma)
c) **Pheochromocytoma**
2) **Type II NF** (**merlin** gene mutation)
→ only get *acoustic neuromas*
Schwannomatosis – multiple schwannomas

Other Skin Lesions
**Merkel cell carcinoma
Neuroendocrine tumor of the skin
**Highly aggressive w/ early regional and systemic spread*
Path
Spreads through **skin** and **lymph nodes**
10% have **mets** (MC bone) and 25% have **lymph node**
spread at Dx
Red to purple papulo-nodules
80% have **Merkel Cell Polyomavirus**
*Have **neuron-specific enolase** (NSE), **cytokeratin,** and
neurofilament protein staining*
Keratin antibodies show **peri-nuclear** pattern
Tx:
All pts need SLNBx or formal lymph node dissection
Resection w/ 2-3 cm margin
Post-op Chemo-XRT
5-YS for all patients – 60%
**Glomus Tumor of Skin (from glomus body, not glomus cells)
Benign painful tumor comprised of **blood vessels and nerves*
MC location –*terminal aspect of digit* near or under fingernail (can
also occur behind eardrum – blanches w/ pressure)
Tx: tumor excision
Not a paraganglioma

Paraganglioma (chemodectoma) – rare malignancy, neural crest cell
    Part of **autonomic nervous system**
        From **glomus cells** (chemo-receptors that regulate blood pressure
           and blood flow to various area of body)
        MC location overall – abdomen
        MC ENT location – carotid body tumor (can also occur in ear)
        MC thoracic location – aortic arch body
        Can secrete **norepinephrine**; highly **vascular**
        Tx: tumor excision
Lipomas – **MC mesenchymal neoplasm** ; rarely malignant liposarcomas;
    often on back, neck, between shoulders;
Keratoses
    Actinic keratosis
        Premalignant; tan, pink, or red
        Sun damaged areas
        Tx: **Diclofenac sodium**, liquid nitrogen, 5-fluorouracil cream
        Excisional biopsy if suspicious
    Seborrheic keratosis
        NOT premalignant (keratinocytes)
        Trunk on elderly pts; can be dark looking or look like warts (can
           be mistaken for melanoma)
    Arsenical keratosis – association w/ squamous cell carcinoma
    Keratoacanthoma - from pilo-sebaceous glands, keratin plug, benign
    Hyperhydrosis - perfuse sweating, especially noticeable in palms
        Tx: Try a variety of antiperspirants over 3 months
        Sympathectomy if affecting lifestyle
           Ligate T2-T4 sympathetic chain (hook cautery)
           Not above T2 ganglion – will get Horner's Syndrome
           Need to get **crossing nerve of Kuntz** on the **2nd rib**
           MC Cx – compensatory sweating in face, trunks,
               and legs (15%)

Hidradenitis
    Apocrine sweat gland infection, more common in women
    MC sites – axilla and groin, MC organisms – Staph/strep
    Tx: abx's, improve hygiene, avoid antiperspirants, drain
        abscesses; resection if refractory (not w/ active infection)
    Chronic axillary hidradenitis – need excision extending from fascia
        to skin (removing apocrine glands)
Benign cysts
    Epidermal inclusion cyst (MC) – completely mature epidermis w/
        creamy **keratin** material; **Tx:** resection
    Trichilemmal cyst – scalp, **keratin** filled cyst from hair follicle; no
        epidermis; **Tx:** resection
    Ganglion cyst – over joints in hand or foot (MC – wrist, 80%)
        Filled with **collagenous synovial type** material
        Tx: aspiration cures 50%, recurrence after resection 5%
           (remove check valve at joint capsule to prevent
           recurrence)
    Pilonidal cysts - congenital sinus or abscess formation over
        sacrococcygeal junction; get **infected**; contain **hair**
        Tx: abx's, drainage, packing if abscess; F/U surgical resection
Xanthoma – yellow cholesterol-rich; near tendons and other areas, contain
    histiocytes, can be associated w/ familial hypercholesterolemia;
    benign. Tx: excision
Warts (verruca vulgaris) – HPV origin, contagious
    Tx: **salicylic acid** *(best Tx)*, liquid nitrogen

Keloids - Autosomal dominant; dark skinned people higher risk
　Collagen (Type I and III) **goes <u>beyond</u> original scar**
　　(main differentiation w/ hypertrophic scar)
　**From failure of collagen breakdown*
　Tx: **Intra-lesional steroid injection after keloid excision** (best
　　Tx); others – silicone gel sheet or injection (preferably before
　　development of keloids), pressure garments
Hypertrophic scar tissue
　Higher risk in dark skinned people
　Often on **flexor surfaces** of upper torso
　Collagen stays within confines of scar
　Often w/ burns or wounds taking a long time to heal
　Tx: **steroids, silicone,** and/or **pressure garments**
Lip lacerations – most important issue is to line up vermillion border

*<u>Sacral Decubitus Ulcer</u> (pressure sores)
　Prevention – pressure relieving beds
　Look to see how deep the wound is on exam

Ulcer Stage	Exam	Tx
I	Erythema, pain, no skin loss	Keep pressure off
II	Partial skin loss w/ yellow debris	Local treatment below, keep pressure off
III	Full-thickness skin loss, has subcutaneous tissue exposure	Sharp debridement necessary, likely need myocutaneous flap
IV	Bone, muscle or tendon exposed	Need myocutaneous flaps

　Tx:
　　Keep pressure off the area → place pt on **kin-air bed**
　　Optimize **nutrition**
　　Consider diverting stool w/ **colostomy** (stage III and IV)
　　Debride wound in OR; moist dressings
　　Bx and send cultures w/ appropriate **Abx's**
　　No flap if the pt has an **active infection**
　　When wound looking good, place **gluteal myocutaneous flap**

*<u>Retroperitoneal fibrosis</u>
　RFs – autoimmune disease, CA, methysergide, hydralazine, previous XRT
　Sx's: usually related to **trapped ureters and hydronephrosis*
　　Can get lymphatic obstruction.
　Dx: **intravenous pyelogram** (best test)* – see compressed ureters
　Tx: **Steroids** + immunosuppression (eg Tamoxifen, Imuran, Infliximab)
　　Surgery if renal function becomes compromised (**free up ureters
　　and wrap in omentum*) – R/O CA
　　Percutaneous nephrostomy tube if pyelonephritis develops (+ abx's),
　　　then free up ureters at later procedure

575. *There were 172,000 new cases of lung cancer diagnosed in 2010. This would be an example of:
    a. Prevalence
    b. Incidence
    c. Mean
    d. Mode

    Answer b. Incidence is the number of new cases in a certain time frame (usually a year). Prevalence would be the current number of people with the disease (or trait).

576. *In an investigational oral agent study for breast CA, pts were randomly assigned to either the experimental drug or Tamoxifen. Pts were not aware of which drug they were receiving however the physicians were aware. This would be an example of:
    a. Cohort study
    b. Retrospective review
    c. Double blind randomized control trial
    d. Single blinded randomized control trial

    Answer d. Because the physicians were aware of whether or not the pts were receiving the drug or placebo, it is only a single blinded randomized control trial.

577. **Combining the data from several independent trials investigating the same subject is an example of
    a. Cohort study
    b. Meta-analysis
    c. Double blind randomized control trial
    d. Single blinded randomized control trial

    Answer b. **Meta-analysis** combines data from many independent trials

578. *Sensitivity of a test reflects:
    a. Ability to detect disease
    b. Ability to say that no disease is present
    c. Rejecting the null hypothesis when it is true
    d. Accepting the null hypothesis when it is false

    Answer a. Ability to detect disease

579. *Specificity of a test reflects:
    a. Ability to detect disease
    b. Ability to say that no disease is present
    c. Rejecting the null hypothesis when it is true
    d. Accepting the null hypothesis when it is false

    Answer b. Ability to say that no disease is present

580. *Type I error reflects:
    a. Ability to detect disease
    b. Ability to say that no disease is present
    c. Rejecting the null hypothesis when it is true
    d. Accepting the null hypothesis when it is false

    Answer c. Rejecting the null hypothesis when it is true

581. *Type II error reflects:

a. Ability to detect disease
b. Ability to say that no disease is present
c. Rejecting the null hypothesis when it is true
d. Accepting the null hypothesis when it is false

Answer d. Accepting the null hypothesis when it is false

582. **Statistical power of a test is:
    a. = 1- probability of Type I error
    b. = 1- probability of Type II error
    c. = 1+ probability of Type I error
    d. = 1+ probability of Type II error

    Answer b. ***The **power** of a test is the probability of making a right conclusion. A large sample size will increase power (by decreasing the likelihood of a Type II error).*

583. The most common cancer death is:
    a. Lung Cancer
    b. Breast Cancer
    c. Prostate Cancer
    d. Pancreatic Cancer

    Answer a. Lung cancer accounts for more deaths than any other cancer.

584. The HPV vaccine given to young women is an example of:
    a. Screening
    b. Primary prevention
    c. Secondary Prevention
    d. Tertiary Prevention

    Answer b. The HPV vaccine is n example of primary prevention.

585. Given a test with a high positive predictive value:
    a. A negative result suggests the pt is very likely to have the disease
    b. Prevalence of the disease in the population has no impact on the test
    c. The false positives for the test are likely very high
    d. A positive result suggests the patient is very likely to have the disease

    Answer d. A positive result suggests pt is very likely to have the disease

586. An epidemiologic study is performed and the odds ratio for smoking and the development of lung cancer are performed. All of the following are true except:
    a. Odds ratio is the odds of an event occurring in one group compared to the odds of that event occurring in another group.
    b. An odds ratio of 9 in the above study would indicate smokers are 9 times more like to get lung cancer compared to non-smokers.
    c. An odds ratio of 1 in a different study would indicate both groups are equally likely to develop the disease
    d. Odds ratio is equivalent to sensitivity

    Answer d. Odds ratio is defined as the odds of an event occurring in one group (group 1) compared to the odds of that event occurring in a separate group (group 2). The higher the odds ratio, the more likely the condition or event is going to occur in the first group.

587. A retrospective study examined the effect of cytomegalovirus infection on the development of chronic rejection in heart transplant patients. Which of the following is true?

a. A students T-test is most appropriate
b. An ANOVA test is most appropriate
c. A chi-squared test is most appropriate
d. There is no good test for this

Answer c. A chi-squared test is most appropriate.

Basic Rules

Type I error - rejects null hypothesis incorrectly (rejecting the null hypothesis when it is true)

Assumed there was a difference when no difference actually exists

*Type II error - accepts null hypothesis incorrectly

Falsely assumed there was no difference when an actual difference exists

MC due to a *small sample size* (ie a larger sample size would have picked up the difference)

Null hypothesis

The hypothesis that no difference exists between groups

A $p < 0.05$ rejects the null hypothesis

$p < 0.05$ =

>95% likelihood that the difference between populations is true

<5% likelihood that the difference is not true and occurred by chance alone

Variance – the spread of data around a mean value

Parameter – a population

Numeric terms – eg 2, 7, 7, 8, 9, 12, 14

Mode – the most frequently occurring value = 7

Mean – the average = 9

This is the best measure of **central tendency** when **values are distributed normally** (ie you do not have outliers)

There are no outliers in the above set of numbers, so the mean value is a good measure of central tendency

Median – the middle value of a set of data (eg 50th percentile) = 8

This is the best measure of **central tendency** when **values are not distributed equally** (ie you have outliers)

Take example above, but add 85 and 86 (eg 2, 7, 7, 8, 9, 12, 14, 85, 86)

The **mean** would now be = 26

This is not a good representation of **central tendency** due to the outliers 85 and 86

The **median** would now be = 9

This is a better representation of central tendency

Any set of numbers (eg INR values, weight loss, WBC counts, Hct's, temp's) can be used for the above

95% confidence interval

Instead of estimating the parameter by a single value (eg mean), this also includes an interval likely to include the parameter

Confidence intervals are used to indicate reliability of an estimate

Example:

Following **lap banding**, mean weight loss for your pts is 125 lb

95% of your pts have a weight loss between 100 - 150 lb

The 95% confidence interval for amount of weight loss in your population is (100,150)

or there is a 95% probability that following gastric bypass, your pt will lose somewhere between 100 - 150 lb

Written as: mean weight loss125 lb [100,150]

The more narrow the confidence interval, the more accurate the estimate Example – for **gastric bypass**, mean weight loss was 130 lb [120,140]; 130 would be a more accurate estimate of weight loss in this population than 125 in the above lap banding population)

Prevalence
    Number of people w/ disease in a population
    (eg number of patients in US w/ lung CA)
    Longstanding diseases will ↑ prevalence
Incidence
    Number of new cases diagnosed over a certain time frame (MC
        annually) (eg number of pt in US newly diagnosed with lung CA in
        2009)
Relative risk = incidence in exposed population / incidence in unexposed
        population
Odds ratio – odds of an event occurring in one group (group 1) compared
        to odds of that event occurring in a separate group (group 2). The
        higher the odds ratio, the more likely the condition or event is going to
        occur in the first group.
**_Power of test_ (probability of making correct conclusion)
        = 1 - probability of type II error
        Likelihood that the conclusion of test is true
        Larger sample size increases power (by decreasing the likelihood
            of a type II error)

Clinical Trials and studies
Randomized controlled trial (prospective study)
        Prospective study w/ random assignment to treatment and non-
            treatment groups
        Avoids treatment bias
Double-blind controlled trial (prospective study)
        A prospective study in which both pt and doctor are blind to treatment
        Avoids observational bias
        Thought to be the best form of trials
Cohort study (prospective study)
        Cohort – a group of people who share a common characteristic
        Cohort study – a prospective study comparing the cohort to either
            the general population of another group that lacks the
            characteristic
        Example: prospectively following teenagers who smoke and
            comparing them to other teenagers who do not smoke in terms
            of developing lung CA
Case–control study (retrospective study)
        Retrospective study in which those w/ the disease are compared to a
            similar population w/o the disease
        The frequency of the suspected risk factor is then compared between
            the two groups
Meta-analysis – _combines the data from **different studies on a
        specific disease process or treatment (eg combining the data from
        multiple studies examining stroke after CABG)_

Quantitative variables (numbers)
Student's t test
        Two independent groups and variable is **quantitative**
        Compares means (eg mean weight between group A and B)
        Eg – a new preservation solution is used a the time of lung transplant
            harvest and pO2 values are measured after transplantation.
            The average pO2 in the experimental group is 350 mmHg. The
            average pO2 in the control group is 250 mmHg. A student's T
            test is used here to figure out if the 2 groups are significantly
            different
Paired t tests
        Variable is **quantitative** w/ **before and after studies**
        (eg mean weight before and after treatment, comparing drug vs.
            placebo)

337

ANOVA (analysis of variance)

Compares **quantitative** variables (eg means) for more than 2 groups (eg mean weight between groups A, B, C, and D)

Qualitative variables

Nonparametric statistics - compare categorical (qualitative) variables (eg race, sex, diseases, meds); Non-numerical categories

Chi-squared test - compares two groups based on **categorical** (eg qualitative) **variables** (eg number of obese pts w/ and w/o development of hyperlipidemia vs. number of non-obese pts w/ and w/o development hyperlipidemia)

Kaplan-Meier estimator –estimates survival

	Positive Test	Negative Test
Pts w/ disease	True-positive (TP)	False-negative (FN)
Pts w/o disease	False-positive (FP)	True-negative (TN)

Sensitivity

Ability to detect disease = TP / (TP + FN)

Indicates number of people who have the disease who test positive

With high sensitivity, a **negative test** result means pt is very unlikely to have disease

Specificity

Ability to state no DZ present = TN / (TN + FP)

Indicates number of people who do not have the disease who test negative

With high specificity, a **positive test** result means patient is very likely to have disease

Positive Predictive Value – proportion of patients with a positive result who actually have the disease. This value does depend on the prevalence of the disease within a population. Tests with a very high positive predictive value have a low false positive rate and a positive result suggests the patient is very likely to have the disease.

PPV = TP / TP + FP

Negative Predictive value – determines the likelihood of not having the disease given a negative result. A test with a high negative predictive value will have a low false negative rate.

NPV = TN / TN + FN

Accuracy = TP + TN / TP + TN + FP + FN

Predictive value – dependent on disease prevalence

Sensitivity and specificity – independent of prevalence

Prevention

Primary Prevention – avoiding DZ altogether (ie vaccinations for HPV)

Secondary Prevention – focuses on early detection of the disease to prevent progression (ie pap smears, stress test, screening colonoscopy, screening mammograms, blood pressure checks)

Tertiary Prevention – decreasing the morbidity related to an established disease (i.e. controlling blood pressure in patients w/ HTN, screening and treatment of diabetics w/ eye, foot, and renal problems; HMG-CoA reductase inhibitors in pts w/ hyperlipidemia)

CPSIA information can be obtained at www.ICGtesting.com
Printed in the USA
BVOW011851090413

317732BV00011B/225/P